ANIMAL MODELS IN BIOLOGICAL PSYCHIATRY

Animal Models in Biological Psychiatry

Allan V. Kalueff
Editor

Nova Science Publishers, Inc.
New York

For permission to use material from this book please contact us:
Telephone 631-231-7269; Fax 631-231-8175
Web Site: http://www.novapublishers.com

Library of Congress Cataloging-in-Publication Data
Available upon request.

ISBN 1-59454-814-5

Published by Nova Science Publishers, Inc. ✦ New York

Contents

Preface

Allan V Kalueff

To Kay Cameron Montgomery
(1921-1956)

Stress plays the main role in pathogenesis of many brain disorders. Anxiety, depression, epilepsy and neurodegeneration are extremely common, dramatic and debilitating multifacetic psychiatric illnesses affecting a substantial portion of the population. The problem of correct diagnosis has always been crucial for psychiatrists fighting these disorders. Other important question to ask in a book about biological psychiatry is why to study neurobiological mechanisms and behavioural manifestations of these disorders in animals? Since it is now becoming recognized that multidisciplinary approaches are the most useful in the modern biomedical science, without a knowledge of both clinical and biological aspects of brain disorders it is impossible to offer effective treatment strategies to the patients.

Over the past decades, there has been intensive study of a variety of neurobiological mechanisms of various brain disorders. The choice of which biological correlates to study is not easy, but it is now widely recognized that all brain disorders are associated with definite specific biological changes. Can mice and other animals assist us to understand normal and pathological human brain? Although mice and humans share more than 90% of their genes, the behavior of mice and humans is apparently very different. However, nowadays animal models seem to be an extremely useful tool in bio-medical sciences, as evidenced by a notable increase in the number of active laboratories working in the field. Finally, the ability to generate transgenic and knockout strains resulted in animal models with extraordinary potential for the study of molecular mechanisms of brain pathologies.

In this book experts from academia introduce the reader to some of the recent new developments in the field of experimental modeling of various brain disorders. Covering data from neuroethology to neurogenetics and psychopharmacology, this book collects a number of outstanding state-of-the-art papers on the topic. They will give us a brief but sound resume of the reasons why it is so important to study biological markers of brain pathology, and in so doing, discuss the various challenges and available opportunities.

This book is dedicated to Kay C. Montgomery (1921-1956) - an outstanding American neuroscientist, whose ideas have inseminated and continued to influence generations of biologists and psychiatrists. Importantly, the present volume will mark Montgomery's 85th anniversary and the 50th anniversary of his death. Montgomery made important contributions at an early age before suffering an untimely death. We should always remember that Science is not merely a collection of findings and interpretations but also a story written by outstanding personalities. Professor Montgomery was one such extraordinary personality, and we are honored here to pay a tribute to his efforts, which have proven so important to advancing experimental and theoretical biological psychiatry and behavioural neuroscience.

Why do we need animal models in biological psychiatry? According to McKinney (1984), we use animal models as "experimental preparations developed in one species for the purposes of studying phenomena occurring in another species". However, general problems with animal models of human psychic disorders include i) the difference between human's and non-human's nervous systems, ii) the difficulty in determining analogous behaviors among species and iii) the need in extrapolation of results from animals to humans. In addition, such problems most likely reflect a significant difference in etiology and complexity of different brain behavioural disorders.

Importantly, we shall all understand that the data derived from animal models are of value only to the extend that the models are valid (Willner, 1997). Moreover, the level of the disorder in animals may not be the level of the disorder in humans we want to model. This book will reveal that our understanding of how various brain disorders occur and co-occur in the brain is still quite limited. That is why one of the current challenges is to utilize the best of both clinical and pre-clinical approaches to biological psychiatry of stress-related disorders.

The authors took their part in bringing this about from their side. The book focuses on a comprehensive and systematic approach to certain biological markers of anxiety, depression, epilepsy and several other disorders. It is intended for graduate students, postdoctoral researchers and established biomedical scientists who have strong interests in biological psychiatry, want to apply their knowledge to practice, or need to understand the subject in order to critically evaluate their own findings. We hope that our efforts will be positively evaluated by the readers, and the book would have a significant value for biomedical research purposes – the way K. Montgomery would have liked it to be.

Allan V. Kalueff, PhD*
Medical School,
University of Tampere, Tampere, Finland

* Present address: National Institute of Mental Health, Bethesda, USA

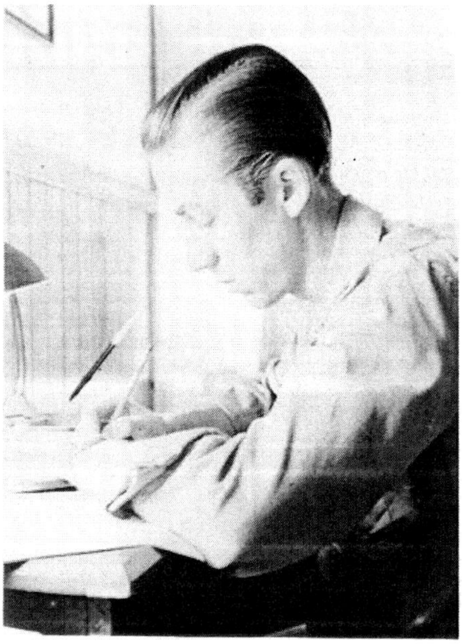

K. Montgomery, late 1940s

Brief Biography of Kay C. Montgomery

13 May 1921: Kay Cameron Montgomery was born in Greensburry (Pa., USA) in the family of Franklin P. Montgomery, an interior decorator, and Elisabeth MacKay, a housewife

March 1943-August 1946: Montgomery serves in the USA Air Forces

Education: University of Florida (1 year); Murray State Teachers College (1 year); Alabama Polytechnic Institute (1 year); University of North Carolina (1 year)

1945-1949: University of Chicago (Psychology): BS (1945), PhD (1949)

15 January 1945: Kay Montgomery marries Shirley Lyons, a Chicago University graduate, at a ceremony in Cincinnati, Ohio

July 1949- July 1950: Instructor of Psychology at Harvard University

July 1950- July 1951: Assistant Professor of Psychology at Cornell University

1 July 1952: Assistant Professor of Psychology at Yale University (teaches Introductory psychology and Experimental psychology courses). Montgomery's major research interests during that time included psychology of learning, motivation, and exploration

7 July 1956: Kay C. Montgomery commits suicide, aged only 35, suffering from a severe depression.

Selected Bibliography

[1] Montgomery, K.C. An experimental investigation of reactive inhibition and conditioned inhibition. *J. Exper. Psychol.* 1951; 41: 39-41.

[2] Montgomery, K.C. "Spontaneous alternation" as a function of time between trials and amount of work. *J. Exper. Psychol.* 1951; 42: 82-92.

[3] Montgomery, K.C. The relation between exploratory behavior and spontaneous alternation in the white rats. *J. Comp. Physiol. Psychol.* 1951; 44: 582-589.

[4] Montgomery, K.C. Exploratory behaviour and its relation to spontaneous alternation in a series of maze exposures. *J. Comp. Physiol. Psychol.* 1952; 45: 50-57.

[5] Montgomery, K.C. The effect of the hunger and thirst drives upon exploratory behavior. *J. Comp. Physiol. Psychol.* 1953; 46: 315-319.

[6] Montgomery, K.C. Concerning the use of analysis of variance on latency data. *Am. J. Psychol.* 1953; 66: 131-135.

[7] Montgomery, K.C. The effect of activity deprivation upon exploratory behavior. *J. Comp. Physiol. Psychol.* 1953; 46: 438-441.

[8] Montgomery, K.C. Exploratory behavior as a function of "similarity" of stimulus situations. *J. Comp. Physiol. Psychol.* 1953; 46: 129-133.

[9] Montgomery, K.C. The role of the exploratory drive in learning. *J. Comp. Physiol. Psychol.* 1954; 47: 60-64.

[10] Montgomery, K.C., Monkman, J.A. The relation between fear and exploratory behavior. *J. Comp. Physiol. Psychol.* 1955; 48: 132-136.

[11] Montgomery, K.C., Segall, M. Discrimination learning based upon the exploratory drive. *J. Comp. Physiol. Psychol.* 1955; 48: 225-228.

[12] Montgomery, K.C. The relation between fear induced by novel stimulation and exploratory behavior. *J. Comp. Physiol. Psychol.* 1955; 48: 254-260.

[13] Zimbardo, P.G., Montgomery, K.C. The relative strengths of consummatory responses in hunger, thirst, and exploratory drive. *J. Comp. Physiol. Psychol.* 1957; 50: 504-508.

In: Animal Models in Biological Psychiatry
Editor: Allan V. Kalueff, pp. 1-26
ISBN 1-59454-814-5

Chapter 1

Overview: Neuroethological Models of Anxiety and Depression

Allan V. Kalueff
Centre for Physiology and Biochemical Research, Moscow, Russia
Tampere University and the University Hospital, Tampere, Finland

I. Introduction

In recent years, a large body of evidence appear to link stressful life events with an increased vulnerability for anxiety and depression disorders (Arborelius et al., 1999) which have long been known to have dramatic impact on behavior. Numerous clinical data show that patients with anxiety and depression differ in their behavioral manifestations, although in many cases mild anxiety and mild depression are clinically very similar. Animals with anxiety and depression share the same "behavioral" problem since many findings show the lack of consistent behavioral effects of animal anxiety and depression (Paterson et al., 2001).

Study of anxiety and depression is a rapidly developing field of biological psychiatry where all contemporary theories and paradigms are based on cross-disciplinary approaches (Fig. 1, 2) and data coming from biology, medicine and psychology. During the past decades, a remarkable link has been formed among psychiatry, physiology, molecular biology, and behavioral biology. Despite human and animal depression or anxiety profiles differ in their cognitive-behavioral aspects, nowadays neuroscientists heavily rely on animals for examining the neurophysiological mechanisms of stress and related pathologies. Animal models are particularly of help in cases where the impact of stress cannot be studied in humans because of ethical and other like reasons.

Behavioral repertoire of animals, especially rodents, has long been used to detect effects on, and impact of, anxiety and depression. A number of animal models, based on animal emotional reactivity, have been designed and proven to be bidirectionally sensitive to stressful manipulations, including those of anxiety and depression (Espejo, 1997; Tables 1-5). Many of these models have been successfully used to test new anxiolytics or antidepressants and understand the underlying neural mechanisms (Salum et al., 2000) by simple, rapid and inexpensive ways of evaluating an animal's condition. Substantial progress has been made in our understanding which stressors may affect behavior and how.

However, there are several key questions in this field we still have to answer. Today, more than 70 years past Hall's classical open field studies in the 1930th, can we really distinguish between animal anxiety and depression? Do we have reliable neurobehavioral tools to assess anxiety and depression in animals? Is altered anxiety/depression behavior a predictive factor of increased sensitivity to anxiety/depression? Do we know robust behavioral markers of anxiety and depression? And, finally, do we always provide correct interpretations of behavioral changes seen in our experiments?

This chapter addresses some of these questions, and is divided into several parts. One part reviews the traditional animal models of anxiety and depression. Another part discusses behavioral measures of anxiety and depression. The topic of the final part of the chapter is the pitfalls of animal models and the ways how to overcome such difficulties.

II. Experimental Modeling Approach to Anxiety and Depression

Classification of experimental animal models of anxiety and depression is a difficult task. For example, it can be based on the nature and type of stressors employed (Tables 1-3). Clearly, the stressfulness of a behavioural test has to be taken into account when analysing the behavior, as it may significantly affect behavioural performance. For example, extreme stressors suppress general activity and result in non-specific alterations in animal performance. Ethologically based paradigms are more sensitive to stress compared to animal conditioned behavior models (Table 3) which usually use strong and often painful stressors like electric shock. This chapter will focus on the first group of models since conditioned response-based models represent "Yesterday" of this field of research.

Papers dealing with modification, validation or refinement of the existing models and introducing the new experimental paradigms appear regularly in the literature. However, are animal anxiety and depression a good approximation of human disorders? Which tests are good models of anxiety or depression? Which particular subtypes of anxiety of depression they model? - These questions are relatively rarely asked, but are fundamentally important.

The use of nearly all animal models from all groups has been extensively criticized in the literature. Firstly, one has to keep in mind that many clinically important symptoms, especially cognitive-based, of anxiety and depression can not be directly modeled in animals. Secondly, it appears that serious modelling problem is that the measures may often be confounded by altered levels of general activity, exploration and anxiety-depressiveness (Rodgers, Cole, 1994; Lapin, 2000; Belzung, Griebel, 2001; File, 2001). Finally, poor correlation between different behavioural measures taken in the same test, or the same measures taken in several different tests, is another problem.

Table 1. Classification of animal behavioural models

Criterion	Types of models	Comments
Behavioural similarity	"basic" animal assays	based on animal behaviors that do not need to be similar to human symptoms
	sophisticated homologous models	share some functional similarity with human behavior, see (Newport et al., 2002) for details
Model complexity	simple	utilize relatively primitive manipulations, see (Sarter, Bruno, 2002, Kalueff, 2003) for details
	complex	incorporate both neurobehavioral and behavioral/cognitive aspects of behaviours
	hybrid	that mechanically combine two working simple models in one new.[1]
Time course	acute	single exposure to stressor
	sub-chronic	2-3 exposures
	chronic	>3 exposures (e.g., modeling depression since it is necessary to use the behavioural symptoms persisting for weeks (Willner, 1997).
Relation to pathology	inducing pathology (active)	by drugs, targeted gene mutations, brain lesions/stimulation or stressful external factors
	measuring existing pathology (passive)	in terms of behavioral and physiological reactions
State-trait	state	measure behaviours displayed by an individual when confronted with a stressful stimulus
	trait	measure reactions that are an enduring feature of the subject, i.e. a stable (geneticly-determined) characteristics
Conditioning	unconditioned	based on unconditioned responses
	conditioned	based on conditioned responses
Naturality of behaviours	natural	based on measuring natural animal behaviors (e.g., stress-sensitive seed-finding behavior in hamsters, King et al., 2002) to reproduce behavioral and pathological aspect of the disorder and assess neurobiological mechanisms that are not easily amendable in human studies, see (Overall, 2000)
	artificial	utilizing behaviors not normally seen in natural conditions (e.g., forced swim or tail suspension)

[1] See an example of the hybrid model of anxiety in (Dere et al., 2002) describing graded anxiety test based on the elevated plus maze and light-dark tests.

Table 1. Classification of animal behavioural models (Continued)

Criterion	Types of models	Comments
Behaviours measured	exploratory	assess exploratory behaviors
	social	assess social behaviors
	agonistic	• assess defensive behaviors,
	novelty	• specifically focus on novelty responses
	conditioning	assess active/passive avoidance
	hedonic	measure the suppression of hedonic behavior
	fear-conditioned	analyze conditioned fear
Number of animals and species per trial	mono-animal	a single animal per trial (Kalueff, 2003)
	poly-animal	several animals in a test [2]
	semi-polyanimal	one adult pregnant animal (Kalueff, 2003)
	mono-species	animals of one species (Kalueff, 2003)
	poly-species	use animals of several different species [3]
Ontogenesis	prenatal	see (Newport et al., 2002) for a review[4]
	neonatal	
	postnatal	

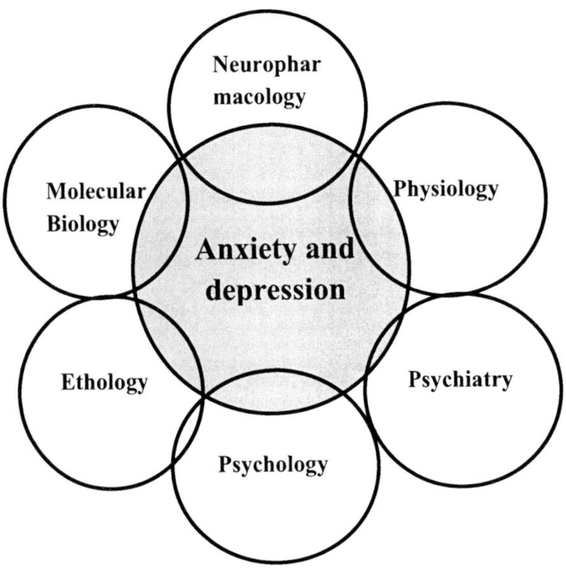

Fig. 1. Biological psychiatry of anxiety and depression

[2] For example, some specific behaviors (rearing, follow, mutual grooming) in social interaction model, known as File's paradigm, are sensitive to anxiolytic drugs and not to antidepressants. Possibly homologous to human "social anxiety" state, it is a valuable behavioral model for testing putative anxiotropic manipulations.

[3] Aggression to infants and adult co-specifics or other species (mice, frogs, cockroaches) is often seen in olfactory bulbectomised rats, and is as a measure of depressiveness sensitive to antidepressants. Exposure to predator is known to be a useful model highly sensitive to anxiolytics and antidepressants.

[4] There are numerous models of anxiety and depression based on prenatal and neonatal manipulations, including acute and chronic exposure to various stressors or different psychotropic drugs, As expected, such experience resulted in long-term behavioral and neurobiological changes similar to those seen in humans having early life stress.

Table 2. Animal models in the study of anxiety and depression

I. Depression:	Acute:	1)Pharmacologic	Reserpine- or clonidine-induced depression
		2) Stress-evoked	Porsolt's test (forced swimming) behavioral despair task, tail suspension test, inclined or vertical screen test
	Chronic:	3) Stress-evoked	Learned helplessness (unsignalled inescapable shock) Vogel and Gellert tests
		4) Social disruption	Maternal or peer separation, Social defeat, altered group hierarchy Reduced submissive behavior *
		5) Sensory models	Olfactory bulbectomy Long-term ZnSO4 anosmia
		6) Anhedonic models	Willner's test (sucrose consumption) Hedonic behavior suppression (feeding, etc)
II. Anxiety:	Acute:	1)Pharmacologic	Convulsant- or stimulant- induced anxiety
		2) Stress-evoked	"Forced" single-factor (novelty) or multi-factor tests (e.g., novelty + aversion): elevated plus or zero-maze, light-dark box, holeboard, inclined or vertical screen test, seed seeking behavior in hamsters, shock-probe defensive burying, etc. Free exploration paradigm.
		3) Social models	Social interaction (File's) paradigm
	Chronic:	4) Stress-evoked	Learned anxiety (Geller conflict test).
		5) Social models	Social interaction (File's) paradigm ("Partition") test
		6) Prenatal models	Prenatal "state" anxiety models
		7) Sensory models	Short-term ZnSO4-induced anosmia Exposure to novel or predator odors Amputation of whiskers
		8) Innate anxiety	Selected "high-anxiety" strains **
III. Transitory models:		Initially anxiety then depression	Developing anosmia-induced anxiety-depressive symptoms Kalueff et al., 2001)
IV. Combination models:	Anxiety and depression states to be measured simultaneously		
V. Comorbidity models:	Allow to model anxiety or depression in comorbidity with other psychiatric illnesses (e.g., addiction, see Rezvani et al., 2002 for details, or epilepsy)		

Comments: * see (Malatynska et al., 2002). ** see (Ohl et al., 2001) for a detailed discussion.

For example, some anxiety-like behaviours detected in the plus-maze test are not detectable by using the two compartment exploratory test or the inner segment ambulation scoring in the open field-test. Likewise, several antidepressants produce effects in the tail suspension test but are not active in the forced swim test (Porsolt, 2000). Furthermore, grooming and defecation can often be seen as the only behaviours that change in the tests designed to measure anxiety behaviours, not grooming, urinations and defecations (Kalueff et al., 2001, 2002). Indeed, scoring of defecation often fails to correlate with any of the parameters in rodent anxiety models. Moreover, depression-like behaviour in the rat cannot be detected by using tests directed to detect anxiety or exploratory motor activity.

Table 3. Summary of animal conditioned response-based models (Flint, 2003)

Two-way avoidance "Shuttle box" conditioning test	Rate of acquisition response
Accoustic startle	Contraction in response to loud
Foot shock induced freezing	Contraction in response to conditioned stimuli
Fear-potentiated startle	Contraction in response to loud noise in conjunction with loud noise
Geller (Geller-Seifnert) conflict test	Frequency of conditioned response coincidental to an electrical shock
Vogel conflict test	Frequency of conditioned licking coincidental to an electrical shock

Moreover, even the simplest task – distinguishing between horizontal exploration and locomotion in the open field, often mistakenly used synonymously in the literature - is also open for further elaboration (Choleris et al., 2001). Thus, since it is difficult to interpret a subjective anxiety or depression level based on a single behavioural measure, proper understanding of animal state is only possible through assessment of interaction between behavioural and physiological variables in the multivariate analysis (Calatayud, Belzung, 2001).

Also importantly, various forms of psychopathologies in animals and humans can be characterized as context-regulation disorders. This means that subjects may sometimes produce "normal" behavior in inappropriate contexts. As such, a special research on behavioural contexts may be needed in the field of animal anxiety or depression biopsychiatry.

Overall, it is important to remember that emotional behavior is not just "plus" or "minus". It is composed of several dimensions including anxiety, exploration, locomotion, risk assessment, general arousal and coping (Salome et al., 2002). These dimensions usually interact with each other and cognitions, giving us, as the outcome, a very "mosaic" picture of animal or human behavior. That is why traditional quantitative behavioural methods (i.e. latency, frequency and duration parameters and their spatial, temporal or sequential patterns) of animal stress are now combined with sophisticated analysis to assess "not just the presence or absence of these behaviours, but also whether or not the … acts, postures and gestures are fully developed in intensity, latency and patterning" (Barrett, Miczek, 2000). In this context, Aguilar et al. (2002) noted frequent incidental rather that relevant relationships among certain behavior indices taken from the same test and common low correlations among variables apparently measuring the same phenomena in different models of anxiety or depression. Because not all significant and robust behavioral changes are in fact meaningful parameters for assessment of animal anxiety and depression, in neurobehavioral science there is a need for clear-cut measures that will be resistant to experimental conditions or apparatus design of particular laboratories but show reliable and predictable changes following experimental manipulations affecting anxiety and depression states (see Crabbe et al., 2002 for a detailed discussion).

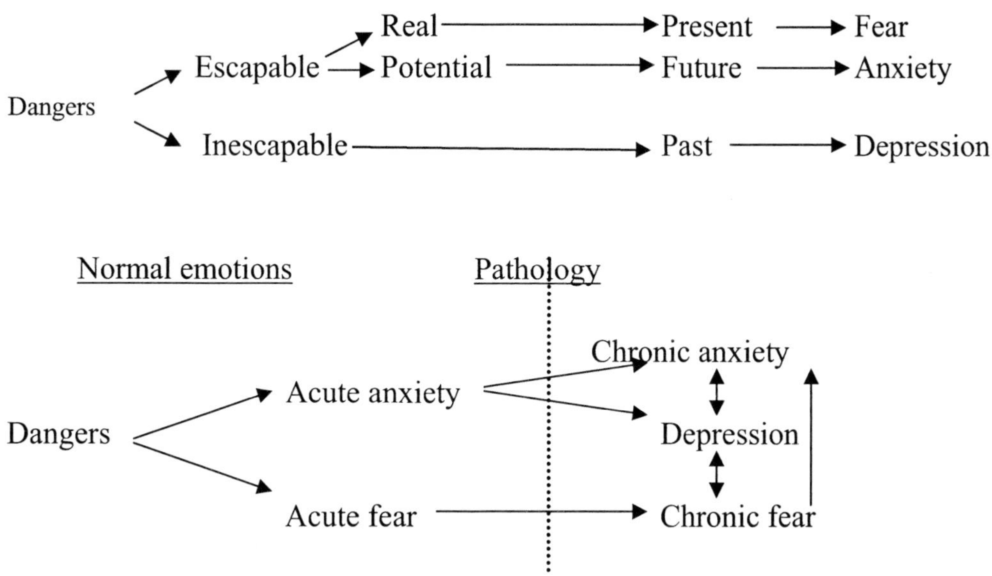

Fig. 2. Biopsychiatry views of stress, anxiety and depression (adapted from Kalueff, 1999)

However, here appears a new cluster of problems. First, can the same model analyze different subtypes of anxiety and depression? For example, distinct subtypes of anxiety can be modeled in the same test, as suggested by (Holmes, Rodgers, 2001) for the elevated plus maze (single vs. repeated testing). A stimulating discussion continues as for whether Porsolt's forced swim test can be a complex model of anxiety and/or depression (see discussion and factor analysis data in Salome et al., 2002). For example, time spent swimming may reflect active or escape-searching behavior as well as anxiety-sensitive exploration of the tank, while passive floating represents animal "despair" (depression). As such, to distinguish between "anxiety" and "depression" in this test, additional approaches are needed. For example, ethological data indicate that not only immobility patterns can be measured in Porsolt's test. Naitoh et al. (1999) described specific stress-induced head twitching behavior which is differentially sensitive to anxiolytics and antidepressants. Other group found that Porsolt's test swimming correlates with open field exploration (Ho et al., 2002) and suggested that this swim test may also be used for studying stress-sensitive exploration (i.e. anxiety) in addition to traditional depression measures. Finally, another group suggested that struggling, but not immobility, is the most reliable and lest subjective measure of antidepressant activity in this test (Armario et al., 1988).

Second, although depression and anxiety are considered to be separate entities according to current diagnostic classifications, in clinical practice these two conditions co-exist. A proper modeling of anxiety or depression in animals presumes that in order to achieve better results we model either pathology separately. The important problem now is whether animals may possibly have comorbidity of depression and anxiety. Theoretically we see no reasons to rule our this possibility, and they indeed may represent certain interest for the researchers. However, relatively few studies of that kind have been conducted and there is a great need in developing specialized models which will allow to detect and study putative comorbidity states in animals. Merited little scrutiny at the moment, this direction of research may be important and fruitful for future studies in biological psychiatry.

Another key question to be asked here is whether we need a single model to be differentially sensitive to anxiety and depression. In other words, can we model pathologies developing one by one in the same experimental test? From neurobehavioral perspective, such "combinational" models may be extremely useful, and therefore will certainly require future elaboration.

Finally, some promising approaches come from behavioral neurogenetics. For example, WKY rats have been recently suggested as an animal model of anxiety and depression (Tejani-Butt et al., 2003) since they demonstrate frequent anxiety-like freezing and depressive-like swim immobility. In line with this, Gass et al. (2001) suggested that mice with targeted mutations of gluco- and mineralocorticoid receptors are the model of anxiety and depression. Perhaps, encouraging can be recent results of Salome et al. (2002) studying high-anxiety HAB rats. These rats are suggested to represent a reliable model of trait anxiety and depression. Thus far, measuring comorbidity of anxiety or depression with other pathologies (addiction, etc), or measuring these states occurring consequently, may present an extremely important field of research. It is however very important to ensure that all such models are being thoroughly validated (see further).

III. Behavioral Parameters Measured

Exploratory behavior is most often studied in the laboratory, in forced (non-escapable) or free (free-choice) situations, as stress-sensitive behavioral parameter to assess anxiety and/or depression level (Cruzio, 2001). In addition, some other behaviors (e.g. self-grooming, see further chapters in this book) are meaningful parameters that can be sensitive to the level of stress but may possess some behavioral "autonomy" (Berrigde, Aldridge, 2000; Galeeva, Tuohimaa, 2001; Kalueff, 2002). As such, one needs to use tests that provide not only independent measures of exploration and motor activity (File, 2001), but also detect changes in "additional" behaviors such as risk assessment, self-grooming, defecation, urination, etc. (Kalueff et al., 2001, 2002), Tables 4 and 5.

For example, an interesting and illustrative case represents measuring of animal urinations. Some researchers measure them as an index of stress, but consider them either as a fear-like "immediate" reaction or anxiety index. Other groups do not measure urinations since they see them as "a highly unreliable behavioral parameter". Third group of scientists measures urinations and defecations separately but later put them together as an integral measure of "vegetative" markers of stress (see criticism in Kalueff et al., 2001). One can use either approach in his own research but it should be clear that other groups (and even other scientists within the same group) may have results which will be different because of the different approaches used. Moreover, some authors even measure stress-induced yawning (e.g., Eguibar et al., 2003) which may be a useful ethological parameter in anxiety/depression research (particularly sensitive, for example, to dopaminergic manipulations).

Risk assessment behavior is another important ethological measure called by the Blanchards in 1989 "anxiety-defensive postures". They include:

1. immobility (freezing),
2. stretched attention (orientation towards the stimulus), and
3. approach to the stimulus, "flatback approach" (Kemble, Bolwahnn, 1997).

Table 4. Summary of principal measures in animal models of anxiety and depression

Behavioral indices	Anxiety	Depression
General locomotion	Activated	Inhibited *
Exploration	Decreased	Decreased
Self-grooming	Activated (frequency)	Activated (duration)
Immobility	Activated (freezing)	Activated (despair)**
Defecation, urination	Activated	?
Aggression	Activated	Activated
Self-aggression	0	Activated
Transitions between behaviors	Increased	Decreased
Risk assessment	Increased or decreased ***	Decreased
Other "specific" behaviors (seed finding, shock-probe defensive burying, etc)	Activated****	0 ?

Comments: ? Unclear or inconsistent effects, 0 – no effects. *activated in the open field in olfactobulbectomy model of depression. **in Porsolt's and tail suspension tests. ***depending on the model. **** see King et al., 2002

Indeed, exploration responses include a large number of behaviors such as walking, approaches, scanning, sniffing, rearing, wall leaning, digging, licking, biting, etc. Risk assessment is particularly specific to stress and can be bidirectionally affected by neurotropic drugs including anxiolytics and antidepressants. However, one has to remember that in a free exploratory paradigm only passive behavioural measures are taken. The presence of passive behavior in an activation paradigm is against the nature of the cognitive component of the task and therefore it complicates the interpretation of any between-task difference in the brain activity. As such, a careful consideration is needed before choosing active/passive behavioural measures in an active/passive behavioural test.

Some of traditional behavioral parameters used in animal models are summarized in Table 5. However, as Crabbe et al. (2002) noted, "different laboratories commonly employ their own idiosyncratic versions of behavioral tests apparatus and protocols, and any laboratory environment has many unique features". One could imagine how true this observation is! Considering animal models first of all as "theories" (see Sarter, Bruno, 2002), we will also agree with Crawley (1999) that a thorough knowledge of behavioral literature is always required to find an optimal test to address the hypotheses in question.

Table 5. Major behavioral measures in experimental models of anxiety and depression

Tests	Parameters	Anxiety	Depression	References
Open field (circular, square or rectangular)	Defecations, urinations number and duration	+	-	
	Total distance traveled or squares crossed	- (a?)	+ *	
	Speed of movements	+	-	
	Distance in the inner area	-		Aguilar et al., 2002 Kalueff et al., 2001 Kalueff, 1999, 2002 Choleris et al., 2001 Mayaho et al., 1995
	Number of squares crossed in the inner area	-		
	Distance in the outer area	-		
	Self-grooming latency	-	+	
	duration	+	+	
	frequency	+	-	
	% of interrupted (aborted) or incorrect grooming	+	+? **	
	Average duration of a single grooming ritual	-	+	
	Rears in the inner/outer areas (including wall leaning)	-	-	
	Stretch Attend postures	+		
	Returns	+	?	
	Latency of 1st and 2nd visits to the central area	+	?	
	Latency to leave the central area	+	?	
	First corner visit / Opposite corner visit	-		
Novel object	Approach latency	+	+	Kalueff et al., 1999, Belzung, 1999 for review
	Number of contacts	-	0	
	Duration of exploration of the novel object	-	0	
Plus maze (also elevated zero-maze, etc)	Latency to leave the centre	+		
	Total arms entries (4 paws criterion)	a	-	Andrade et al., 2003 Aguilar et al., 2002 Kalueff et al., 2001 Kalueff, 1999, 2002 Lapin, 2000
	Enclosed arms entries	+(a?)		
	Open arms entries (4 paws) and rears (2 paws)	-		
	Time spent in the open arms	-		
	Time spent in the enclosed arms	+		
	% Open arms entries	-		
	% Time spent in the open arms	-		
	Head dips (protected and unprotected ***)	-		
	Defecations, urinations	+	+	
	Self-grooming latency	+	-	
	duration	+	+	
	frequency	+	-	
	Central platform crossings and time spent	- b	?	

Table 5. Major behavioral measures in experimental models of anxiety and depression (Continued)

Tests	Parameters	Anxiety	Depres-sion	References
Hole board test (with or without walls)	Head dipping (hole poking) latency number duration Defecations, urinations, total distance traveled/squares crossed, distance/squares crossed in the inner area, distance in the outer area, self-grooming, rears – as in the open field test	+ - -	+ - -	Aguilar et al., 2002 Kalueff et al., 2001 Kalueff, 1999,2002
Light/dark box	Light box entries number (4 paws criterion) Light box time spent Light box rears number (2 paws criterion) Duration of light box rears Latency of the first rear and entry Vertical activity in the light box © Urinations, defecations, grooming	- (a?) - - - - + +	- - - - - ? ?	Kalueff et al., 2001 Kalueff, 1999, 2002
Free exploratory test	Number of entries to the novel compartment Time spent in the novel environment Latency to enter the novel compartment Stretch attention, rearing to the novel box	- - + -	? ? ? ?	Chapillon et al., 1999
Porsolt's forced swim test	Immobility latency (until first floating) Immobility duration Swimming average speed Swimming distance Additional measures: horizontal and vertical rotation, vibrissae clean, struggling (d), floating (immobility with only occasional slight movements), sliding, diving, head-diving and wagging head, defecation Head twitching	? ? ? +? 0	- + - - +	Magalhaes et al., 2002 Kalueff, 1999 Salome et al., 2002 Hedou et al., 2001 Naitoh et al., 1999
Tail suspension test	Immobility latency Immobility duration Number of tail-climbing and % of animals that climbed their tails up	+? +? -	+ + -	Kalueff, 1999 Mayora, Lucki, 2001
Inclined screen	Time spent on the screen (falling latency) Urinations, defecations	- +	- - (?)	Kalueff, 1999
Pinch-induced catalepsy	Duration of catalepsy Required number of pinches	+? +?	+? +?	Fundarro, 1998

Table 5. Major behavioral measures in experimental models of anxiety and depression (Continued)

Tests	Parameters	Anxiety	Depression	References
Stress hyperthermia	The amplitude of hyperthermia The duration of hyperthermia	+ +	? ?	Mercier et al., 2002 Bowknecht et al., 2002
Hyponeophagia	Latency to start eating	+	?	Flint, 2003

Comments: + activated, - inhibited, ? unclear or inconsistent effects, a – considered as a general activity measure, b - considered as a traditional decision index (decision-making behavior), c – is not a traditional measure in the test but can be useful to measure, d – are recorded when animals move strongly all four limbs with the front paws breaking the water surface or scratching the walls. *in olfactory bulbectomy model only. **Different effects of anxiety (shortening, reversals) and depression (prolonged rituals, stereotypy). *** unprotected dips if scan-like dipping of the head and shoulders over the side of the arms.

The discussion focusing on different aspect of animal models validity is another important issue in biological psychiatry. In general, validation is defined as the process by which the reliability and relevance of a method are established for specific purposes. Reliability is characterized by the reproducibility of a test within and between laboratories and over time. Also, data shall be concordant for different methods of registration (i.e. manual vs. automated).

Since numerous differences exist between laboratories, good reproducibility at least between the same laboratory has to be established. Relevance of a model is strongly related to the specificity of the test. Many types of validity have been defined for animal anxiety/depression models so far, including predictive, construct, concurrent or convergent, discriminant, etiological and face validity (Geyer, Markou, 2000). This problem has been commented extensively in the literature and we will only address this question briefly. At present, three principal and some additional validity criteria have been formulated and substantiated for animal models of anxiety and depression (Sarter, Bruno, 2002; Table 6).

- Based of this validity classification, animal models can be:
- correlational (based on predictive validity),
- isomorphic (based on face validity) and
- homologous (based on construct validity).

Ideally, a model shall fulfill all 3 criteria in order to be good model (Clement et al., 2002) which means to be correlational, isomorphic and homologous at the same time. However, this situation is not seen in animal modeling very often. For example, as noted by Bai et al. (2001), traditional models of depression such as Porsolt's swimming and tail suspension tests both lack face and construct validity but are extremely good at predictive validity. Moreover, many rodent anxiety models have poor construct validity, their predictive validity often fails and there is a disconnect between predictive validity and face validity, especially when compared with human data (Overall, 2000).

Furthermore, there are numerous models which work consistently in animals but may not always be appropriate for humans. Consider, for example, olfaction-based behavioural models. Olfaction plays an important role in the regulation of normal and pathological behavior in animals and humans (Makarchuk, Kalueff, 2000) and therefore deserves special attention in this chapter. Exposure to novel and/or aversive (various natural predator and non-predator odors) stimulates "innate" or neophobic animal anxiety, increases risk-assessment behavior (stretched attention and flat back approach duration and frequency) and evokes anxiety-like states that are bidirectionally sensitive to anxiolytic or anxiogenic drugs (Kemble, Bolwahnn, 1997). However, these stimuli may not necessarily work in humans who are generally much less reliant of their olfaction.

Our experiments (Makarchuk, Kalueff, 2000) using ZnSO4 intranasal application have shown that acute olfactory sensory deficit increases the degree of uncertainty and causes anxiety in anosmic animals. Removal of the olfactory bulbs (central anosmia) in rodents produces endocrinal and behavioral depression-like effects including behavioral hyperactivity in the novel environment, muricidal/infanticidal aggression and deficits in avoidance learning. These behavioral changes have been shown to be reversed by chronic antidepressant treatment (McGraugh, Norman, 1999), and are consistent with clinical findings in depressed patients (Bilkei-Gorzo et al., 2002).

Although the brain mechanisms underlying such behavioral changes in anosmia are far from being understood (Kalueff et al., 2001), they can be at least partially explained by i) sensory deficit per se and ii) the role of emotional behavior controlled by some brain areas involved in olfactory processing (e.g., limbic system). Positive olfactory-based stimuli may also be successfully used in anxiety and depression research. For example, specific seed-finding behavior in Golden hamsters was increased by anxiolytics and appeared to be a sensitive behavioral measure of anxiety (King et al., 2002). Note, however, that humans are microsmatic mammals, and the role of olfaction in their functioning is far less crucial, compared to macrosmatic mammals such as rodents (Makarchuk, Kalueff, 2000).

Interestingly, the discussion is ongoing as for which criteria shall be the most important. For example, Porsolt (2000) states that models of depression "should attenuate the behavioral symptoms, which should remain unaffected by other kind of agents such as antipsychotics or anxiolytics". However, this limitation in not in line with predictive validity requirements, since several anxiolytics have positive effects in depression, and no easy and clear-cut differentiation is possible in the clinical conditions. Construct validity seems to be the most important for the animal model, since so many objective limitations exist for predictive validity. They are based on the fact that most of the models are sensitive to certain classes of psychotropic drugs and insensitive to others. For example, the elevated plus maze and the light-dark anxiety models respond to benzodiazepine anxiolytics but are not sensitive to chronic antidepressant administration known to produce anxiolytic effects in humans (Borsini et al., 2002).

However, acute and chronic drug treatments may not be the only options since differential effects can be caused by the anxiolytic and/or antidepressant drugs administered sub-chronically (2 or 3 doses). In addition, it is possible to assume that animal models may have different validities for each type of drugs administrations. Finally, despite apparent favoring construct validity criterion in the literature, we shall note that etiology and pathophysiology of psychiatric diseases are still largely unknown. It therefore seems difficult to suggest an "ideal" animal model of the illness that fully meets even construct validity criterion.

Table 6. Validity of animal models of anxiety and depression

Validity	Importance	Details
Face	-	Reflects phenomenological similarities (isomorphism) between the model and human pathology to be modeled
Predictive	+	Based on ability to predict drugs or manipulations effective in animal models to be effective in humans. May be limited to the drugs or manipulations it has been designed for
Construct	++	Based on similar theoretical rationale (homology) behind the pathology in animals and humans. May be limited to the extend of our knowledge of pathological mechanisms[5]
Discriminant	-	Degree to which a test measures aspects of a phenomenon that are different from other aspects of the phenomenon that other tests assess
Convergent	-	Degree to which a test correlates with other tests to measure the same construct
Etiological	-	Degree of similarity of etiology of animal and human states
Genetic	+	Degree of similarity of the genes involved in anxiety or depression induced in a particular test

Comments: Genetic validation is based on behavioural phenotyping approach; "behavioural phenotype" refers to the specific and characteristic behavioural repertoire exhibited by animals with a specific genetic/chromosomal disorder, see (Flint, 2003) for a detailed discussion. For example, mutations in chromosome 4 affected mice locomotion and mutated chromosomes 1 and 15 affected anxiety measures. In rats, only one locus in chromosome 5 influenced emotionality, while mutations in chromosomes 1, 4, 7, 15, 18 and 19 largely affected activity measures. As such, finding sets of "anxiety" or "depression" chromosomes involved in traditional experimental models in some cases will assist in genetic validation of novel putative models of anxiety or depression. However, the question as for whether certain behaviours shall be a part of behavioural phenotype, is far from being clearly understood (especially since not always an association between behavior and syndrome, and between the syndrome and the gene, is clear-cut and linear).

[5] While Sarter and Bruno (2002) insist on the recognition of animal models as theories, we would disagree that this is always true. See for example (Boyer, 2000; Newport et al., 2002): because the pathophysiology of anxiety and depression remains unclear, the majority of the models do not meet all construct validity requirements, and therefore the homology of an animal model to a human illness can not be fully demonstrated.

IV. Pitfalls and Problems of Animal Models

Considerable attention has been focused on the pitfalls and weaknesses of anxiety and depression animal models. Lapin (2000) listed the following key factors that are often neglected in neurobehavioral studies of anxiety and depression:

- vehicle pH monitoring,
- handling control,
- false injection control,
- body temperature control,
- general activity control (false positives and negatives),
- injection effect,
- time of the day,
- light conditions,
- pre-test manipulations.

Ignoring these factors will almost certainly result in obtaining conflicting data. As more drugs become available and are used concominantly in different psychopharmacological assays, the potential for drug interaction increases and needs to be taken into consideration.

Additional possible significant test problems may include:

- strains/species differences,
- sex and age differences,
- sensitivity to pre-test manipulations (e.g. housing, transportation),
- construction of apparatus,
- conditions prior behavioral testing (lighting, cycle),
- scoring method (manual vs. automated video recording),
- acclimation of animals before and after the testing.

Importantly, even minor variations between laboratories in any of these factors may sometimes lead to great discrepancies in the results (Crabbe et al., 2002). Previous housing regime (individual vs. grouped) is also an important biosocial factor able to affect anxiety and depression-related behaviors (Palanza, 2001). For example, it has been noted that socially isolated animals tend are more active in the novel conditions (engage in more exploratory and escape-oriented behaviors) than the group-housed animals. \

Also notably, rodents used in biomedical research are usually reared in small cages that lack key features of their natural habitat (Wurbel, 2001). It is now becoming evident that animals need to be reared in enriched conditions in order to be able to produce normal behaviors. Rearing conditions may therefore, and in fact do so, strongly affect behavioral reactions seen in animal models of anxiety and depression, also influencing memory, attention, agonistic behaviors and other important aspects of normal brain-behavior interaction (Wurbel, 2001). The differences between laboratories and the lack of general standards of rearing may cause conflicting and even false results (Crabbe et al., 2002).

Table 7. Factor analysis of anxiety-sensitive behaviors in traditional animal models

Factors	References
I Exploration, II grooming, III defecation (emotionality)	Cruzio, 2001
I Activity ("female" factor), II exploration ("male" factor)	File, 2001
I Anxiety, II Motor activity, III risk assessment, IV decision-making, V Vertical activity, VI Exploration	Rodgers, Johnson, 1996
I Exploration, II Motor activity, III Displacement activity, IV Risk assessment	Espejo, 1997
I Learned fear, II Emotional reactivity, III Fear of aversive stimuli	Aguilar at al., 2002
I Anxiety, II Locomotion, III Escape*	Salome et al., 2002

Comments: * Active coping strategy (found only in Porsolt's test)

Timetable and intensity of the experiments is another practical issue to consider. Many workers often ignore this factor and would be surprised to know how critical it is for obtaining correct and reliable data. Since rodents are very sensitive to the rhythm of activity of the researchers and animal house staff (usually much higher from Mondays to Friday), after relatively "easy" weekend days animals will behave differently on Monday than on the rest of the week (Belzung, 1999). Perhaps, a brave scientist working 7 days a week, has more chances to get more reliable data, and after getting Nobel Prize one sunny day would be able to enjoy long and deserved holidays. Alternatively, he may prefer working during weekends only, spending the rest 5 days per week with his family, traveling or doing many other exciting things. In addition, a significant amount of total variability of the behavioral indexes could be attributed to 24-h variation (Andrade et al., 2003). Indeed, all major behavioral parameters in rodents appear to be largely affected by light/dark phases. Generally, scores are much higher during the dark time of the day. This again makes clear the importance of standardization of all experimental procedures (Andrage et al., 2003) especially in their timing aspect. The major challenge, however, lies in determining which factors need to be standardized (Chesler et al., 2002). For example, this group has recently established that experimenter identity has extremely important role in animal behaviors and may overweight all other key factors studied (in the order of importance: season, cage density, time of the day, sex, humidity and the order of testing).

Moreover, individual differences between animals contribute significantly to the discrepancies and conflicting findings available in the literature (Ho et al., 2002). Further important problem arises when it became evident that anxiety and depression are heterogeneous and each may be divided in various forms. Wehner et al. (2001) noted that heterogeneity of anxiety reflects its polygenic regulation and many behavioral models are used to study its nature. Discussing its evolutionary rationale, Marks and Nesse (2001) write that for anxiety "subtypes exist because of the benefits of having responses specialized to deal with particular dangers or threats", yet they agree that subtypes of anxiety are not completely distinct as multiple dangers and thereat are common.

Various subtypes of anxiety and depression include (Blanchard et al., 1998; Calatayud, Belzung, 2001; Belzung, Griebel, 2001; File, 2001; Palanza, 2001):

- state (inductive) and trait (constitutive),
- "male-like" and "female-like",
- acute and chronic,
- normal[6] and pathological,
- innate and evoked,
- mild and severe subtypes (see also Table 2).

It is now clear that all these forms are not only neuroethologically and physiologically different but also possess differential sensitivity to stressors. Importantly, a common factor does not emerge from numerous factor analytical studies and common animal models do not measure the same type of phenomena (Aguilar et al., 2002; Table 7). Perhaps even more interesting data come from factor analysis of strain differences (Ohl et al., 2001) showing that different strains have different sets of factors controlling their behavior in the same model, and playing different roles within this model (Table 8).

Clearly, genetic factor may play a key role in producing such inconsistent results. The availability of an increasing number of transgenic and knockout animal models as well as integration of emerging tools and technologies for genetic analysis will provide the groundwork for the genetic dissection of anxiety, depression and related disorders (Crabbe et al., 1999). Numerous data report abnormal social, reproductive, parental, eating behaviors, aggression, learning and memory deficits, anxiety- and depression-like alterations as well as abnormal sensitivity to all major classes of psychotropic drugs (Crawley, 1999, Wehner et al., 2001; Bilkei-Gorzo et al., 2002) associated with different genetic modifications. As estimated, up to 80% of behavioral differences between strains may be due to polygenetic factors. However, not only several genes regulate a certain behavior, but a single gene can control several different behaviors, including those which may be opposite. For example, the same genes regulate activity and defecation in the open field in the mice of certain strains (Wehner et al., 2001). Again, this makes animal behavioral modeling even more complicated. In line with this, variability in the response to anxiolytic/antidepressant drugs may also be related to genetic factors underlying sensitivity to pharmacological treatments (Belzung, 2001).

What exactly do the existing models reflect? Despite the fact that most of the widely available animal models use state pathological condition, one has to show more logical interest in further study of more pathological (and clinically relevant) "trait" anxiety and depression in animals. For this, genetic approach may be very useful (also see further chapters in this book). Importantly, although common genes regulate general aspects of emotionality (see comments by Marks and Nesse, 2001), a unique set of genes may regulate certain specific emotionality measures, and it is now clear that different groups of genes

---

[6] True for anxiety, but not for animal depression

regulate baseline (trait) and state anxiety behaviors (Wehner et al., 2001). The same basic principle is most likely to be true for different depression subtypes. Clearly, "pathological" anxiety is not always an excess of normal "anxiety", and in many cases may represent a new qualitative variation. Thus far, the researcher has to remember that simple increase of normal anxiety in the model may not produce "pathological" anxiety! And behavioural changes observed in the models could be the result of not fully recognized species-typical normal response.

Terminology issue is another reason for experimental problems and further difficulties with data analysis and interpretation. Often the same term is used for different behaviors (e.g. "rears" which can be either vertical activity or horizontal "looks to" or "looks from" behaviors) as well as different terms are used for the same behaviors (consider, for example, "immobility" in Porsolt's test which some authors describe as "floating movements or making only those movements necessary to keep its head above the water" while other groups explain them as "complete motionless with no movements of limbs").

It must, however, be emphasized that we can not ask animals how they feel in a model, what exactly they are doing, or why they react in a certain way. As already mentioned, problems with data interpretations are common and well-documented in neurobehavioral studies. Interpretation of the behavior is critically important since it may be "more in the eye of the researcher than in the brain of the animal" (Overall, 2000).

Table 8. Factors controlling behaviors in different rat strains (Ohl et al., 2001)

Factors	Low anxiety	Normal Wistar	High anxiety
Locomotor activity	+++	++++	+
Anxiety	++++	++	+++
Exploration	+	++	++
Risk assessment	++	-	++++
Arousal	+	+	+

Additional disadvantage of many ethological models is that in experiments it is sometimes difficult to distinguish certain different meaningful behaviors. For example, novelty often used in anxiety research is known to be both anxiety-provoking and attractive. As such, approach to one stimulus (attraction) will be difficult to distinguish from avoidance of another (aversion). That is why detailed analyses and correct terming and interpretation of behaviors are crucial issues for biological psychiatry of anxiety and depression.

Here we will give one meaningful example. Let us suppose that one scientist observed the simplest single behavior - freezing (immobility) in rats or other laboratory rodents. In general, freezing can be defined as a motionless behavior and can be registered in animals or humans who have just been exposed to an aversive stimulus. However, is it a mere temporal "absence of behavior", inhibition of meaningful ongoing behaviors or, in contrary, activation of a meaningful adaptive behavior with complex allied stress-sensitive reflexes? Does it mean increased anxiety or, perhaps, depression? In our case, for "immobility" one has to consider at least several distinct possible behavioral subtypes; (see also: Whishaw et al., 2000; Davies, Whalen, 2001; Drai et al., 2001 for details):

1. sleep or resting (no body movements and postural support, closed eyes, small movements of the whiskers),
2. catalepsy (lost capacity to move and retained postural support),
3. learned "pseudocatalepsy" as a specific behavioral response to low doses of neuroleptics (see Ferre et al., 1990),
4. certain forms of horizontal exploration (e.g. rear-like postures, normally inhibited by anxiety),
5. fearful freezing (retained capacity to move and postural support, often seen in anxiety) with or without facial expression of fear, eye-blink reflex, sonic/ultrasonic vocalization,
6. restrained-induced (tonic) immobility or "animal hypnosis" (phenomenon seen in many animal species),
7. heat-loss posture (sprawling, immobility without tone),
8. heat-gain posture (immobility with muscle tone),
9. stereotypic freezing (often seen in depression),
10. decision-making behavior,
11. risk-assessment behaviors (with or without head movements, active breathing, gnawing, licking, sniffing and/or vibrissae micro-movements),
12. "stopping" state (a pause which might normally occur between two distinct behavioral bouts),
13. part of normal self-grooming ritual,
14. false "immobility" during defecation or urination,
15. element of hiding or escape behaviors,
16. immobility as a part of normal agonistic rituals (usually in subordinant animals),
17. illness-induced (seen with bad general appearance),
18. drug-induced non-specific behavioral inhibition (sedation),
19. "sit", type of animal normal behavior (Choleris et al., 2001),
20. predator-induced "tonic-like" immobility (Olsen et al., 2002), a terminal defense response when there is a physical contact between pray and predator.

That speaks to the great difficulty in behavioural research and reading animals minds! It also appears that each of these twenty subtypes has its own causes, own controlling neural networks, differentially sensitive to anxiety and depression, and cannot be therefore interpreted by observer as a simple non-specific unitary act. In addition, they may be differentially sensitive to different psychotropic drugs and manipulations. With this in mind, do we really always know that in our experiments we picked the right explanation and interpretation? Perhaps, the most important conclusion from this is that one parameter is not enough to judge and interpret animal anxiety or depression. Thus, we would question the idea that finding a model with a good and sensitive single parameter may be an ideal solution. Although several extremely useful single-parameter models have appeared recently (see King et al., 2002 for details), simplicity is desirable from the practical reasons but is not the major requirement for the model per se. In other words, simplicity of the model does not necessarily mean having a good and reliable model. The latter is especially important since some key phenomena (e.g., fast occurring positive changes or "overnight" recovery in human depression, as mentioned in Broekkamp (1997)) are not accounted in the traditional models.

V. Concluding Remarks

As stated by Sarter and Bruno (2001), "animal models may not only generate data with very limited validity but also deprive the researcher from achieving the main goal of research using animal models, i.e. to test and extend a theory about the disorder of interest". Therefore, the key issue will be to know how to use the right animals in the right animal models and, following the right protocols, receive behavioral data for their correct interpretation within the right model of the right pathology. For this, we have formulated several essential principles to be used for a proper animal modeling of anxiety and depression (also see Crawley, 1999 for details).

1. Use a battery of tests vs. a single paradigm.
2. Make sure animals have unimpaired motor activity and sensory abilities.
3. Study sex-related differences. Use male and female animals vs. one-sex trials.
4. Avoid models based on strong stressors, try to use more "naturalistic" models.
5. Always care about animal housing conditions to be standard and appropriate.
6. Use ethologically "rich" multi-parameter models vs. single-measure tests (remember, however, that the more complex test you use, the more difficult is to standardize it and control fully for variations in test performance).
7. Analyze all behavioral data as a whole integral complex, do not rely on a limited number of "traditional" measures.
8. Avoid where possible test-test interactions or animal re-test, since Trial 1 may not only quantitatively but qualitatively differ from Trial 2.
9. Consider factors which may cause conflicting data (transportation, handling, housing).
10. Try to assess different subtypes of anxiety and/or depression, use both acute and chronic stressors of different strength and origin.
11. Consider hyper/hypo locomotion problem (false positives and negatives) and baseline aspects (ceiling and floor effects).

We shall also note that when combining several behavioral models in the multiple study, one has to remember the time course dilemma existing in neurobehavioral research. Namely, some important behavioral differences may be absent immediately after the stress but develop later (after the behavioral testing). There is no general rule as for when such effects may appear and disappear. Some behavioral effects last several minutes, others can last for weeks. Some effects appear fast (within 30 min. after exposure to stress) while others may be visible only 24 h later. In these cases, the risk of false negatives is very high if the wrong checkpoint time is selected. The risk of false positives can be high too if one uses a battery of tests which the most likely strategy of neuroethological research nowadays. The behavioral effects induced by earlier tests may overlap with the effects seen after the current stress exposure. Clearly, prior test history has to be carefully controlled in all behavioural experiments.

The bad news to our fellow colleagues is that only a routine ethological time-course analysis has to be done to overcome such experimental problem. Also, the behavioral changes produced in the stressed animals by different stressors may interact with each other and produce long-lasting biological changes which may affect behaviors and will make the results even more complicated and difficult to interpret. Thus, step-by-step and factor-by-factor analysis may be needed to eliminate this unwanted overlapping. Quite predictably, relatively simple, activity-based tests may not be of much help for these purposes.

Finally, a careful observation of general health state, sensory and motor functions shall be performed in animals to avoid false positives or negatives (Crawley, 1999). A variety of measures have to be taken (Weiss et al., 1998) to ensure that physical properties (robustness) of animals are similar in each group. Thus, size, weight, weight gain, food intake, home cage activity (daily spontaneous ambulation), day cycle shall be carefully monitored.

After all this, invention of the new models and re-validation and sophistication of the existing tests will allow us to move further, from what Borsini et al. (2002) ironically called "models of benzodiazepine pharmacology" to the models which will demonstrate sensitivity to all major factors affecting anxiety and depression. As already mentioned, animal model is generally seen as an attempt to reproduce a psychiatric disorder in a laboratory animal. However, since the symptoms of psychiatric disorders are often being revised and re-defined (Geyer, Markou, 2000), some caution is needed before claiming or using an animal model of anxiety or depression. With this in mind, we shall remember that, as McKiney (2001) incredibly timely and rightly notes, generating the perfect animal model does not represent a separate goal of research in biological psychiatry, rather the model and its constant evolution represents an integral part of biological psychiatry. And, of course, modelling proceeds most effectively when scientists who are experts in the phenomena in question join forces with scientists who know and understand available modelling tools (Davidson et al., 2002).

Acknowledgements

This study was supported in parts by CPBR, CIMO, Tampere University and the Medical Research Council EVO (Finland)

References

[1] Aguilar R., Flint J., Gray J.A. et al. (2002) Learned fear, emotional reactivity and fear of heights: a factor analytic map from a large F2 intercross of Roman rat strains. *Brain Research Bulletin*, 57, 1, 17-26.

[2] Andrade M.M.M., Tome M.F., Santiago E.S. et al. (2003) Longitudinal study of daily variation of rats' behavior in the elevated plus maze. *Physiology and Behavior*, 78, 125-133.

[3] Arborelius L., Owens M.J., Plotsky P.M., Nemeroff C.B. (1999) The role of corticotropin-releasing factor in depression and anxiety disorders. *Journal of Endocrinology*, 160, 1-12.

[4] Armario A., Gavalda A., Marti O. (1988) Forced swimming test in rats: effects of desipramine administration and the period of exposure to the test on struggling behavior, swimming, immobility and defecation rate. *European Journal of Pharmacology*, 158, 207-212.

[5] Bai F., Li X., Clay M. et al. (2001) Intra- and interstrain differences in models of "behavioral despair". *Pharmacology Biochemistry and Behavior*, 70, 187-192.

[6] Barrett J.E., Miczek K.A. (2000) Behavioral techniques in preclinical neuropsychopharmacology research In: Psychopharmacology – The forth generation of the progress. The American College of Neuropsychopharmacology. (ACNP website http:www.acnp.org/g4).

[7] Bilkei-Gorzo A., Racz I., Michel K., Zimmer A. (2002) Diminished anxiety- and depression-related behaviors in mice with selective deletion of the Tac1 gene. *Journal of Neuroscience*, 22, 22, 10046-10052.

[8] Blanchard R.J., Nikulina J.N., Sakai R.L. et al. (1998) Behavioral and endocrine change following chronic predatory stress. *Physiology and Behavior*, 63, 4, 561-569.

[9] Belzung C. (1999) Measuring rodent exploratory behavior In: Handbook of Molecular genetics for brain and behavior research. Eds. Cruzio W.E., Gerlai R.T. Elsevier, NY, 738-749.

[10] Belzung C. (2001) The genetic basis of the pharmacological effects of anxiolytics: a review based on rodent models. *Behavioural Pharmacology*, 12, 451-460.

[11] Belzung C., Griebel G. (2001) Measuring normal and pathological anxiety-like behaviour in mice: a review. *Behavioural Brain Research*, 125, 141-149.

[12] Berridge K.C., Aldridge J.W. (2000) Super-stereotypy I: Enchancement of a complex movement sequence by systemic dopamine D1 agonists. Synapse, 37, 194-204.

[13] Bilkei-Gorzo A., Racz I., Michel K., Zimmer A. (2002) Diminished anxiety- and depression-related behaviors in mice with selective deletion of the Tac1 gene. *Journal of Neuroscience*, 22, 22, 10046-10052.

[14] Borsini F., Podhorna J., Marazziti D. (2002) Do animal models of anxiety predict anxiolytic-like effects of antidepressants? *Psychopharmacology*, 163, 2, 121-131.

[15] Bouwknecht J.A., Hijzen T.H., van der Gugten J. et al. (2000) Stress-induced hyperthermia in mice: effects of flesinoxan on heart rate and body temperature. *European Journal of Pharmacology*, 400, 59-66.

[16] Boyer P. (2000) Do anxiety and depression have a common pathophysiologica mechanism? *Acta Psychiatrica Scandinavica Supplement*, 406, 24-29.

[17] Broekkamp C. (1997) Predictive validity and the robustness criterion for animal models. *Psychopharmacology*, 134, 341-343.

[18] Calatayud F., Belzung C. (2001) Emotional reactivity in mice, a case of nongenetic heredity? *Physiology and Behavior*, 74, 355-362.

[19] Chapillon P., Manneche C., Belzung C., Caston J. (1999) Rearing environment enrichement in two inbred strains of mice: 1. Effect of emotional reactivity. *Behavioral Genetics*, 29, 1, 41-46.

[20] Chesler E.J., Wilson S.G., Lariviere W.R. et al. (2002) Infliences of laboratory environment on behavior. *Nature Neurosciences*, 5, 11, 1101-1102.

[21] Choleris E., Thomas A.W., Kavaliers M., Prato F.S. (2001) A detailed ethological analysis of the mouse open field test: effects of diazepam, chlordiazepoxide and an extremely low frequently pulsed magnetic field. *Neuroscience and Biobehavioral Reviews*, 25, 235-260.

[22] Clement EY., Calatayd F., Belzumg C. (2002) Genetic basis of anxiety-like behaviour: a critical review. *Brain Research Bullettin*, 57, 1, 57-71.

[23] Crabbe J.C., Wahlstein D., Dudek B.C. (2002) Genetics of mouse behavior: interaction with laboratory environment. Science, 284, 1670-1672.

[24] Crawley J.N. (1999) Behavioral phenotyping of transgenic and knockout mice: experimental design and evaluation of general health, sensory functions, motor abilities, and specific behavioral tests. *Brain Research*, 835, 18-26.

[25] Cruzio W.E. (2001) Genetic dissection of mouse exploratory behavior. *Behavioural Brain Research*, 125, 127-132.

[26] Davidson R.J., Lewis D.A., Alloy L.B. et al. (2002) Neural and behavioral substrates of mood and mood regulation. *Biological Psychiatry*, 52, 478-502.

[27] Dalvi A., Lucki I. (1999) Murine models of depression. *Psychopharmacology*, 147, 14-16.

[28] Davis M., Whalen P.J. (2001) The amygdala: vigilance and emotion. *Molecular Psychiatry*, 6, 13-34.

[29] Drai D., Kafkali N., Behjamini Y., Elmer G., Golani I. (2001) Rats and mice share common ethologically relevant parameters of exploratory behavior. *Behavioural Brain Research*, 125, 133-140.

[30] Dere E., Topic B., De Souza M.A. et al. (2002) The graded anxiety test: a novel test of murine unconditioned anxiety based on the principles of the elevated plus-maze and light-dark test. *Journal of Neuroscience Methods*, 122, 65-73.

[31] Eguibar J.R., Romero-Carbente J.C., Moyaho A. (2003) Behavioral differences between selectively bred rats: D1 versus D2 receptors in yawning and grooming. *Pharmacology Biochemistry and Behavior*, 6837, 1-6.

[32] Espejo E.F. (1997) Structure of the mouse behaviour on the elevated plus-maze test of anxiety. *Behavioural Brain Research*, 86, 105-112.

[33] Ferre S., Guix T., Prat G. et al. (1990) Is experimental catalepsy properly measured? *Pharmacology Biochemistry of Behavior*, 35, 4, 753-757.

[34] File S.E. (2001) Factors controlling measures of anxiety and responses to novelty in the mouse. *Behavioural Brain Research*, 125, 151-157.

[35] Flint J. (2003) Animal models of anxiety and their molecular dissection. *Seminars in Cell and Developmental Biology*, 14, 37-42.

[36] Fundarro A. (1998) Pinch-induced catalepsy in mice: a useful model to investigate antidepressant or anxiolytic drugs. *Progress in Neuro-Psychopharmacology and Biological Psychiatry*, 22, 147-158.

[37] Gaas P., Reinghart H.M., Strekalova T. et al. (2001) Mice with targeted mutations of glucocorticoid and mineralocorticoid receptors: Models for depression and anxiety? *Physiology and Behavior*, 73, 811-825.

[38] Galeeva A., Tuohimaa P. (2001) Analysis of mouse plus-maze behavior modulated by ovarían steroids. *Behavioural Brain Research*, 119, 41-47.

[39] Geyer M., Markou A. (2000) Animal models in psychiatric disorders. In: Psychopharmacology – The forth generation of the progress. The American College of Neuropsychopharmacology. (ACNP website http:www.acnp.org/g4).

[40] Hedou G., Pruce C., Di Iorio L. et al. (2001) An automated analysis of rat behavior in the forced swim test. *Pharmacology Biochemistry and Behavior*, 70, 65-76.

[41] Ho Y.J., Eichendorf J., Schwarting R.K. (2002) Individual response profiles of male Wistar rats in animal models for anxiety and depression. *Behavioral Brain Research*, 136, 1-12.

[42] Holmes A., Rodgers R.J. (2003) Prior exposure to the elevated plus-maze sensitizes mice to the acute behavioral effects of fluoxetine and phenelzine. *European Journal of Pharmacology*, 459, 221-230.

[43] Kalueff A.V. (1999) Problems of the study of stress-related behavior. *Kiev, KSF*, 136 p.

[44] Kalueff A.V., Makarchuk N.E., Samokhvalov V.P., Deryagina M.A. (2001) Urination and behavior. *Kiev, KSF*, 148 p.

[45] Kalueff A.V. Makarchuk N.E., Deryagina M.A., Shishkin S.L. (2001) The role of defecation in human and animal behavior. *Kiev, KSF*, 134p.

[46] Kalueff A.V., Maisky V.A., Pilyavskii A.I., Makarchuk N.E. (2001) Persistent c-fos expression and NADPH-d reactivity in the medulla and the lumbar spinal cord in rat with short-term peripheral anosmia. *Neuroscience Letters*, 301, 131-134.

[47] Kalueff A.V. (2002) Grooming and stress. Moscow, *Avix*, 138 p.

[48] Kalueff A.V. (2003) Today and tomorrow of anxiety research. Proceedings of the 7th Stress and behavior Multidisciplinary conference, Moscow, Russia.

[49] Kemble E.D., Bolwahnn B.L. (1997) Immediate and long-term effects of novel odors on risk assessment in mice. *Physiology and Behavior*, 61, 4, 543-549.

[50] King J.A., Messenger T., Ferris C.F. (2002) Seed finding in golden hamsters: a potential animal model for screening anxiolytic drugs. *Neuropsychobiology*, 45, 3, 150-155.

[51] Lapin I.P. (2000) Models of anxiety in mice: experimental verification and critical methodology. *Experimental and Klinical Farmacology*, 63, 3, 58-62.

[52] Magalhaes A., Tavares M.A., De Sousa L. (2002) Postnatal cocaine: effects on behavior of rats in forced swim test. *Annals of the NY Academy of Sciences*, 965, 529-534.

[53] Makarchuk N.E., Kalueff A.V. (2000) Olfaction and behavior. *Kiev, KSF*, 148 p.

[54] Malatynska E., Goldenberg R., Shuck L. et al. (2002) Reduction of submissive behavior in rats: a test for antidepressant drug activity. *Pharmacology*, 64, 1, 8-17.

[55] Marks I., Nesse R. (2001) The evolutionary analysis of anxiety disorders. In: Understanding Mental health. On-line information center. www.Depression.org.uk.

[56] Mayorga A.J., Lucki I. (2001) Limitation on the use of C57BL/6 mouse in the tail suspension test. *Psychopharmacology*, 155, 110-112.

[57] McGraugh C., Norman T.R. (1999) (+)-S-20499 – a potential antidepressant? A behavioural and neurochemical investigation in the olfactory bulbectomised rat. *European Neuropsychopharmacology*, 9, 21-27.

[58] McKinney W.T. (1984) Animal models of depression: an overview. *Psychiatry*, 2, 77-96.

[59] McKinney W.T. (2001) Overview of the past contributions in animal models and their changing place in psychiatry. *Seminars in Clinical Psychiatry*, 6, 68-78.

[60] Moyaho A., Eguibar J.R., Diaz J.L. (1995) Induced grooming transitions and open field behavior differ in high- and low-yawning sublines of Sprague-Dawley rats. *Animal Behavior*, 50, 61-72.

[61] Naitoh H., Nomura S., Kunimi Y., Yamaoka K. (1992) "Swimming-induced head twitching" in rats in the forced swimming test induced by overcrouding stress: a new marker in the animal model of depression? *Keio Journal of Medicine*, 41, 4, 221-224.

[62] Newport D.J., Stowe Z.N., Nemeroff C.B. (2002) Parental depression: animal models of an adverse life event. *American Journal of Psychiatry*, 159, 8, 1265-1283.

[63] Ohl F., Toschi N., Wigger A. et al. (2001) Dimensions of emotionality in a rat model of innate anxiety. *Behavioral Neuroscience*, 115, 2, 429-436.

[64] Olsen C.K., Hogg S., Lapiz M.D. (2002) Tonic immobility in guinea pigs: a behavioural response for detecting an anxiolytic-like effects? *Behavioural Pharmacology*, 13, 4, 261-269.

[65] Overall K.L. (2000) Natural animal models of human psychiatry conditions: assessment of mechanisms and validity. *Progress in Neuro-Psychopharmacology and Biological Psychiatry*, 24, 727-776.

[66] Palanza P. (2001) Animal models of anxiety and depression: how are females different? *Neuroscience Biobehavioral Reviews*, 25, 3, 219-233.

[67] Paterson A., Whitting P.J., Gray J.A., Flint J., Dawson G.R. (2001) Lack of consistent behavioural effects of Maudsley reactive and non-reactive rats in a number of animal tests of anxiety and activity. *Psychopharmacology*, 154, 336-342.

[68] Porsolt R.D. (2000) Animal models of depression: utility for transgenic research. *Reviews in the Neurosciences*, 11, 53-58.

[69] Rezvani A.H., Parsian A., Overstreet D.H. (2002) The Fawn-Hooded (FH/Wjd) rat: a genetic animal model of comorbid depression and alcoholism. *Psychiatric Genetics*, 12, 1, 1-16.

[70] Rodgers R.J., Cole J.C. (1994) The elevated plus maze: pharmacology, methodology and ethology. In: Cooper S.J., Hendrie C.A. (eds) *Ethological Pharmacology*, Willey, New York, 9-44.

[71] Rodgers R.J., Johnson N.J.T. (1996) Factor analysis of spatiotemporal and ethological measures in the murine elevated plus maze test of anxiety. *Pharmacology Biochemistry and Behavior*, 52, 297-303.

[72] Rodgers R.J. (2001) Anxious genes, emerging themes. *Behavioural Pharmacology*, 12, 471-476.

[73] Salome N., Viltart O., Darnaudery M. et al. (2002) Reliability of high and low anxiety-related behaviour: influence of laboratory environment and multifactorial analysis. *Behavioral Brain Research*, 136, 227-237.

[74] Salum C., Morato S., Roque-da-Silva A.C. (2000) Anxiety-like behavior in rats: a computational model. *Neural Networks*, 13, 21-29.

[75] Sarter M., Bruno J.P. (2002) Animal models in biological psychiatry. In: D'haenen H., den Boer J.A., Willner P. (eds) *Biological psychiatry*, Willey and Sons, New York, 1-8.

[76] Tejani-Butt S., Kluczynski J., Pare W.P. (2003) Strain-dependent modification of behavior following antidepressant treatment. *Progress in Neuro-Psychopharmacology and Biological Psychiatry*, 27, 7-14.

[77] Wall P.M., Messier C. (2001) Methodological and conceptual issues in the use of the elevated plus-maze as a psychological measurement instrument of animal. *Neuroscience and Biobehavioral Reviews*, 25, 275-286.

[78] Wehner J.M., Radcliffe R.A., Bowers B.J. (2001) Quantitative genetics and mouse behavior. *Annual Reviews in Neuroscience*, 24, 845-867.

[79] Weiss Y.M., Cierpial M.A., West C.H.K. (1998) Selective breeding of rats for High and Low motor activity in a swim test: toward a new animal model of depression. *Pharmacology Biochemistry and Behavior*, 61, 1, 49-66.

[80] Willner P. (1997) Validity, reliability abd utility of chronic mild stress model of depression: a 10-year review and evaluation. *Psychopharmacology*, 134, 319-329.

[81] Whishaw I.Q., Haun F., Kolb B. (2000) Analysis of behavior in laboratory rodents.

[82] Wurbel H. (2001) Ideal homes? Housing effects on rodent brain and behavior. *Trends in Neurosciences*, 24, 4, 207-211.

In: Animal Models in Biological Psychiatry
Editor: Allan V. Kalueff, pp. 27-42
ISBN 1-59454-814-5

Chapter 2

Protocol: Ethological Analysis of Grooming for Stress-Oriented Research in Mice – The Grooming Analysis Algorithm

Allan V. Kalueff and Pentti Tuohimaa
Medical School, University of Tampere,
Tampere University Hospital, Tampere, Finland

I. Introduction

Self-grooming is an ancient innate behaviour that is represented across most animal species and is a particularly important part of rodent behavioural repertoire (review: Kalueff, 2002). In rodents, a general pattern of self-grooming cephalocaudal progression is observed as follows: paw licking, nose and face wash, head wash, body wash and fur licking, leg licking, tail/genitals licking and wash (Inbox 1, also see further chapters in this book). Rodent grooming is also known to be bidirectionally sensitive to various psychotropic drugs and genetic manipulations (Eguibar et al., 2003; Moyaho et al., 1995; Moyaho and Valencia, 2002; van Erp et al., 1994), and is often studied in mice (Bolivar et al., 1996; Cromwell et al., 1998; Dunn et al., 1984; Gerlai et al., 1998; Greer and Capecci, 2003; Strazielle and Lalonde, 1998).

It has long been known that rodents' grooming activity can be generally increased in two opposite situations: in high and low stress (Kalueff, 2000; Kalueff and Tuohimaa, 2004). Low-stress comfort grooming is a spontaneous body care ritual which occurs as a transition from rest to activity; it is a typical behavioural marker of low or no stress and usually goes in a "relaxed fashion" from paw licking to tail/genitals wash (Fentress, 1977; Kalueff, 2000). Similarly, stress has long been known to induce grooming in rodents (Eguibar and Moyaho, 1997; Moyaho et al., 1995; van Erp et al., 1994, 1995). However, this stress-evoked grooming is ethologically different from low-stress grooming, and characterised by frequent bursts of rapid short grooming (Fentress, 1997; Kalueff, 2002; Moyaho et al., 1995).

Inbox 1.

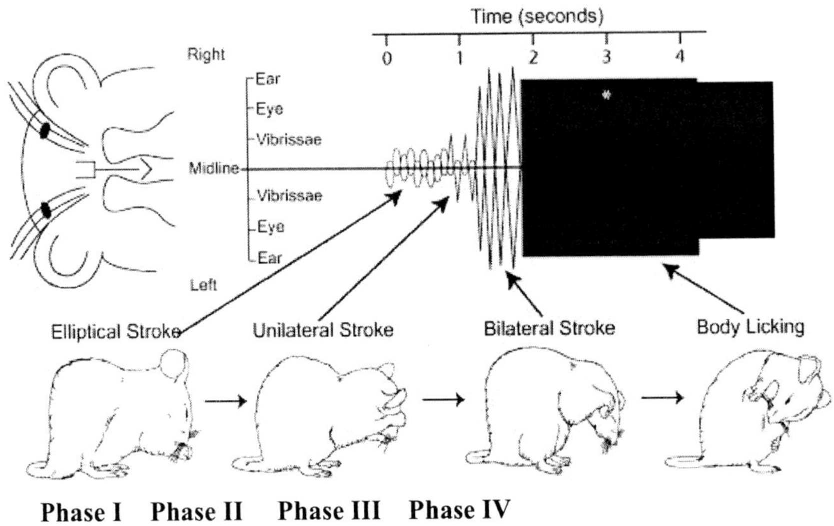

Figure I. Prototypical syntactic grooming chain pattern in mice (adapted from Berridge et al., 2005, with permission). Phase I: series of ellipse-shaped strokes tightly around the nose (paw, nose grooming). Phase II: series of unilateral strokes (each made by one paw) that reach up the mystacial vibrissae to below the eye (face grooming). Phase III: series of bilateral strokes made by both paws simultaneously. Paws reach back and upwards, ascending usually high enough to pass over the ears (head grooming). Phase IV: body licking, preceded by postural cephalocaudal transition from paw/head grooming to body grooming.

Grooming is an ancient behavior that is represented (with a striking homology) across most vertebrate species, including humans. Its biological functions include care of body surface, removal of ectoparasites, thermoregulation, chemo-communication, sensory stimulation of skin, displacement, de-arousal, maternal and social interaction. Both self- and heterogrooming behaviors are commonly seen in the wild and laboratory rodents. Self-grooming is common in mice, representing approximately 10-15% of all waking time, and the longest (after sleep) activity in their repertoire. It can be induced in animals by various factors, such as novelty, misting with water, swimming, exposure to predators or their odors, and pain. It is also often seen during pregnancy, as a "transitional element" between rest and exploration, or as a part of sexual behavior.

Many endogenous substances, including neuromediators such as dopamine, γ-amino butyric acid (GABA), serotonin, and hormones (adrenocorticotropin, vasopressin, oxytocin, prolactin, substance P, somatostatin, bombesin, corticotrophin releasing hormone, opioids, cholecystokinin) as well as multiple brain regions (especially basal ganglia and hypothalamus) are involved in the regulation of rodent self-grooming. Various psychotropic drugs also affect rodent grooming, collectively making its analysis a useful tool in behavioral neuroscience.

Mouse grooming appears in early ontogenesis, confirming the evolutionary "old" age of this behavior. Usually more frequent in the homecage, self-grooming is also seen in stressful situations such as novelty-based anxiety tests (e.g., elevated plus maze, open field and holeboard tests), implying that this behavior is not only important to assess, but can interfere with the primary behavior being assessed, and thus easily become a confounding factor, if neglected.

Nevertheless, in many studies this behavior has merited little scrutiny. Surprisingly, there are no grooming data in the extensive Mouse Phenome Database (MPD), nor in many recent comprehensive studies. Some authors assessed several grooming patterns but reported only one global behavioral score. Others compared different strains but analyzed only cumulative scores, or even combined grooming data in "overall activity scores" with horizontal and vertical exploration. In some other studies, several grooming indices were assessed in different strains cursorily among other measures, mostly including gross activity characteristics such as the latency, frequency and duration of grooming.

However, there is a growing understanding that only "quantitative" measures alone of mouse grooming may be insufficient for correct data interpretation and analysis. Rodent grooming is a complex, ethologically rich ritual, which normally proceeds in a cephalocaudal direction (Fig. I); Berridge et al., 2005. Dissectible at a number of levels, ranging from individual organ kinematics to the sequencing of grooming patterns, their habituation and association with non-grooming behaviors, such complex patterned structure is particularly attractive for behavioral phenotyping. Importantly, this approach can be used not only to assess "normal" mouse behaviors and their patterning, but also a source for ethologically-oriented experimental models of human stereotypic behavioral disorders. For example, the utility of grooming assessment has recently been suggested for mouse models of obsessive-compulsive disorder (OCD) and Tourette syndrome (Berridge et al., 2005). Consistent with this, psychotropic drugs that exacerbate OCD in patients have been reported to elicit robust rodent grooming (Graf et al., 2003), suggesting that grooming phenotyping may also be extensively used in behavioral pharmacology (also see Kalueff and Tuohimaa, 2005b for discussion), Fig. II.

Since rodents' self-grooming is increased by both stress and comfort conditions (Kalueff, 2000, 2002), the major problem with grooming behavioural analysis is that its traditional cumulative "gross" measures (the latency to onset, the number of bouts and the duration) may not be valid for correct data interpretation and analysis. As such, there is a great need for a tool which will make it possible to ethologically dissect different types of grooming activity. For this, we have designed the present Grooming Analysis Algorithm based on the above mentioned ethological differences between comfort- and stress-evoked groomings (Kalueff and Tuohimaa, 2004).

Our approach is based on differential registration and analysis of grooming behavioural microstructure, including 1) transitions between self-grooming patterns and 2) interruptions of grooming bouts in mice exposed to different stressors. Here we will review this method in detail and discuss its potential practical applications in mice, including neurobehavioural stress research and behavioural genetics.

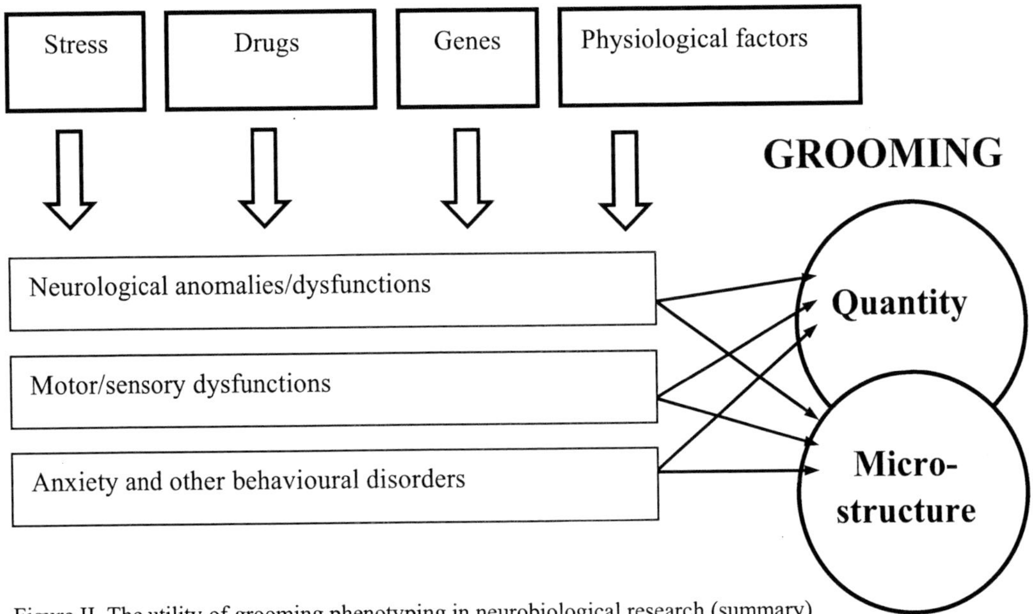

Figure II. The utility of grooming phenotyping in neurobiological research (summary)

II. Details of the Protocol

Brief Procedure

a) Observe animal self-grooming behaviours in the actimeter for 5 min. Record the number and the duration of grooming bouts. Include paw licking, nose/face grooming (strokes along the snout), head washing (semicircular movements over the top of the head and behind the ears), body grooming/scratching (body fur licking and scratching the body with the hind paws), leg licking and tail/genitals grooming (licking of the genital area and tail) as components of grooming behaviour, according to (Kalueff and Tuohimaa, 2004).
b) Record all instances of interruption of grooming activity; interruptions longer than 5 s determine separate grooming bouts.
c) Identify and register separately all grooming patterns and transitions between them using the following scaling system:
    - no grooming (stage 0),
    - paw licking (stage 1),
    - nose and face wash (stage 2),
    - head wash (stage 3),
    - body grooming (stage 4),
    - leg licking (stage 5),
    - tail/genitals grooming (stage 6).

d) Analyze all "correct" and "incorrect" transitions between grooming stages, as well as interruptions in grooming activity using the transition matrix (see Table 1 for details).
    - Correct transitions between grooming stages include the following progressive transitions: 0-1, 1-2, 2-3, 3-4, 4-5, 5-6, 6-0.
    - Incorrect transitions are chaotic and characterized by skipped (e.g. 0-6, 1-6, etc.) or reversed (e.g. 3-2, 4-1, 5-2, etc.) stages.

e) The percentage of incorrect transitions (of total transitions) and the percentage of interrupted grooming bouts (of total number of bouts) are used as behavioural indices of stress.

Animals and Behavioural Testing

Adult male 129S1, BALB/c and NMRI mice (25-30 g, n=10 in each group; University of Tampere, Finland) aged 20-24 weeks were maintained in a virus/parasite-free facility under conditions of controlled temperature (22±2 °C), humidity (60%), and exposed to a 12-h light, 12-h dark cycle. Lights were turned off at 18.00 h and on at 6.00 h. The animals were experimentally naïve and housed 3-4 per cage, with food and water freely available (except food finding experiments, when in order to increase hunger, animals were food deprived for 14 h prior to testing).

Table 1. An example of grooming transitions matrix for two mice from different experimental groups (adapted from Kalueff and Tuohimaa, 2004)

Stages of grooming	Control mouse # 3							Mouse # 12 (experimental group)						
	0	1	2	3	4	5	6	0	1	2	3	4	5	6
0	-	3	2	1	1			-	2	1		1	2	
1	2	-	2					2	-		1		1	
2	1		-	1				3	1	-				
3				-	1						-	1		
4		1			-	1			1			-		1
5	1					-	1	1	1			1	-	2
6	0						-	0	1	1			1	-
Interruption		1							1	2				

Sample of data summary:
Mouse 3 (Control): incorrect transitions - 9 (50%), total – 18; interrupted grooming bouts – 1 (12,5%), total – 8.
Mouse 12 (Experimental group): incorrect transitions - 16 (76%), total – 21; interrupted grooming bouts – 3 (50%), total – 6.

Behavioural testing was always conducted between 14.00 and 18.00 h. On the day of the experiments, animals were transported to the dimly lit room and left undisturbed for 3 h prior to testing. To induce spontaneous novelty-induced grooming, the mice were placed individually in a clean unfamiliar plastic actimeter box (30 x 30 x 30 cm) for 10 min. In all experiments, the animals were observed by an experienced investigator (reliability >0.9). During the testing sessions, the experimenter remained standing in front of (and 2 m away from) the testing boxes scoring mouse grooming and non-grooming behaviours using a specially designed register. Between subjects, the apparatus was thoroughly cleaned (wet and dry cloths). All experimental procedures were conducted in accordance with the European legislation (86/609/EEC) and the guidelines of the National Institutes of Health. All animal experiments reported here were approved by the Ethical Committee of the University of Tampere.

Rows are preceding stages; columns are following stages (see Detailed procedure for the grooming scaling system used in this protocol). “Correct” transition fields are marked by grey colour.

Behavioural Analysis of Novelty-Induced Behaviours in the Actimeter Test

Non-Grooming Measures

Vegetative behaviours (the number of fecal boli deposited and the number of urination spots) were scored as the conventional emotionality indices in the present study. We also assessed general vertical activity (vertical rears; the number of times an animal stood erect on its hind-legs with forepaws in the air or against the wall) and the latency to the first vertical rear (s) - as conventional behavioural measures of exploratory motor activity. Additional non-grooming behavioural parameters were displacement activity, including the number of jumping, tail-rattling episodes and manipulatory activity directed at the fecal boli (touching, pushing, lifting with the forepaws, eating and relocation by mouth).

Grooming Activity Measures

Four ethological measures of grooming activity were evaluated in all these tests:

- latency to start grooming (s);
- frequency (the number of grooming bouts);
- total time (s) spent grooming,
- average duration of a single grooming bout (s), calculated as total time spent grooming divided by the number of bouts.

Analysis of Grooming Behavioural Microstructure

The following patterns of grooming activity were recorded for each individual bout, as described earlier (Kalueff and Tuohimaa, 2004): forepaw licking, nose/face grooming (strokes along the snout), head washing (semicircular movements over the top of the head and behind ears), body grooming/scratching (body fur licking and scratching the body with the hind paws), hind-leg licking and tail/genitals grooming (licking of the genital area and tail). The 6-point scaling system was used in the present study, as described above.

Grooming behavioural microstructure was assessed using the grooming analysis algorithm, and the percentages of interrupted bouts and incorrect transitions were calculated for all mouse stains. A grooming bout was considered "interrupted" if at least one interruption was recorded within its stages; interruptions > 6 s determined separate grooming bouts. Transition between grooming patterns were analysed using the transition matrix (Table 1). In addition, the occurrence of atypical "vertical grooming" (the number and duration of episodes when an animal self-groomed standing *erect/semi-erect* on its hind-legs) was analysed in this study. This displacement behaviour included forepaw grooming bouts frequently seen in NMRI mice following vertical rears. Notably, this specific grooming pattern differed markedly from more common "non-vertical" forepaw grooming (displayed by all mouse strains and characterised by a typical flexed body position).

Data Analysis

All results are expressed as means ± S.E.M. Behavioural data were analysed by Mann-Whitney U-test for independent samples. To evaluate differences between strains in the actimeter test, analysis of variance (one-way ANOVA) was performed with the post-hoc U-test. A probability of less than 0.05 was considered statistically significant in all tests.

III. Results and Discussion

Non-Grooming Behaviours

Table 2 summarizes non-grooming behavioural data obtained in NMRI, BALB/c and 129S1 mice. Using one-way ANOVA to compare behaviours of mice tested in the actimeter test, we found significant strain differences for all non-grooming measures except urination. Further analysis using U-test revealed that the NMRI mice displayed maximal vertical activity scores (78±6 vs. 43±6 (129S1) and 61±4 (BALB/c); $P<0.05$) and the shortest latency to the first vertical rear (12±2 s vs. 32±5 s (129S1) and 40±6 s (BALB/c); $P<0.05$). In contrast, the 129S1 mice deposited significantly fewer boli (4±0.4) compared to both BALB/c (12±2) and NMRI (8±1) groups, while no changes were seen in the number of urination episodes in this test (Table 2). Another striking finding, as can be seen in Table 2, was that all mouse groups markedly differed in their strain-specific displacement activity, including tail rattling (BALB/c), jumping activity (129S1) and manipulations with own fecal boli (NMRI).

Table 2. Non-grooming behaviours in NMRI, BALB/c and 129S1 mice subjected to actometer test. Strains sharing common letters are statistically different (P<0.05, U-test; adapted from Kalueff and Tuohimaa 2005a)

Behaviours	129S1	BALB/c	NMRI
Vertical activity F(2,27) = 10.44; P < 0.0004	43 ± 6 a	61 ± 4 b	78 ± 6 ab
Latency to the first vertical rear (s) F(2,27) = 9.6; P < 0.001	32 ± 5a	40 ± 6 b	12 ± 2 ab
Number of tail rattling episodes F(2,27) = 123.45; P < 0.0001	0 a	2 ± 0.2 ab	0 a
Manipulations with own fecal boli * F(2,27) = 100; P < 0.0001	0 a	0 b	10 ± 1 ab
Defecation boli deposited F(2,27) = 9.14; P < 0.001	4 ± 0.5 ab	12 ± 2 a	8 ± 1b
Urination F(2,27) = 1,23; P < 0.28 (NS)	0.4 ± 0.1	0.4 ± 0.1	0.2 ± 0.1
Number of jumping episodes F (2,27) = 100; P < 0.0001	1 ± 0.1 ab	0 a	0 b

NA - data not available. * Touching, lifting, eating, moving with forepaws, relocating by with mouth. Between-groups difference was analysed by one-way ANOVA test (factor: strain)

Novelty-Induced Grooming Behaviours

Table 3 shows grooming activity of mice tested in the actimeter test. Using one-way ANOVA test, we found significant strain differences in the following grooming measures: time spent grooming; average duration of a single bout; percent of incorrect transitions, number of interruptions of grooming activity, percent of interrupted bouts; number and duration of vertical grooming episodes. Further analysis using post-hoc U-test showed that the BALB/c mice spent significantly more time grooming (34±4 s) than did their 129S1 (19±2 s) and NMRI (23±3 s) counterparts. The number of grooming bouts in all three strains was similar, although the 129S1 mice showed a tendency to display more bouts. The average duration of a single bout was significantly longer in the BALB/c group (8.1±1 s) compared to the 129S1 (3.2±0.3 s) and NMRI (5.2±2 s) groups. As can be seen in Table 3, the latency to start grooming was not statistically different in all three mouse strains, although the NMRI mice showed a clear tendency to earlier onset of grooming, compared to both 129S1 and BALB/c strains.

Table 3. Grooming behaviours in NMRI, BALB/c and 129S1 mice tested in a 10-min actimeter test. Between-groups difference was analysed by one-way ANOVA test (factor: strain) followed by a post-hoc U-test. Strains sharing common letters are statistically different (P<0.05, U-test; adapted from Kalueff and Tuohimaa, 2005a)

Grooming behaviours / F (one-way ANOVA) test	129S1	BALB/c	NMRI
General cumulative measures			
Number of bouts F(2,27) = 0.91; P < 0.41 (NS)	5.8 ± 1	4.2 ± 1	4.4 ± 0.7
Time spent grooming (s) F (2,27) = 6.24; P < 0.006	19 ± 2 a	34 ± 4 ab	23 ± 3 b
Latency to start grooming (s) F(2,27) = 1.38; P < 0.27 (NS)	130 ± 23	146 ± 19	100 ± 17
Average duration of a single bout (s) F(2,27) = 11.52; P < 0.0002	3.2 ± 0.3 a	8.1 ± 1 ab	5.2 ± 0.7 b
Behavioural microstructure of grooming			
Total number of transitions between patterns F(2,27) = 1.34; P < 0.28 (NS)	14 ± 2	16 ± 4	21 ± 3
% Incorrect transitions F(2,27) = 5.65; P < 0.008	64 ± 5 ab	43 ± 4 a	47 ± 5 b
Number of interruptions F(2,27) = 54.32; P < 0.0001	1.4 ± 0.1 ab	0.2 ± 0 ac	0.7 ± 0.1 bc
Average transitions per bout F(2,27) = 2.85; P < 0.07 (NS)	2.4 ± 0.5	3.8 ± 1	4.7 ± 0.4
% Interrupted bouts F(2,27) = 14.63; P < 0.0001	28 ± 5 ab	5 ± 1 a	10 ± 2 b
Number of vertical grooming episodes F(2,27) = 891.00; P < 0.0001	0 a	0 b	2 ± 0 ab
Time spent vertical grooming (s) F(2,27) = 25.00; P < 0.0001	0 a	0 b	5 ± 1 ab

Analysis of grooming behavioural microstructure in these strains (Table 3) shows that 129S1 mice tend to display fewer transitions between patterns but show significantly higher percentages of incorrect transitions (64±5% vs. 43±4% (BALB/c) and 47±5% (NMRI) and interrupted grooming bouts (28±5% vs. 5±1% (BALB/c) and 10±2% (NMRI). The average number of transitions per bout was similar in all groups, while the NMRI mice displayed specific vertical grooming activity completely lacking in the BALB/c and 129S1 groups (Table 3).

IV. Discussion

129S1, NMRI and BALB/c mouse strains were chosen for their importance in genetic and behavioural research, and for their marked strain differences in several features that might be related to grooming (Kalueff and Tuohimaa, 2005a). Moreover, this situation when one strain is always different from the other two (activity: 129S1; anxiety: NMRI; aggression: BALB/c; brain anatomy: NMRI; displacement activity: NMRI; Table 2) allows pair-wise comparisons between the strains and one-by-one dissection of possible factors influencing their grooming. Here we show that mice from these strains exhibit contrasting behavioural patterns in their spontaneous (novelty-induced) grooming (Table 3).

Analysing behavioural profiles of 129S1, BALB/c and NMRI mice, we first noted that these strains differ markedly in their baseline activity (review: Kalueff and Tuohimaa, 2005a). Thus, it was possible to assume that the strain differences in grooming seen in the present study may be merely due to different levels of activity in these strains. However, analysis of grooming and motor activity shows no clear correlation between these behaviours (Tables 2 and 3). Indeed, the two strains with low-grooming phenotypes show markedly different activity profiles (low: 129S1; high: NMRI, Table 2) while both active strains show different grooming activity (low: NMRI; high: BALB/c, Table 3). Finally, grooming sequencing was also different in the 129S1 vs. BALB/c and NMRI mice (Table 3), consistent with earlier findings showing that the organisation of behaviour in mice varies independently of the amount of activity (Paulus et al., 1999). Taken together, these findings suggest that the contrasting grooming phenotypes reported here are not determined by different levels of activity in these three mouse strains.

Notably, 129S1, BALB/c and NMRI mice differ markedly in their aggressiveness (BALB/c>129S1>>NMRI). Since grooming is often seen as a part of agonistic behavioural repertoire in mice (Spruijt et al., 1992), it was possible to assume that the strain differences in grooming reported here may be due to different levels of aggression. However, our data show no clear correlation between grooming and aggression. Indeed, while both non-aggressive strains (NMRI, 129S1) show markedly different patterning of grooming, the strains with different levels of aggression (BALB/c and NMRI) show similar unimpaired grooming microstructure (Table 3). Collectively, these observations negate the idea that the contrasting grooming phenotypes reported in the present study are due to different aggressiveness of these mouse strains.

Finally, all three strains have been reported to possess different baseline levels of anxiety (Kalueff and Tuohimaa, 2005a). As already mentioned in the Introduction, grooming has long been known to be a behavioural marker of stress in rodents, raising the possibility that more grooming in BALB/c mice may be due to more anxiety in this strain, compared to low-grooming NMRI and 129S1 mice. The fact that defecation scores - a traditional marker of stress in rodents - were maximal in the BALB/c and minimal in the 129S1 mice (Table 2) seems to support this notion. However, this hypothesis clearly contradicts numerous earlier findings (see review: Kalueff and Tuohimaa, 2005a) and our present data (Table 2), demonstrating more anxiety in 129S1 compared to BALB/c and particularly NMRI mice. The fact that non-anxious NMRI mice also showed high defecation levels indicates that defecation index is only one of several types of stress measures, and different mouse strains display some but not all stress-related behaviours.

Importantly, it has long been recognised that the interaction of grooming and anxiety is rather complex, and that rodent grooming is increased in both high and low stress situations (Kalueff 2000, 2002). Therefore, its cumulative measures may not reflect the level of stress, if taken alone. Consistent with this, anxious BALB/c mice showed more grooming than non-anxious NMRI mice, while low grooming levels were seen in both anxious 129S1 and non-anxious NMRI mice (Table 3). Given the low-anxiety profile of NMRI mice, we can suggest that their non-grooming behaviours (such as high vertical activity) may confound their grooming, thus, showing a clear low-anxiety low-grooming response. Moreover, grooming may represent a displacement activity and/or a "self-directed form of coping" in these mice, serving to alleviate anxiety, as has already been suggested for NMRI mice (Pardon et al., 2004). Indeed, grooming is a common displacement activity in rodents, including mice. In line with this, our NMRI mice frequently displayed displacement "vertical" grooming and another interesting displacement activity - manipulations with fecal boli (behaviour that cannot be expected in high-anxiety states and, predictably, was not seen in anxious 129S1 and BALB/c mice), Tables 2 and 3. Some other strain-specific non-grooming behaviours may also explain the low grooming activity of 129S1 mice seen in the present study. For example, these mice frequently display anxiogenic-like "freezing" behavioural response to stressors as well as a tendency to more escape-like behaviours (jumping). It is therefore possible that these behaviours may affect the grooming phenotypes reported here.

In contrast to cumulative measures of grooming, its behavioural microstructure shows consistent increase in abnormalities in more anxious strains (NMRI<BALB/c<129S1 mice; as reported here). Taken together, these data support our hypothesis that shifts in the behavioural microstructure of grooming (the percentages of interrupted bouts and incorrect transitions between patterns) are highly sensitive behavioural markers of stress (Kalueff and Tuohimaa, 2004). Thus, a dramatic difference between non-anxious NMRI, moderately anxious BALB/c and anxious 129S1 mice in their grooming microstructure (Table 3) may be explained by different levels of anxiety in these strains. Moreover, the behavioural microstructure of rodent grooming is very sensitive to the level of stress, known to disrupt its cephalocaudal pattern and increase the percentage of interrupted and incomplete bouts (Kalueff, 2002). Indeed, our observations that 129S1 mice generally display extra-short (1-2 patterns) incomplete and frequently interrupted grooming bouts with more incorrect transitions (Table 3) are in line with our non-grooming data (Table 2) and previously published studies (review: Kalueff and Tuohimaa, 2005a) describing the anxious behavioural phenotype of this strain.

V. General Assessment and Potential Applications of the Protocol

Overall, understanding strain differences in the patterning of complex behaviours, such as grooming, may assist us in the search for better animal models of specific behavioural disorders. Given our data on impaired patterning of grooming in 129S1 mice, it can be suggested that BALB/c mice are a better choice to study the effects of mutations or drugs likely to impair motor coordination and patterning of complex behaviours. In contrast, 129S1 mice may be useful to assess genetic or other manipulations likely to improve such performance. Overall, our results, establishing contrasting grooming behavioural phenotypes in NMRI, 129S1 and BALB/c mice, may provide valuable information for discriminating between the effects in question and the effects of mouse strain-specific phenotypes.

In summary, our data reveal different grooming profiles in 129S1, BALB/c and NMRI mouse strains in novelty stress (Table 4), which appear to be unrelated to the strain differences in general activity levels, sensory abilities, brain anatomy or aggressiveness. The results of this study suggest that the strain differences in grooming may be a result of complex interplay between anxiety, motor and displacement activity (Table 4), perhaps reflecting different behavioural stress-coping strategies in these mice. We suggest that contrasting grooming phenotypes may be attributed to a high anxiety low activity phenotype of 129S1 mice, compared to anxious BALB/c and non-anxious NMRI active mouse strain. In addition, NMRI mice showed frequent displacement behaviours, including specific manipulatory activity and "vertical" grooming, suggesting that animals of this non-anxious strain make extensive use of displacement activity as an effective stress-coping strategy (see also Pardon et al., 2004)). Given the increasing use of NMRI, BALB/c and 129S1 mice in behavioural research, the results of the present study emphasise the importance of understanding the differences between grooming patterns in these mouse strains for correct ethological analyses of behavioural data. Thus, as has already been speculated (Fentress, 1988), an in-depth analysis of mouse grooming (especially using our protocol) may sufficiently contribute to our understanding of some human behavioural disorders,

Table 4. Summary of behavioural strain differences in the novelty situation between NMRI, BALB/c and 129S1 mice (adapted from Kalueff and Tuohimaa, 2005a)

Behaviour	**129S1**	**BALB/c**	**NMRI**
General activity	Low	High	High
Anxiety	High	High	Low
Self-grooming activity	Low	High	Low
Grooming patterning (sequencing)	Impaired	Unimpaired	Unimpaired
Vertical (displacement) grooming	None	None	High
Non-grooming displacement activity	None	Low*	High *

* Tail rattling (BALB/c mice) and manipulations with own fecal boli (NMRI mice), see Table 2 for details.

Several aspects may explain why this protocol can be a novel alternative method of behavioural analysis, and a valuable tool in behavioural research, used to complement or even replace more traditional gross measures.

The idea of analysing grooming separately instead of focusing on grooming demonstrated only during other behavioural tests (e.g., the open field or elevated plus maze, as done in the majority of studies) can be a clear advantage. Indeed, grooming scores taken during these tests are generally low (being masked by alterations in other, non-grooming behaviours), and their analysis can therefore be extremely difficult. In contrast, more specific analysis of mouse grooming in an actimeter test following testing in these paradigms not only enables higher grooming scores, but also the identification of more "pure" stress-evoked grooming, not confounded by other (non-grooming) behaviours. This approach allows obtaining several parallel sets of data, including: a) behavioural measures taken in these initial behavioural tests, and b) grooming measures obtained in the subsequent testing using this current protocol, which can then both be used for a detailed behavioural analysis.

The data presented here show that alteration in grooming microstructure itself can be used as a sensitive behavioural index, which is at least as useful as traditional grooming measures. This observation further confirms the utility of the protocol as a universal method for analysing potential changes in grooming produced by different factors in question.

We may also suggest that the present protocol is able to detect stress-evoked alterations in grooming in different genetically modified animals (e.g., Kalueff and Tuohimaa, 2004), implying the utility of our approach to study behavioural phenotypes of various mutant mice, especially those displaying abnormal emotional behaviours. In addition, since some mutant mice may have abnormal sequencing of behavioural patterns including grooming (which may occur with or without changes in grooming gross measures), our protocol based on sequential analysis of grooming may be a useful tool in the detection of such behavioural abnormalities.

In general, our results show that a detailed analysis of grooming behaviour according to this protocol appears to be a useful tool for the study of mouse behaviours in the field of stress research and behavioural neurogenetics. Furthermore, we suggest that the protocol is also suitable for use with rats and other laboratory rodents given the similarity in their grooming behaviours. The protocol can also be used in psychopharmacology research, in the search of novel anxiolytic antistress drugs. Given the results of our study, this protocol will be especially useful in assisting with more accurate interpretation of other (non-grooming) behavioural data, especially in situations when conflicting data have been obtained, and there is a need for more detailed and in-depth behavioural analysis. For example, it may be extensively used when studying different manipulations with mixed or unclear effects, interpreting the behaviour of novel mutant mice with unknown or unclear behavioural phenotype, or screening drugs with unclear profile.

Finally, although not directly tested in this study, it is possible to speculate that our protocol may not only detect stress-evoked alterations in grooming microstructure, but also (after some modification) actually measure the degree of stress evoked by different tests. Clearly, this promising research direction will almost certainly require further investigation, and may represent an important potential application of our protocol.

VI. Methodological Considerations

Numerous studies confirm that grooming is the initial behavioural response to stressful situations and is used by the animals to lower arousal. The finding that grooming microstructure is sensitive to stressors suggests good predictive validity for the current protocol as a powerful tool to detect stress in animal behaviour. However, we should point out that stress-evoked non-grooming behavioural activity (e.g. risk assessment, freezing, and urination/defecation) can be a possible confounding factor, because alterations in these behaviours may reciprocally affect animal grooming. Since all non-grooming behaviours are more obvious when mice are first exposed to the actimeter test, their grooming is easily affected by minimal changes in environmental conditions. Thus, it is crucial that the experimenters handle the mice for 5 min./day for 5 days and expose them to the actimeter for 5 min./day 2-3 times before the first experiment, in order for them to become familiar with environmental stimuli (Kalueff and Tuohimaa, 2004).

Since grooming response is known to habituate after repeated exposures to stress, we have noted that experimentally naïve animals on Test 1 usually show clearer and more robust results. If, however, a battery of several stressors has to be used in the same animals (which is nowadays the most common situation in behavioural research), the mice should be allowed at least 7 days for acclimation between the tests. We have also noted that the present grooming analysis algorithm works better if the battery includes 3 or fewer tests. The timetable and intensity of the experiments is another related practical issue which may be critical for obtaining correct and reliable data (Belzung, 1999; Clement et al., 2002; Crawley et al., 1997; Crawley, 1999). Since rodents are very sensitive to the rhythm of activity of the researchers and animal house personnel (usually higher from Monday to Friday), all their behaviours can be affected by this factor (Belzung, 1999). This also relates to grooming: for example, we have noted that animal grooming scores are different on Monday than during the rest of the week. Although this is a common problem with all behavioural studies (Belzung, 1999), it is advisable to consistently avoid, or, alternatively, prefer, weekends when scheduling the experiments aiming to assess animals' grooming behaviours (Kalueff and Tuohimaa, 2004).

Another common behavioural problem that may be encountered during the experiments is that mice sometimes display an unusually low activity level. This also relates to specific grooming activity. For example, some mice may fail to groom during the test, while others may display frequent extra-short (1-2 stages) bouts or have unusual long latencies to start grooming (Kalueff, 2002; Kalueff and Tuohimaa, 2004). Although usually the percentage of these animals is <5-10%, which usually does not affect the results, this potential problem should be considered when performing analysis of animal grooming. There is neither a simple explanation nor a simple solution for this phenomenon. As one possible solution, it can be recommended to carefully check homecage behaviours before the testing and, if necessary, exclude mice with very low general motor and/or grooming activity from the experiments. In addition, the observation room conditions (ventilation, temperature, humidity, soundproofing, lights, etc.) and even experimenter identity may affect animal grooming performance, known to be very sensitive to all environmental conditions. As such, these factors have to be carefully controlled in the experiments.

Acknowledgements

This study was supported in parts by CPBR, Tampere University and the Medical Research Council EVO (Finland).

References

[1] C. Belzung. Measuring rodent exploratory behavior. In: *Handbook of molecular genetics for brain and behavior research*. Eds. Cruzio W.E., Gerlai R.T. Elsevier, NY (1999), 738-749.

[2] K.C. Berridge, J.W. Aldridge, K.R. Houchard, X. Zhuang, Sequential super-stereotypy of an instinctive fixed action pattern in hyper-dopaminergic mutant mice: a model of obsessive compulsive disorder and Tourette's. *BMC Biol. 3* (2005) 1-16.

[3] V.J. Bolivar, W. Danilchuk, J.C. Fentress, Separation of activation and pattern in grooming development of weaver mice, *Behav Brain Res*. 75 (1996) 49-58.

[4] Y. Clement, F. Calatayud, C. Belzung, Genetic basis of anxiety-like behaviour: a critical review. *Brain Res Bull*. 57 (2002) 57-71.

[5] J.N. Crawley, J.K. Belknap, A. Collins, J.C. Crabbe, W. Frankel, N. Henderson, R.J. Hitzermann, S.C. Maxson, L.L. Miner, A.J. Silva, J.M. Wehner, A. Wynshaw-Boris, R. Paylor, Behavioural phenotypes of inbred mouse strains: implications and recommendations for molecular studies, *Psychopharmacol*. 132 (1997) 107-124.

[6] J.N. Crawley, Behavioural phenotyping of transgenic and knockout mice: experimental design and evaluation of general health, sensory functions, motor abilities, and specific behavioural tests, *Brain Res*. 835 (1999) 18-26.

[7] H.C. Cromwell, K.C. Berridge, J. Drago, M.S. Levine, Action sequencing is impaired in D1A-deficient mutant mice, *Eur J Neurosci*. 10 (1998) 2426-2432.

[8] A.J. Dunn, C.W. Berridge, Y.I. Lai, T.L. Yachabach, CRF-induced excessive grooming behavior in rats and mice, Peptides. 8 (1987) 841-844.

[9] J.R. Eguibar, A. Moyaho, Inhibition of grooming by pilocarpine differs in high- and low-yawning sublines of Sprague-Dawley rats, *Pharmacol Biochem Behav*. 58 (1997) 317-322.

[10] J.R. Eguibar, J.C. Romero-Carbente, A. Moyaho, Behavioral differences between selectively bred rats: D1 versus D2 receptors in yawning and grooming, *Pharmacol Biochem Behav*. 74 (2003) 827-832.

[11] J.C. Fentress, The tonic hypothesis and the patterning of behaviour, *Ann NY Acad Sci*, 290 (1977) 370-394.

[12] R. Gerlai, J.F. Henderson, J.C. Roder, Z. Jia, Multiple behavioural anomalies in GluR2 mutant mice exhibiting enchanced LTP, *Behav Brain Res*. 95 (1998) 37-45.

[13] M. Graf, S. Kantor, Z.E. Anheuer, E.A. Modos, G. Bagdy, m-CPP-induced self-grooming is mediated by 5-HT2C receptors, *Behav Brain Res*. 142 (2003) 175-179.

[14] J.M. Greer, M.R. Capecci, Hoxb8 is required for normal grooming behaviour in mice, *Neuron*. 33 (2003) 23-34.

[15] A.V. Kalueff, Measuring grooming in stress and comfort, *Proc Measur Behav*. 3 (2000) 148-149.

[16] A.V. Kalueff, Grooming and stress, KSF, Kiv, 2002, 148 pp.

[17] A.V. Kalueff, P. Tuohimaa, Grooming analysis algorithm for neurobehavioural stress research, Brain Res. *Protocols*. 13 (2004) 151-158.

[18] A.V. Kalueff, P. Tuohimaa, Contrasting grooming phenotypes in three mouse strains markedly different in their anxiety and activity (129S1, BALB/c and NMRI), *Behav Brain Res.* 160 (2005a) 1-10.

[19] A.V. Kalueff, P. Tuohimaa, Mouse grooming microstructure is a reliable anxiety marker bidirectionally sensitive to GABAergic drugs, *Eur J Pharmacol.* 508 (2005b) 147-153.

[20] Moyaho, J.R. Eguibar, J.L. Diaz, Induced grooming transitions and open field behaviour differ in high- and low-yawning sublines of Sprague-Dawley rats, *Anim Behav.* 50 (1995) 61-77.

[21] Moyaho, J. Valencia, Grooming and yawning trace adjustment to unfamiliar environments in laboratory Sprague-Dawley rats (Rattus norvegicus), *J Comp Psychol.* 116 (2002) 263-269.

[22] M.C. Pardon, D.A. Kendall, F. Perez-Diaz, M.S. Duxon, C.A. Marsden, Repeated sensory contact with aggressive mice rapidly leads to an anticipatory increase in core body temperature and physical activity that precedes the onset of aversive responding, *Eur J Neurosci* 20 (2004) 1033-1050.

[23] M.P. Paulus, S.C. Dulawa, R.J. Ralph, M. Geyer, Behavioural organization is independent of locomotor activity in 129 and C57 mouse strains, *Brain Res*, 835 (1999) 27-36.

[24] B.M. Spruijt, J.A. van Hooff, W.H. Gispen, Ethology and neurobiology of grooming behavior, *Physiol Rev*, 72 (1992) 825-852.

[25] Strazielle, R. Lalonde, Grooming in Lurcher mutant mice, *Physiol Behav.* 64 (1998) 57-61.

[26] A.M. van Erp, M.R. Kruk, W. Meelis, D.C. Willekens-Bramer, Effect of environmental stressors on time course, variability and form of self-grooming in the rat: handling, social contact, defeat, novelty, restraint and fur moistening, *Behav Brain Res.* 65 (1994) 47-55.

[27] A.M. van Erp, M.R. Kruk, D.C. Willekens-Bramer, P.C. Fermont, M.J. Nijsen, PVH lesions do not inhibit stressor-induced grooming in the rat, *Physiol Behav.* 57 (1995) 887-892.

In: Animal Models in Biological Psychiatry
Editor: Allan V. Kalueff, pp. 43-57
ISBN 1-59454-814-5

Chapter 3

Grooming Analysis Algorithm for Neurobehavioural Stress Research in Rats

Allan V. Kalueff and Pentti Tuohimaa
Tampere University and the University Hospital, Tampere, Finland

I. Introduction

Self-grooming is an ancient innate body care behaviour that is represented across most animal species (Fentress, 1977; Spruijt et al., 1992; Greer and Capecci, 2003). Grooming is a frequently performed behaviour by small felids, bovids, cervids and primates (Eckstein and Hart, 2000; Hart and Pryor, 2004), and is an important part of rodent behavioural repertoire (Berridge et al., 1987; Berridge and Whishaw, 1992; Van Erp et al., 1995). In rodents, grooming is a complex, ethologically rich ritual which normally proceeds in a cephalocaudal direction and consists of several stages, including licking the paws, washing movements over the head, fur licking, and tail/genitals cleaning (Fentress, 1977; Eguibar et al., 1997; Berridge and Aldridge, 2000a,b). Many neuromediators and hormones as well as multiple regions in the brain appear to be involved in the regulation of grooming behaviours (Van Erp et al., 1995; Bolivar et al., 1996; Cromwell and Berridge, 1996; Cromwell et al., 1996; Bressers et al., 1998). Grooming is highly sensitive to various stressors, psychotropic drugs and genetic manipulations (Dunn et al., 1987; Spruijt et al., 1992; Gerlai et al., 1998; Choleris et al., 2001), and has long been studied in laboratory rodents, including mice and rats (Van Erp et al., 1995; Crawley et al., 1997; Van de Weerd et al., 2001; Jarbe et al. 2002; Kalueff et al., 2004a,b). In rodents, grooming plays an important role in behavioural adaptation to stress, including stress-coping and de-arousal (Kametani, 1988; Sachs, 1988; Spruijt et al., 1992; Eguibar et al., 2003).

Overall, rodents' grooming can be dissected at a number of levels, ranging from individual limb segment kinematics to the sequencing of grooming patterns and their association with other (non-grooming) behaviours (Moyaho et al., 1995; Bolivar et al., 1996; Komorowska and Pisula, 2003). Although many studies have analysed different aspects of grooming and its behavioural organization (Van Erp et al., 1994, 1995; Cromwell and Berridge, 1996; Cromwell et al., 1996; Bressers et al., 1998), the exact role of grooming behaviour in stress is still not well understood (Homberg et al. 2002; Komorowska and Pellis, 2004). Indeed, it has long been known that rodents' grooming activity can be generally increased in two opposite situations: in high and low stress (Katz and Roth, 1979; Kalueff, 2002). "Comfort" grooming is a ritual occurring as a transition from rest to activity, and under spontaneous or low stress conditions following a cephalocaudal rule (Fentress, 1977; Spruijt et al., 1992; Kalueff, 2000). However, mild stress such as exposure to novel environment has also been known to induce grooming in rats (Moody et al., 1988; Van Erp et al., 1994; Eguibar and Moyaho, 1997; Escorihuela et al., 1999). Notably, this stress-evoked "displacement" grooming is ethologically different from no-stress grooming, and characterised by frequent and rapid short bursts (Fentress, 1977; Kalueff, 2000; Moyaho and Valencia, 2002). As such, it is becoming necessary to assess in more detail stress-evoked grooming behaviours and their behavioural microstructure in rodent species commonly used in neurobehavioural research, such as mice and rats.

Although grooming in rodents plays a very important role in various behavioural models of stress (Van Erp et al., 1994, 1995), in many studies this behaviour has merited little scrutiny, frequently addressed only cursorily among other measures (e.g., Ohl et al., 2001; Van de Weerd et al., 2001; Aguilar et al., 2003, Hossain et al., 2004; but: Jarbe et al., 2002). In most studies, general characteristics of grooming behaviour (latency to onset, frequency and duration) have been described (Moody et al., 1988; Barros et al. 1994; Espejo, 1997), however, few reports analyse the organization (patterning) of grooming in different stressful situations (Kametani, 1988; Komorowska and Pisula, 2003). Since rodents' self-grooming is increased by both stress and comfort conditions (File et al., 1988; Lawler et al., 1988; Moody et al., 1988), the traditional "quantitative" measures of grooming may be insufficient for correct data interpretation and analysis (Kalueff, 2000, 2002).

Indeed, although stress elicits grooming activity in rodents, there are many data showing that reduced levels of stress may also lead to this phenomenon. For example, "anxiolytic" sudden darkness (Nasello et al., 2003) in rats is seen together with increased time spent grooming. Some anxiolytics (ethanol, muscimol) have been reported to increase, while anxiogenics (bicuculline) to inhibit grooming in rats (File et al., 1988; Osborne et al., 1993; Perier et al., 2002). In mice, anxiolytic chlordiazepoxide and diazepam activated grooming in the elevated plus maze (Rodgers et al., 2002) and in the central area of the open field (Choleris et al., 2001), respectively. Furthermore, our recent studies also found no clear correlation between grooming scores and anxiety in mice. For example, lower grooming activity was seen in more anxious 129S1 vs. non-anxious C57BL/6 mice (Kalueff and Tuohimaa, 2004b, also see similar results in Hossain et al., 2004). C57BL/6 mice demonstrated similar degree of grooming activation in both low-stress (novel box) and high-stress (social encounter with an unfamiliar male) tests (Kalueff and Tuohimaa, 2004a). Finally, more stressful situation (exposure to the elevated plus maze) produced less grooming in these mice than did a relatively weak stressor (exposure to a familiar box) (Kalueff and Tuohimaa 2004a). Taken together, these data indicate that grooming "quantitative" measures in rodents may not always reliably reflect the level of stress, and that additional grooming measures (such as its "qualitative", or patterning characteristics) are also necessary in order to assess animals' stress-evoked behaviours.

The patterned structure of rodent grooming makes it particularly attractive for neurobehavioural stress research (Komorovska and Pellis, 2004). It has been recently suggested that grooming behavioural microstructure undergoes predictable changes in stressful situations (Kalueff, 2000; Komorowska and Pellis, 2004), thus making it possible to ethologically dissect different types of rodents' grooming activity. For this, we have previously designed the mouse grooming analysis algorithm based on the ethological differences between comfort- and stress-evoked grooming (Kalueff and Tuohimaa, 2004a). This "qualitative" approach used differential registration and analysis of grooming behavioural microstructure, including 1) transitions between self-grooming patterns and 2) interruptions of grooming bouts in mice exposed to different stressors. In a striking contrast to grooming "activity" measures, this algorithm worked consistently in all experimental models, demonstrating clear impairments of grooming patterning in anxious animals (129S1 vs. C57BL/6 mice, stressed vs. non-stressed C57BL/6 mice) and showing no such alterations in low or no-stress situations (Kalueff and Tuohimaa, 2004a,b).

Importantly, although mice and rats share many common behavioural features, including grooming (Whishaw et al. 2001), it was unclear whether this approach may be used for stress-oriented research in rats. Indeed, some differences have been reported for various behaviours in these two species, including grooming. For example, rats generally display complex and organized grooming patterns, with more symmetrical movements and transitions between stages (Berridge, 1990). Together, this suggests that grooming microstructure in mice may be much simpler than that in rats, see (Whishaw et al., 2001) for details. Given these findings, it was possible to assume that stress sensitivity of grooming microstructure in rats may markedly differ from that previously reported in mice (Kalueff and Tuohimaa, 2004a).

In our subsequent study, we wanted to examine whether shifts in grooming behavioural microstructure (detected by our grooming analysis algorithm) can be used to assess different levels of stress in rats (Kalueff and Tuohimaa, 2005). To induce different (high and low) levels of stress, we used the light-dark paradigm (Crawley, 1999), validated for rats and widely used in behavioural neuroscience (Salome et al., 2002). This two-chambered test consists of two different compartments – highly aversive "light" compartment (brightly lit box with transparent walls) and more protective "dark" compartment (black box). In our study, we first randomly exposed rats to the light or dark box (to induce high or low stress, respectively), and then assessed their stress-evoked grooming in the actimeter test. We showed that behavioural microstructure of rat grooming is indeed very sensitive to the level of stress, and that stress-induced alterations in rat grooming activity are in many ways similar to those previously reported in mice (Kalueff and Tuohimaa, 2004a, 2005). Overall, our study shows that this method allows detection of stress by measuring alterations in grooming patterns (microstructure), and can be a useful tool for neurobehavioural stress research in rats (Kalueff and Tuohimaa, 2005).

II. Materials and Methods

Subjects:

Twenty two male Wistar rats (2 months old, 220-240 g, University of Tampere, Finland) were maintained in a virus/parasite-free facility under conditions of controlled temperature (22±2 °C), humidity (60%), and a 12:12-h light–dark cycle (lights on 7:00 am). The animals were housed in pairs in standard laboratory cages, with water and food available ad libitum.

Apparatus and Procedure:

All testing was conducted between 1700 and 1900 h. On the day of the experiments, animals were transported to the dimly lit laboratory and left undisturbed for 2 h prior to exposure to the light-dark test. The light-dark test was a Plexiglas box consisting of two compartments – the transparent (light) box and the black (dark) box (30×30×30 cm each). The light box was brightly lit (75-w lamp, 10 cm above the top) and connected to the dark box by a sliding door (this door was not used in the present study). Each rat was placed separately in the light (high stress group, n=11) or dark (low stress group, n=11) box for 5 min. Immediately after this exposure, each rat was placed separately in the actimeter test where its behavior was recorded for 5 min. The actimeter test was a glass cylinder (20 cm in diameter; 40 cm in length). During the testing sessions, the experimenter remained standing in front of (and 2 m away from) the testing boxes. Between subjects, each apparatus was thoroughly cleaned (wet and dry cloths); to remove olfactory stimuli, each apparatus was cleaned with a 10% ethanol solution and dried with paper towelling. All animal experiments were performed in full compliance with the Finnish laws on animal experimentation and approved by the Ethical Committee of the University of Tampere.

Behavioural Analysis

Non-Grooming Behaviours:

Defecation and urination index (DU, the sum of two visceral behaviours: the number of boli deposited and urination spots) was scored as the conventional emotionality index in all animal groups in the light-dark and the actimeter tests. In addition to measuring grooming and visceral behaviours in the actimeter test, we also assessed general vertical exploratory activity (VR, the number of vertical rears) as the conventional stress-sensitive behavioural measure (Kalueff and Tuohimaa, 2005).

Grooming Ethological Analysis:

Three gross measures of grooming activity were evaluated in this study: (i) the latency (s) to start grooming, LG, (ii) the number of grooming bouts, NB (the number/frequency of grooming episodes), and (iii) total time (s) spent grooming, TS. A bout consisted of a single pattern (single-area bout, SAB) or was composed of several patterns (multiple-area bout, MAB): 1 - paw licking; 2 - nose/face grooming (strokes along the snout); 3 - head washing (semicircular movements over the top of the head and behind the ears); 4 - body grooming/scratching (body fur licking and scratching the body with the hind paws); 5 - leg licking and tail/genitals grooming (licking of the genital area and tail), according to (Kalueff and Tuohimaa, 2004a; 0 indicated no grooming). The number of grooming patterns (NP) and the number of interruptions (NI) were calculated for all groups (interruptions longer than 5 s determined separate, independent grooming bouts). A grooming bout was considered "interrupted" (IB) if at least one interruption was recorded within its transitions. The number (NIB) and the percentages of interrupted bouts (%IB = NIB/NB) were assessed in this study. A "complete" bout (CB) consisted of the following sequence of patterns: 0-1-2-3-4-5-6-0; all other bouts were considered "incomplete" (ICB). The number (NICB) and the percentages of incomplete bouts (%ICB = NICB/NB) were assessed in this study (Kalueff and Tuohimaa, 2005).

Transitions between grooming patterns were assessed using the transition matrix as described earlier (Kalueff and Tuohimaa, 2004a). "Correct" transitions (CT) adhered to the cephalocaudal progression: (0-1), (1-2), (2-3), (3-4), (4-5), (5-6), and (6-0); "incorrect" transitions (IT) included all other possible transitions between grooming patterns. Total number of transitions (T) was the sum of correct and incorrect transitions (T = CT + IT). Four main types of IT were analysed in this study: (i) aborted, IT(a) (prematurely terminated, e.g. 3-0, 4-0); (ii) skipped, IT(s) (e.g. 1-6, 2-5); (iii) reversed, IT(r) (e.g. 3-2, 4-1, 5-2) and (iv) incorrectly initiated, IT(i) (e.g. 0-4, 0-5). The percentages of incorrect transitions (%IT) were calculated for both groups of rats (%IT = IT/T). The numbers of incorrect transitions (total and for each category) were assessed in this study, and the percentages of incorrect transitions of each type reversed IT(r), skipped IT(s), aborted IT(a) and incorrectly initiated IT(i) of total transitions (T) were calculated in this study (%IT(...) = IT(...)/T).

The grooming analysis algorithm also included a set of ethological indices derived from the following calculations: average durations of a single bout (ADB) and pattern (ADP) were calculated as total time spent grooming divided by the number of bouts (ADB = TS/NB) and patterns (ADP = TS/NP), respectively. Average number of transitions per bout (ATB) and pattern (ATP) were calculated as the number of transitions divided by the number of bouts (ATB = T/NB) and patterns (ATP = T/NP), respectively. Average number of interruptions per bout (AIB) was calculated as the number of interruptions divided by the number of bouts (AIB = NI/NB), (Kalueff and Tuohimaa, 2005).

Regional Distribution of Grooming:

In order to assess the regional distribution of grooming in rats, we separately analysed their grooming activity directed to the following five anatomic areas: forepaws, head, body, hind legs and tail/genitals (caudal grooming). Rostral grooming included forepaw (preliminary rostral grooming, according to (Komorowska and Pellis, 2004)) and head grooming. The percentages of (i) total grooming patterns, (ii) time spent grooming, and (iii) interruptions were calculated for each anatomic area. In addition, each grooming bout was categorised as being directed to (i) multiple regions or (ii) a single region, according to

(Eckstein and Hart, 2000), and the percentage of grooming bouts and the percentage of time spent grooming were calculated for both categories.

Statistical Analysis:

All data are presented as mean ± S.E.M. Data were analyzed by Mann-Whitney two-tailed U-test. In all tests, a probability of less than 0.05 was considered statistically significant.

III. Results

In the light box, the rats demonstrated significantly more defecations and urinations, compared to the dark-exposed animals (Table 1). In the actimeter test, the light-exposed group demonstrated significantly less vertical rears and more defecation and urination scores (although this did not reach significance, P = 0.07) (Kalueff and Tuohimaa, 2005).

Table 1. Non-grooming behaviours in male Wistar rats exposed to the light/dark box and the actimeter test (n = 11 in each groups). Data are expressed as mean ± S.E.M. P - difference between the groups (U-test), adapted from (Kalueff and Tuohimaa, 2005).

Behavioural measures	Light-induced stress group	Dark-induced stress group	P
Light/dark exposure test			
Defecation and urination index, DU	0.8 ± 0.2	0.1 ± 0.1	<0.05
Actimeter test (following the light/dark exposure)			
Defecation and urination index, DU	0.5 ± 0.3	0.1 ± 0.1	NS
Number of vertical rears, VR	14 ± 4	26 ± 5	<0.05

DU index in the sum of defecation boli deposited and urination spots.

Table 2 shows grooming activity of rats after their exposure to the light or dark boxes of the light-dark test. Following exposure to high stress evoked by the light box (novelty + open lit arena), the traditional gross measures of grooming (the number and the duration of grooming bouts) in the actimeter increased significantly compared to the group exposed to a low-stress test (dark box). As can be seen in Table 1, the latency to start grooming was predictably shorter in more anxious light-exposed rats, while the average duration of a single bout was similar in both groups.

Analysis of grooming patterns using our grooming analysis algorithm shows that anxious light-exposed rats display significantly more patterns and more interruptions of grooming activity, compared to the low-stress group (Table 2). However, average duration of a single pattern was unaltered in both groups (Kalueff and Tuohimaa, 2005).

Table 2. Behavioural alterations in grooming activity in the actimeter test in the light- and the dark-exposed Wistar rats. Data are expressed as mean ± S.E.M. P - difference between the groups (U-test), adapted from (Kalueff and Tuohimaa, 2005.

Grooming measures	Light-induced stress group	Dark-induced stress group	P
Traditional gross measures			
Latency to start grooming (s), LG	201 ± 50	360 ± 58	<0.05
Total number of bouts, NB	4.8 ± 0.8	2.4 ± 0.5	<0.05
Total time spent grooming (s), TS	53 ± 8	24 ± 5	<0.05
Average duration of a single bout (s), ADB = TS/NB	11 ± 2	10 ± 2	NS
Patterns			
Total number of patterns, NP	14 ± 2	8 ± 1	<0.05
Number of interruptions of grooming, NI	1.6 ± 0.5	0.2 ± 0.1	<0.05
Average duration of a single pattern (s), ADP = TS/NP	3.8 ± 0.6	3 ± 0.7	NS
Transitions between patterns			
Total number of transitions, T	18 ± 3	9 ± 1	<0.05
Average transitions per pattern, ATP = T/NP	1.3 ± 0.4	1.1 ± 0.1	NS
Percent of incorrect transitions (IT), %IT (of total transitions, T)			
% Reversed IT, %IT(r)	13 ± 2	2 ± 1	<0.05
% Skipped IT, %IT(s)	6 ± 1	6 ± 1	NS
% Aborted IT, %IT(a)	20 ± 3	13±1	<0.05
% Incorrectly initiated, %IT(i)	8 ± 1	7 ± 1	NS
% Total, %IT = IT/T = %IT(r+s+a+i)	47 ±5 (100)	28 ±3 (100)	<0.05
Bouts			
Number of interrupted bouts, NIB	1.2 ± 0.4	0.2 ± 0.1	<0.05
% Interrupted bouts, %IB = NIB/NB	25 ± 8	8 ± 4.8	<0.05
Number of incomplete bouts, NICB	4.5 ± 0.4	1.8 + 0.2	<0.05
% Incomplete bouts, %ICB = NICB/NB	94 ± 5	75 ± 9	NS
Average number of patterns per bout, APB = NP/NB	2.9 ± 0.4	3.3 ± 0.4	NS
Average number of transitions per bout, ATB = T/NB	3.8 ± 0.6	3.8 ± 0.4	NS
Average interruptions per bout, AIB = NI/NB	0.4 ± 0.1	0.1 ± 0	NS

Analysis of transitions between grooming patterns again shows that following exposure to the light box, the number of transitions increased significantly (Table 2) compared to their less stressed (dark-exposed) counterparts. While average number of transitions per pattern was only slightly higher in the first group, we found a marked increase in the percentage of incorrect transitions in more stressed group. The use of grooming analysis algorithm also revealed the increase in reversed and aborted incorrect transitions in these rats, compared to their less stressed counterparts.

As can be seen in Table 2, a detailed analysis of grooming bouts in both groups shows that the light-exposed rats generally display more interrupted bouts and a clear tendency to more incomplete bouts. Average numbers of patterns and transitions per a single bout were similar in both groups, also showing a tendency to more interruptions per bout.

Table 3. Regional distribution of grooming in the actimeter test in the light- and the dark-exposed Wistar rats. Data are expressed as mean ± S.E.M. P - difference between the groups (U-test), adapted from (Kalueff and Tuohimaa, 2005).

Regional distribution	Light-induced stress group	Dark-induced stress group	P
Grooming patterns (% of total number of patterns, NP)			
Forepaws	38 ± 5	26 ± 4	NS
Face/head	31 ± 8	31 ± 7	NS
Rostral grooming (paws+face/head)	69 ± 7	57 ± 5	NS
Body	18 ± 4	17 ± 3	NS
Hindlegs patterns	7 ± 1	10 ± 1	NS
Tail and genitals (caudal grooming)	7 ± 1	16 + 2	<0.05
Grooming duration (% of total time spent grooming, TS)			
Forepaws	45 ± 6	33 ± 5	<0.05
Face/head	26 ± 4	24 ± 3	NS
Rostral grooming (paws+face/head)	71 ± 5	57 ± 4	<0.05
Body	15 ± 4	17 ± 4	NS
Hindlegs	6 ± 1	6 ± 1	NS
Tail and genitals (caudal grooming)	8 ± 1.5	20 + 3	<0.05
Interruptions of grooming (% of total number of interruptions, NI)			
Forepaws	50 ± 11	33 ± 3	<0.05
Face/head	32 ± 5	0	<0.05
Rostral grooming (paws+face/head)	82 + 7	33 + 3	<0.05
Body	6 ± 1.5	0	<0.05
Hindlegs	6 ± 2	33 ± 3	NS
Tail and genitals (caudal grooming)	6 ± 2	0	<0.05

Table 3. Continued

Regional distribution	Light-induced stress group	Dark-induced stress group	P
Regional characteristics of grooming bouts, % of total bouts (NB) or time spent (TS)			
Single-area bouts, %SAB	34 ± 5	34 ± 7	NS
Single-area duration, %SAD	66 ± 9	66 ± 7	NS
Multiple-area bouts, %MAB	17 ± 4	16 ± 5	NS
Multiple-area duration, %MAD	83 ± 7	84 ± 11	NS

%SAB = number of single-area bouts/NB; %SAD = single-area bouts duration/TS; %MAB = number of multiple-area bouts/NB; %MAD = multiple area bouts duration/TS.

Moreover, our experiments also show that the regional distribution of grooming behaviours was markedly affected by stress, manifest in more paw grooming patterns and less tail and genitals grooming in the high stress group (Table 3). Consistent with this, these stressed rats spent significantly more time grooming paws and less time grooming tail and genitals, compared to their dark-exposed counterparts. Furthermore, analysis of the regional distribution of interruptions clearly shows the rostral character of grooming interruptions in more stressed rats. Finally, both rat groups displayed essentially the same percentages of single- and multiple-area bouts and time spent grooming (Table 3).

IV. Discussion

The results of this study show that, in line with traditional interpretation of the light-dark paradigm (Crawley et al., 1997; Crawley, 1999), this procedure induced two different levels of stress, as assessed by the number of urination spots and defecation boli deposited (Table 1). This confirms that the rats subjected to the light box in this study were more anxious than their counterparts subjected to the dark box. Consistent with this, the rats from the first group showed fewer vertical rears in the actimeter test – the behavioural response traditionally considered as a reliable marker of stress in rodents (Crawley et al., 1997; Espejo, 1997; Belzung, 1999). Furthermore, this group demonstrated shorter latencies to start grooming, and a dramatic increase in grooming frequency and duration (Table 2). These alterations in rats' grooming have long been considered as behavioural markers of stress (Kalueff, 2000; Moyaho and Valencia, 2002). Taken together, this allowed us to conclude that the two groups of rats used in the present study exhibited different levels of the induced stress.

We then applied our grooming analysis algorithm in order to assess in detail the behavioural microstructure of the rat stress-evoked grooming. In general, the idea of analysing the rat grooming in the actimeter test after the exposure to the light-dark apparatus was useful for two main reasons. Firstly, as already mentioned, the light-dark test is a convenient standard paradigm in which two different levels of stress can easily be produced and assessed. Secondly, more specific analysis of stress-induced grooming behaviours in the subsequent relatively simple actimeter test enables higher grooming scores and minimizes possible confounding effects of other (non-grooming) behaviours. As expected, the grooming analysis algorithm revealed a marked shift in grooming behavioural patterns, significantly increasing the percentage of incorrect transitions and interrupted bouts in more anxious rats. Finally, our present data show that these stress-evoked alterations in grooming microstructure in rats parallel changes in their gross grooming measures, thus further supporting the validity of our results. Together, this shows that the present method may be particularly effective in detection of stress-evoked abnormal grooming patterns in rats tested in different experimental models of stress.

Does the behavioural organization of stress-evoked grooming activity differ in mice and rats? Comparing our results with previously published own grooming data in mice (Kalueff et al., 2004a; Kalueff and Tuohimaa, 2004a,b), we note that stressed rats and mice spent similar amount of test time engaged in self-grooming (~8-14%). Likewise, mice and rats exposed to low stress situations, also demonstrated similar (although much lower) levels of grooming activity. However, in line with the previously published observations (Berridge, 1990), we also found that grooming behaviour in rats appeared to be more complex and better organized, showing fewer but longer bouts, and lower percentages of incomplete and interrupted bouts. In addition, essentially the same increase in incomplete and interrupted bouts occurred in stressed mice and rats, compared to their non-stressed controls (Kalueff and Tuohimaa, 2004a; Table 2). Collectively, these observations not only confirm common behavioural organization of stress-evoked grooming in these two species, but also prove the potential utility of ethological analysis of rodent grooming microstructure for the detection of stress-induced behavioural alterations in mice and rats.

At first glance, the dark box exposure used in this study is similar to the sudden darkness test (Nasello et al., 2003) known to reduce anxiety and activate grooming in rats. Clearly, this phenomenon supports the notion that increased grooming activity does not always reflect higher levels of stress (Kalueff, 2000; Kalueff and Tuohimaa, 2004a). However, it is possible that the dark exposure used here differs from the sudden darkness procedure, especially since we did not find increased grooming activity in the dark-exposed rats (Table 2). However, we did find a significantly higher level of tail/genital grooming – the effect similar to that induced by the sudden darkness (Nasello et al., 2003). Although these interesting phenomena need further investigation, they are generally consistent with the idea of low stress in the dark-exposed rats (Nasello et al., 2003, Tables 1-3). Moreover, this "anxiolytic" interpretation of the increased caudal grooming in both studies is in line with predominantly "rostral" nature of rodent grooming evoked by stress (van Erp et al., 1995; Komorowska and Pisula, 2003; Kalueff and Tuohimaa, 2004a). Consistent with this, we found that rostral grooming (paws, face and head) was significantly higher in more anxious light-exposed group (~70%) compared the dark-exposed rats (~57%), Table 3.

Furthermore, since interruptions in grooming activity are considered as behavioural markers of stress in rodents (Kalueff, 2000; Kalueff and Tuohimaa, 2004a), the fact that the light-exposed rats displayed 8-fold more interrupted grooming bouts, especially while grooming rostrally (Tables 1 and 3), further confirms their higher anxiety profile compared to the dark-exposed rats. Moreover, since high anxiety in rats has long been associated with frequent prematurely terminated (aborted) grooming bouts (Komorowska and Pisula, 2003), the increased percentage of incorrect aborted transitions in the light-exposed group (Table 2) clearly supports the idea that grooming behavioural microstructure in rats is very sensitive to the level of stress. In line with this conclusion, we also found a dramatic increase in the number of reversed transitions (another behavioural marked of stress-evoked grooming; Kalueff, 2002) in the light-exposed group. Finally, all these alterations in grooming microstructure appear to parallel non-grooming stress-related behaviours (Table 1), further strengthening the validity of our approach. Taken together, the results of the present study in rats confirm that alterations in rodents' grooming microstructure can be used as reliable behavioural markers of stress.

In summary, given the similarity of mouse and rat grooming behaviours (Berridge, 1990; Berridge and Aldridge, 2000a,b), our findings further support the idea of common principles of behavioural organization of stress-evoked grooming in small laboratory rodents, such as mice and rats. Importantly, the data presented in Tables 2 and 3 show that in high and low stress situations our algorithm in rats was able to detect the level of stress, as assessed by increased percentages of (i) incorrect transitions between different patterns; (ii) duration of incorrect patterns; (iii) interrupted bouts; and (iv) altered regional distribution of grooming (more rostral, less caudal grooming). Importantly, these findings are consistent with several recent studies (Komorowska and Pisula, 2003; Komorowska and Pellis, 2004) which, using different ethological approaches, also demonstrated the disruption of the cephalocaudal grooming progression in rats subjected to novelty stress In general, the results presented here show that a detailed grooming analysis based on the algorithm previously designed for mice (Kalueff and Tuohimaa, 2004a) may be a valuable tool in neurobehavioural stress research in rats.

What can be the potential practical applications of this method? First, it is possible to speculate that this method may not only detect stress-evoked alterations in rat grooming microstructure, but also measure the degree of stress evoked by different tests. Clearly, the idea of grooming-based "stress-meter" in rodents needs further investigation to be confirmed, but, if true, may represent an important practical application of our algorithm. To some extend, the results of the present study and our recent data on mice (Kalueff et al., 2004b; Kalueff and Tuohimaa, 2004a,b), showing consistent stress-dependent shifts in grooming microstructure, indirectly support thus contention. Second, given similar behavioural organisation of grooming in mice and rats, and also our recent findings in mutant mice (Kalueff and Tuohimaa, 2004a), we can suggest that this method may be able to detect stress-evoked alterations in grooming in different rat strains used in behavioural neuroscience research. Although not directly studied here, this also implies the potential utility of our method for behavioural phenotyping of various mutant rats, especially those displaying abnormal emotional behaviours and/or grooming (e.g. Kobayashi et al., 1996). Third, since various physiological (Spruijt et al., 1992) and genetic manipulations (Kobayashi et al., 1996) in rats may impair their behavioural organization, including grooming, the sequential analysis of grooming according to our protocol is also likely to detect various motor/coordination anomalies in such animals.

Another potential application of our method may be ethological analysis of age-related behavioural alterations in rats. Our general knowledge of the age-related progression of motor and stress-related emotional disorders indicates that this aspect, although not directly tested in the present study, may be especially important to consider further. For example, interesting data on rats (Kametani et al., 1984; Kametani, 1988) clearly show age-related alterations in grooming activity and its behavioural microstructure. Therefore, it is possible to assume that an in-depth analysis of grooming in rats tested at different ages, using our present algorithm, may allow detection of age-related motor/coordination and affective disorders. If successful, this possibility may have an important clinical relevance, especially considering the growing number of such disorders in the elderly. Finally, given high sensitivity of rat grooming and its microstructure to various pharmacological manipulations (Barros et al., 1992, 1994; Eguibar and Moyaho, 1997; D'Aquila et al., 2000; Choleris et al., 2001), we suggest that ethologically-oriented analysis of grooming in rats, such as reported here, may be successfully used in the field of psychopharmacology research, including screening of compounds with mixed or unclear properties, or testing novel psychotropic anxiolytic and antidepressant drugs.

Acknowledgements

This research was supported by grants from CIMO Finland, the University of Tampere, the Medical Research Council of Tampere University Hospital (EVO) and the Academy of Finland.

References

[1] Aguilar R, Gil L, Gray JA, Driscoll P, Flint J, Dawson GR, Gimenez-Llort L, Escorihuela RM, Fernandez-Teruel A, Tobena A. Fearfulness and sex in F2 Roman rats: males display more fear though both sexes share the same fearfulness traits. *Physiol. Behav.*, 2003; 78:723-732.

[2] Barros HM, Tannhauser SL, Tannhauser MA, Tannhauser M. Effect of sodium valproate on the open-field behavior of rats. Braz. *J. Med. Biol.* Res., 1992; 25:281-287.

[3] Barros HM, Tannhauser SL, Tannhauser MA, Tannhauser M. The effects of GABAergic drugs on grooming behaviour in the open field. *Pharmacol. Toxicol.*, 1994; 74:339-344.

[4] Belzung C. Measuring rodent exploratory behavior. In Cruzio WE, Gerlai RT, editors. Handbook of Molecular genetics for brain and behavior research Elsevier: New York, 1999; 738-749.

[5] Berridge KC, Fentress JC, Parr H. Natural syntax rules control action sequence of rats. *Behav. Brain Res.*, 1987; 23: 59-68.

[6] Berridge KC. Comparative fine structure of action: rules of form and sequence in the grooming patterns of six rodent species. *Behavior.*, 1990; 113: 21-56.

[7] Berridge KC, Whishaw IQ. Cortex, striatum and cerebellum: control of serial order in a grooming sequence. *Exp. Brain Res.,* 1992; 90: 275-290.

[8] Berridge KC, Aldridge JW. Super-stereotypy I: enhancement of a complex movement sequence by systemic dopamine D1 agonists. *Synapse.*, 2000; 37: 194-204.

[9] Berridge KC, Aldridge JW. Super-stereotypy II: enhancement of a complex movement sequence by intraventricular dopamine D1 agonists. *Synapse.*, 2000; 37: 205-215.

[10] Bolivar VJ, Danilchuk W, Fentress JC. Separation of activation and pattern in grooming development of weaver mice. *Behav. Brain Res.*, 1996; 75: 49-58.

[11] Bressers WM, Kruk MR, Van Erp AM, Willekens-Bramer DC, Haccou P, Meelis E. The hypothalamus: cross-roads of endocrine and behavioural regulation in grooming and aggression. Neurosci. *Biobehav. Rev.*, 1998; 23: 163-177.

[12] Choleris E, Thomas AW, Kavaliers M, Prato FS. A detailed ethological analysis of the mouse open field test: effects of diazepam, chlordiazepoxide and an extremely low frequency pulsed magnetic field. *Neurosci. Biobehav. Rev.*, 2001; 25: 235-260.

[13] Crawley JN, Belknap JK, Collins A, Crabbe JC, Frankel W, Henderson N, Hitzermann RJ, Maxson SC, Miner LL, Silva AJ, Wehner JM, Wynshaw-Boris A, Paylor R. Behavioural phenotypes of inbred mouse strains: implications and recommendations for molecular studies. *Psychopharmacol.,* 1997; 132: 107-124.

[14] Crawley JN. Behavioural phenotyping of transgenic and knockout mice: experimental design and evaluation of general health, sensory functions, motor abilities, and specific behavioural tests. *Brain Res.*, 1999; 835: 18-26.

[15] Cromwell HC, Berridge KC. Implementation of action sequences by a neostriatal site: a lesion mapping study of grooming syntax. *J. Neurosci.*, 1996; 16: 3444-3458.

[16] Cromwell HC, Berridge KC, Drago J, Levine MS. Action sequencing is impaired in D1A-deficient mutant mice. *Eur. J. Neurosci.*, 1998; 10: 2426-2432.

[17] D'Aquila PS, Peana AT, Carboni V, Serra G. Exploratory behaviour and grooming after repeated restraint and chronic mild stress: effect of desipramine. *Eur. J. Pharmacol.*, 2000; 399: 43-47.

[18] Dunn AJ, Berridge CW, Lai YI, Yachabach TL. CRF-induced excessive grooming behavior in rats and mice. *Peptides.*, 1987; 8: 841-844.

[19] Eckstein RA, Hart BL. Grooming and control of fleas in cats. Appl. Anim. Behav. Sci., 2000;68: 141-150.

[20] Eguibar JR, Moyaho A. Inhibition of grooming by pilocarpine differs in high- and low-yawning sublines of Sprague-Dawley rats. *Pharmacol. Biochem. Behav.*, 1997; 58: 317-322.

[21] Eguibar JR, Romero-Carbente JC, Moyaho A. Behavioral differences between selectively bred rats: D1 versus D2 receptors in yawning and grooming. *Pharmacol. Biochem. Behav.*, 2003; 74: 827-832.

[22] Escorihuela RM, Fernandez-Teruel A, Gil L, Aguilar R, Tobena A, Driscoll P. Inbred Roman high- and low-avoidance rats: differences in anxiety, novelty-seeking, and shuttlebox behaviors. *Physiol. Behav.*, 1999; 67: 19-26.

[23] Espejo EF. Structure of the mouse behaviour on the elevated plus-maze test of anxiety. *Behav. Brain Res.*, 1997; 86: 105-112.

[24] Fentress JC. The tonic hypothesis and the patterning of behaviour. *Ann. NY Acad. Sci.*, 1977; 290: 370-394.

[25] File SE, Mabbutt PS, Walker JH. Comparison of adaptive responses in familiar and novel environments: modulatory factors. *Ann NY Acad. Sci.*, 1988; 525: 69-79.

[26] Gerlai R, Henderson JF, Roder JC, Jia Z. Multiple behavioural anomalies in GluR2 mutant mice exhibiting enchanced LTP. *Behav. Brain Res.,* 1998; 95: 37-45.

[27] Greer JM, Capecci MR. Hoxb8 is required for normal grooming behaviour in mice. *Neuron.,* 2003; 33: 23-34.

[28] Hart BL, Pryor PA. Developmental and hair-coat determinants of grooming behaviour in goats and sheep. *Animal. Behav.*, 2004; 67: 11-19.

[29] Homberg JR, van den Akker M, Raaso HS, Wardeh G, Binnekade R, Schoffelmeer AN, de Vries TJ. Enhanced motivation to self-administer cocaine is predicted by self-grooming behaviour and relates to dopamine release in the rat medial prefrontal cortex and amygdala. *Eur. J. Neurosci.*, 2002; 15: 1542-1550.

[30] Hossain SM, Wong BK, Simpson EM. The dark phase improves genetic discrimination for some high throughput mouse behavioral phenotyping. *Genes Brain Behav.*, 2004; 3: 167-177.

[31] Jarbe TU, Andrzejewski ME, DiPatrizio NV. Interactions between the CB1 receptor agonist Delta 9-THC and the CB1 receptor antagonist SR-141716 in rats: open-field revisited. *Pharmacol. Biochem. Behav.*, 2002; 73: 911-919.

[32] Kalueff AV. Measuring grooming in stress and comfort, *Proc. Int. Conf. Measur. Behav. 2000*; 3, 148-149.

[33] Kalueff AV. Grooming and stress, KSF: Kiv, 2002: 148.

[34] Kalueff AV, Lou YR, Laaksi I, Tuohimaa P. Increased grooming phenotype in mice lacking Vitamin D receptors. *Physiol. Behav.,* 2004a; 82: 405-409.

[35] Kalueff AV, Lou YR, Laaksi I, Tuohimaa P. Grooming microstructure in mice is affected by genetic ablation of vitamin D receptors, *Proc. FENS Forum*. 2004b; P353.

[36] Kalueff AV, Tuohimaa P. Grooming analysis algorithm for neurobehavioural stress research. *Brain Res. Protocols.*, 2004a; 13: 151-158.

[37] Kalueff AV, Tuohimaa P. Contrasting grooming phenotypes in C57BL/6 and 129S1 mice. *Brain Res.*, 2004b; 1028, 75-81.

[38] Kalueff AV, Tuohimaa P. The grooming analysis algorithm discriminates between different levels of anxiety in rats: potential utility for neurobehavioural stress research. *J. Neurosci. Methods.*, 2005; 143, 169-177.

[39] Kametani H, Osada H, Inoue K. Increased novelty-induced grooming in aged rats: a preliminary observation. Behav. *Neural. Biol.*, 1984; 42: 73-80.

[40] Kametani H. Analysis of age-related changes in stress-induced grooming in the rat. Ann *NY Acad. Sci.*, 1988; 525: 101-113.

[41] Katz RJ, Roth KA. Stress-induced grooming in the rat – an endorphin mediated syndrome. *Neurosci. Lett.*, 1979; 13: 209-212.

[42] Kobayashi S, Ohta M, Miyasaka K, Funakoshi A. Decrease in exploratory behavior in naturally occurring cholecystokinin (CCK)-A receptor gene knockout rats. *Neurosci. Lett.*, 1996; 214:61-64.

[43] Komorowska P, Pisula W. Does changing levels of stress affect the characteristics of grooming behaviour in rats? *Int. J. Comp. Psychol.,* 2003; 16: 237-246.

[44] Komorowska J, Pellis SM. Regulatory mechanisms underlying novelty-induced grooming in the laboratory rat. *Behav. Processes*, 2004; 67: 287-293.

[45] Lawler CP, Cohen PS. Pawgrooming induced by intermittent positive reinforcement in rats. *Ann NY Acad. Sci.*, 1988; 525: 417-419.

[46] Moody TW, Merali Z, Crawley JN. The effects of anxiolytics and other agents on rat grooming behaviour. *Ann NY Acad. Sci.*, 1988; 525: 281-290.

[47] Moyaho JR, Eguibar JL, Diaz A. Induced grooming transitions and open field behaviour differ in high- and low-yawning sublines of Sprague-Dawley rats. *Anim. Behav.*, 1995; 50: 61-77.

[48] Moyaho A, Valencia J. Grooming and yawning trace adjustment to unfamiliar environments in laboratory Sprague-Dawley rats (Rattus norvegicus). *J. Comp. Psychol.*, 2002; 116: 263-269.

[49] Nasello AG, Sassatani AS, Ferreira FS, Felicio LF, Tieppo CA. Modulation by sudden darkness of apomorphine-induced behavioral responses. *Physiol. Behav.*, 2003; 78: 521-528.

[50] Ohl F, Toschi N, Wigger A, Henniger MS, Landgraf R. Dimensions of emotionality in a rat model of innate anxiety. *Behav. Neurosci.*, 2001; 115: 429-436.

[51] Osborne PG, Mataga N, Onoe H, Watanabe Y. Behavioral activation by stimulation of a GABAergic mechanism in the preoptic area of rat. *Neurosci. Lett.*, 1993; 158: 201-204.

[52] Perier C, Tremblay L, Feger J, Hirsch EC. Behavioral consequences of bicuculline injection in the subthalamic nucleus and the zona incerta in rat. *J. Neurosci.*, 2002; 22: 8711-8719.

[53] Rodgers RJ, Davies B, Shore R. Absence of anxiolytic response to chlordiazepoxide in two common background strains exposed to the elevated plus-maze: importance and implications of behavioural baseline. *Genes Brain Behav.*, 2002; 1: 242-251.

[54] Sachs BD. The development of grooming and its expression in adult animals. Ann. NY *Acad. Sci.*, 1988; 525:1-517.

[55] Salome N, Viltart O, Darnaudery M, Salchner P, Singewald N, Landgraf R, Sequeira H, Wigger A. Reliability of high and low anxiety-related behaviour: influence of laboratory environment and multifactorial analysis. *Behav. Brain Res.,* 2002; 136: 227-237.

[56] Spruijt BM, van Hooff JA, Gispen WH. Ethology and neurobiology of grooming behavior. *Physiol Rev.*, 1992; 72: 825-852.

[57] Van de Weerd HA, Bulthuis RJ, Bergman AF, Schlingmann F, Tolboom J, Van Loo PL, Remie R, Baumans V, Van Zutphen LF. Validation of a new system for the automatic registration of behaviour in mice and rats. *Behav Processes.*, 2001; 53: 11-20.

[58] Van Erp AM, Kruk MR, Meelis W, Willekens-Bramer DC. Effect of environmental stressors on time course, variability and form of self-grooming in the rat: handling, social contact, defeat, novelty, restraint and fur moistening. *Behav. Brain Res.*, 1994; 65: 47-55.

[59] Van Erp AM, Kruk MR, Willekens-Bramer DC, Fermont PC, Nijsen MJ. PVH lesions do not inhibit stressor-induced grooming in the rat. *Physiol. Behav.*, 1995; 57: 887-892.

[60] Whishaw IQ, Metz GA, Kolb B, Pellis SM. Accelerated nervous system development contributes to behavioral efficiency in the laboratory mouse: a behavioral review and theoretical proposal. *Dev. Psychobiol.*, 2001; 39: 151-170.

In: Animal Models in Biological Psychiatry
Editor: Allan V. Kalueff, pp. 59-73
ISBN 1-59454-814-5

Chapter 4

The Genetic Cataleptic (GC) Rat Strain as a Model of Depressive Disorders

Alexander V. Kulikov, Victor G. Kolpakov and Nina K. Popova
Institute of Cytology and Genetics, Novosibirsk, Russia

I. Introduction

Existence of a considerable individual variability in predisposition to depression is beyond any doubt. Numerous studies have established an essential genetic component determining individual risk of affective psychoses, in particular, depressions (Gershon et al., 1987; Mendlewicz et al., 1992). Elucidation of the sequence of molecular events linking changes at the level of genome with psychopathology is impossible without the use of genetic animal models of depression. These models are also necessary to study mechanisms of action of antidepressant drugs, since it is well known that some of them (e.g., tricyclic antidepressants) are effective in depressive patients but do not act on healthy people (Willner, 1990).

Several rat strains have been suggested as genetic animal models of depression, allowing us to simulate some symptoms and mechanisms of depression (Overstreet, 1992). However, since practically all models of psychopathology are incomplete, for a better understanding of genetic, molecular and physiological mechanisms of depression and for modeling all the diversity of its forms, creation of new genetic models of depression is undoubtedly very important.

One of candidates for being a new genetic model of depression is the rat strain called GC (initials of "Genetics" and "Catalepsy"). Breeding of this strain for a high expression of cataleptic freezing reaction was started at the Institute of Cytology and Genetics of the Siberian Branch of the Russian Academy of Sciences (Novosibirsk) more than 20 years ago from a random-bred Wistar stock (Barykina et al., 1983), and currently counts over 50 generations. GC rats are characterized by a considerably increased frequency and intensity of freezing (Fig. 1) as compared to the parental Wistar stock (Kolpakov et al., 1996). Long-term studies have established that, in addition to exaggerated passive defense reaction such as cataleptic freezing, GC rats have many other behaviours similar to those seen in depression. The present review will demonstrate the fact that selective breeding for a high expression of defensive behavior has produced depression-like traits, allowing us to suggest GC rats as a valid and feasible animal model of depression.

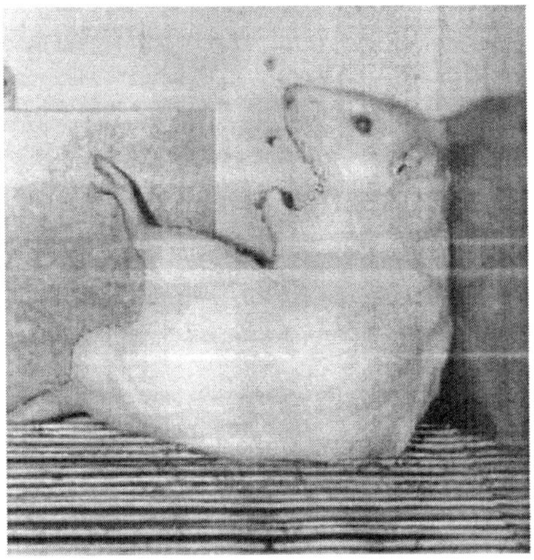

Fig. 1 Cataleptic immobility in GC rat

Since animal models of psycho- or neuropathology must meet at least 3 criteria:

1. face validity,
2. predictive validity and
3. construct validity (Willner, 1984; 1990; 1991; Geyer, Markou, 1995),

We will demonstrate that GC rats are characterized by symptoms corresponding to all these criteria, including such features that are considered as most important characteristics of animal models of depression.

II. Face Validity of the Model

This criterion means similarity of behavioral and physiological characteristics of the model to the symptoms of the prototype (in our case, depression). Willner (1990) states that in animal models one can simulate the following symptoms of depression: anhedonia, appetite disturbance or weight change, sleep disturbances, psychomotor retardation, or agitation. This list should be supplemented with disturbances of hormonal functions which are often observed in depressive patients (Muselman, Nemeroff, 1996; Schweiger et al., 1999; Michael et al., 2000).

Psychomotor Disturbances (Retardation and Agitation)

This category may include most manifestations of depression, from a decrease of interest in new objects to prevalence of passive reactions and decrease of general activity. A mental and motor inhibition varying from a slight torpidity to stupor is the most specific and important symptom of depression (Weitbrecht, 1960; Abrams et al., 1979; Leonhard, 1980; Nuller, Mikhalenko, 1988). In addition to increased predisposition to catatonic stupor, GC rats are characterized by lower general motor activity compared to Wistar rats. This decrease strongly correlates with the expression of catalepsy, since the individuals with the most intense cataleptic reactions display the lowest spontaneous motor and exploration activity (Barykina et al., 1983; Shtilman et al., 1988; Petrova, 1990; Barykina et al., 2002). GC rats are characterized also by a considerably higher immobility in the Porsolt's forced swimming test than Wistar rats (Nikulina et al., 1987). This "behavioural despair" has been regarded by some authors as an important proof of depression-like state (Porsolt et al., 1977) corresponding to some other models of depression (Pare, 1992, 1993; Overstreet, 1993).

Besides the psychomotor retardation, a pronounced psychomotor agitation is also a characteristic of depressions; often, these two states alternate. A distinctive feature of GC rats is jumpiness and "nervousness". The acoustic startle reflex amplitude in GC rats is about twice as high as in Wistar, and the startle reflex habituation in repeated exposures to acoustic stimuli is much less (Popova et al., 2000). About 90% of GC rats react to manipulations with fright reactions, aggression and vocalization, while the overwhelming majority of Wistar rats behave quietly under similar conditions (Nikulina et al., 1987; Kolpakov et al., 1996). GC rats display a 3-fold higher foot shock aggression than Wistar rats (Nikulina et al., 1987). One may suppose that catalepsy and "nervousness" are two manifestations of the same abnormality, i.e. psychomotor disturbance.

Sleep Disturbances

GC rats are characterized by a delta-sleep deficit (Oganesian et al., 1990; Karmanova, Oganesian, 1994), also common in human depression (Bondy et al., 1988; Van Delft et al., 1988; Kupfer et al., 1989; Ammon et al., 1990).

Endocrine Disorders

Depression is often accompanied by disturbances of the hypothalamic-pituitary-adrenal and hypothalamic-pituitary-thyroid systems (Musselman, Nemeroff, 1996). In GC rats a lowered blood corticosterone level was found (Amstislavsky et al., 2000). This seems to contradict the elevated corticosteroid level found in human depression (Nuller, Mikhalenko, 1988). However, many depressive patients have normal levels of cortisol (Carroll et al., 1976). Besides, there are reports showing antidepressant effect of hydrocortisone administration (DeBattista et al., 2000), which may point to a compensatory, but not a pathogenic, role of the elevation of corticosteroid level in depression. In GC males, testosterone level is decreased (Shul'ga et al., 1997) similar to the androgen deficit observed in depressive men (Schweiger et al., 1999; Michael et al., 2001). GC rats have a significantly lowered total blood plasma thyroxine concentration with respect to Wistar rats (37.4 ± 1.9 nM vs. 47.5 ± 2.3 nM, respectively, $P<0.001$) (Barykina et al., 2002). This is in a good accordance with the clinical data on hypothyroidism in some depressive patients (Haggerty et al., 1993; Howland, 1993; Clear et al., 1995; Duval et al., 1999; Frye et al., 1999).

Taken together, all these abnormalities (i.e. stupor, psychomotor, sleep and endocrine disturbances, i.e. hypothyroidism and androgen deficit), are similar to those frequently seen in depressive patients. One may assert that GC rats simulate the majority of symptoms observed in human depression which can be objectively modeled on animals and therefore meet the requirements of face validity.

III. Predictive Validity of the Model

This requirement means that the model must react to factors enhancing depression and to antidepressants in the same manner as does depression (Willner, 1984, 1990). At the same time, positive response to antidepressants is a desirable but not at all indispensable criterion of the model (Willner et al., 1990), since about 20% of depressive patients are insensitive to antidepressant treatment (Klein et al., 1980).

Antidepressants

There are numerous publications suggesting that classical antidepressants attenuate catalepsy in rats and mice. Imipramine and amitryptiline attenuate haloperidol-induced (Worms et al., 1987; Al-Katib et al., 1989; Khisti et al., 1989) and histamine-induced (Onodera, 1991) catalepsy. Imipramine, amitryptiline and fluoxetine attenuate pinch-induced catalepsy in mice (Fundaro, 1998). Since there is an association between the haloperidol-induced, pinch-induced catalepsy and that elicited by imposing an uncomfortable posture in genetically predisposed GC rats (Kolpakov et al., 1999), one may expect that antidepressants may affect GC rats.

Our preliminary experiments indicate that only chronic, but not acute, imipramine administration decreases catalepsy expression in GC rats (Kulikov et al., 2004). This result is in accordance with the time course of clinical effect of the drug (Willner, 1990; Borsini, 1994; Blier, de Montigny, 1994). **A** non-specific 5-HT_2 receptor antagonist cyproheptadine which displays a clinical antidepressant effect (Greenway et al., 1995), considerably shortened the duration of cataleptic freezing in GC rats (Kulikov et al., 1995). It was also found that a 5-HT_{1A} receptor agonist flesinoxane which also possesses a clinical antidepressant effect (Grof et al., 1993; Baumann, Bertschy, 1997) significantly and dose-dependently decreased immobility time in GC rats (Kulikov et al., 1994; Popova, Kulikov, 1995).

Thyroid Hormones

Numerous clinical observations unambiguously confirm that a deficit of thyroid hormones is an essential risk factor for occurrence of depression (Clear et al., 1995; Musselman, Nemeroff, 1996). Treatment with thyroxine succeeded in some cases in attenuating considerably the degree of depression in patients (Bauer, Whybrow, 1990; Clear et al., 1996). Triiodothyronine is widely used in clinic to potentiate the effect of antidepressants (Joffer et al., 1995; Prange, 1996). Thyroid hormone deficit produced by thyroidectomy provokes catalepsy in Wistar rats and enhances the expression of catalepsy in GC rats (Barykina et al., 2002; Kulikov et al., 2002a). A chronic administration of a therapeutic dose of thyroxine attenuated catalepsy in GC rats (Kulikov et al., 2002a). The cataleptogenic effect of thyroid hormone deficit and the anticataleptic effect of thyroxine are in a good accordance with the clinical observations.

IV. Construct Validity of the Model

The construct validity means similarity of physiological, neurobiological and neurochemical mechanisms between the model and the prototype (depression). However, since the mechanisms of depression are not quite clear, practically the requirement of construct validity is reduced to correspondence of physiological, biochemical and molecular changes found in the model to the present notions of the mechanism of depression. All the existing hypotheses of depression mechanisms underline the key role of brain biogenic amines – serotonin, norepinephrine and dopamine (Maes, Meltzer, 1995; Willner, 1983, 1995; Harro, Oreland, 1996; Duman et al., 1997).

Dopamine

Hypofunction of mesocorticolimbic dopaminergic system may lead to anhedonia and loss of interest for environment which are the core symptoms of depression (Sampson et al., 1991; Willner, 1983, 1995). There are data on brain dopamine deficit in patients with depressive illness (Lambert et al., 2000). Catalepsy is also traditionally considered to be associated with reduced dopaminergic transmission (Sanberg et al., 1988; Klemm, 1989). Indeed, D_2 receptor antagonists are the strongest cataleptogens. Catalepsy is also elicited in rats after intracerebral administration of an antisense sequence for the gene of D_2 receptors (Zhang, Creese, 1993; Qui et al., 1995; Davidkova et al., 1998). Moreover, a linkage between the predisposition to haloperidol-induced catalepsy and the gene coding for D_2 receptors has been found (Kanes et al., 1996; Patel, Hitzemann, 1999). D_2 receptor antagonist haloperidol and chlorpromazine elicited a stronger cataleptogenic effect on GC than on Wistar rats (Nikulina et al., 1987; Kolpakov et al., 1995), suggesting altered brain dopaminergic system in GC rats. Although at early stages of breeding no differences either in dopamine or its metabolite DOPAC in the striatum or n. accumbens was found between GC and Wistar rats (Nikulina et al., 1987), the studies carried out on later generations found lower dopamine and DOPAC levels in the striatum and amygdala, and a lower dopamine content of n. accumbens in GC as compared to Wistar rats (Alekhina et al., 1994; Kolpakov et al., 2001).

Norepinephrine

The noradrenergic system of locus coeruleus is believed to be the key circuit in the regulation of fear and stress reactions (Charney et al., 1995) and to be associated with pathological anxiety and posttraumatic syndrome (Charney et al., 1993, 1995). Anxiety and fear often accompany depression and are its symptoms. Finding a considerably lower norepinephrine level in the frontal cortex, striatum and hypothalamus of GC as compared with Wistar rats (Alekhina et al., 1994; Kolpakov et al., 2001) is in a good accordance with the notion of decreased noradrenergic transmission in depressive patients (Van Praag, 1982; Harro, Oreland, 1995; Anand, Charney, 2000; Frazer, 2000; Lambert et al., 2000).

Serotonin (5HT)

Theories suggesting the key role of serotonin in the mechanisms of depression are based on the following clinical observations: 1) drugs which deplete the serotonin store (reserpine) provoke relapses of depression, 2) tricyclic antidepressants are inhibitors of serotonin reuptake and increase its concentration in the synaptic cleft, and 3) 5-HT_{2A} receptor density is shown to be increased in suicides` brain cortex and chronic antidepressant treatment to decrease density of cortical 5-HT_{2A} receptors (Maes, Meltzer, 1995). In GC rats, a considerable decrease of serotonin content of the frontal cortex as compared to Wistar rats has been found (0.6 ± 0.03 μg/mg in Wistar vs 0.42 ± 0.03 μg/mg in GC, $P<0.01$). The concentration of serotonin metabolite 5-HIAA was lowered in the cortex found (0.28 ± 0.04 μg/mg in Wistar vs. 0.18 ± 0.01 μg/mg in GC, $P<0.05$) and hypothalamus found (1.74 ± 0.18 μg/mg in Wistar vs. 1.47 ± 0.19 μg/mg in GC, $P<0.05$) (Kolpakov et al., 2001). Another important peculiarity of the serotonin system of GC rats is the decreased number of centers of (3H) ketanserin binding to 5-HT_{2A} receptors in the striatum (Kulikov et al., 1995; Popova, Kulikov, 1995).

Although no changes in the intensity of specific binding of (3H)ketanserin to 5-HT_{2A} receptors in the brain cortex of GC rats were found (Kulikov et al., 1995; Popova, Kulikov, 1995), the frequency of head shakes provoked by administration of serotonin precursor – 5-hydroxytryptophan was lower in GC rats (Popova et al., 1985a; Popova, Kulikov. 1995). Since head shakes are produced by stimulation of 5-HT_{2A} receptor activity (Green, Heal, 1985) and its frequency is correlated positively with the density of 5-HT_{2A} receptors in the brain cortex (Popova et al., 1985b) it may expect a decrease in 5-HT_{2A} receptors functioning in the brain cortex of GC rats (Popova, Kulikov, 1995). This suggestion is in a good agreement with the decreased level of mRNA coding for 5-HT_{2A} receptors in brain cortex of GC rats (Kulikov et al., 2002b). A similar decrease of 5-HT_{2A} receptor mRNA expression has been found in the brain cortex of FSL rats proposed as a biological model of depression (Osterlund et al., 1999).

It is commonly accepted that depression is associated with activation of 5-HT_{2A} receptors in brain cortex. This idea is based on the fact that the number of specific centers of binding of 5-HT_{2A} receptors with their antagonists in brain cortex is increased in depressive suicides (Arora et al., 1989; Hrdina et al., 1993), and a chronic administration of tricyclic antidepressants decreases the specific binding of receptor antagonists (Lafaille et al., 1991; Burnet et al., 1994). However, this hypothesis does not account for such observations as a decreased function of 5-HT_{2A} receptors in depressive patients suffering from hypothyroidism (Clear et al., 1995, 1996), the increase of cortical 5-HT_{2A} receptor density after electroconvulsive treatment (Kellar et al., 1981), and the lack of changes in 5-HT_{2A} receptor mRNA expression after a chronic administration of tricyclic antidepressants (Burnet et al., 1994; Spurlock et al., 1994). Probably, there are certain forms of depression linked with hypothyroidism which are accompanied by a decrease of 5-HT2A receptor (Kulikov, Jenningros, 2000; Kulikov et al., 2002a,b).

Our present data indicate that another type of serotonin receptors – 5-HT_{1A} receptors – also plays an important role in the mechanisms of depression and its pharmacological correction (Blier, de Montigny, 1994; Borsini, 1994). It has been demonstrated that this type of receptors is involved in the regulation of catalepsy in GC rats, and that their activation by selective agonists shortens considerably and dose-dependently the time of cataleptic freezing in GC rats (Kulikov et al., 1994). The decreased specific binding of (3H)8-OH-DPAT to 5-HT_{1A} receptors in the brain cortex in GC rats (B max = 41.9 ± 5.2 fmol/mg in GC vs. 101.1 ± 8.3 fmole/mg in Wistar, $P<0.001$) (Popova et al., 1998) is in a good accordance with pharmacological data and currently accepted views of the role of these receptors in the regulation of catalepsy.

Borsini (1994) hypothesizes that in depression a relative increase of 5-HT_{2A} receptor levels (with respect to 5-HT_{1A} receptor level) occurs in the brain cortex. In GC rats, the 5-HT_{2A}/5-HT_{1A} ratio is by more than two times higher than in Wistar rats, which, according to Borsini`s hypothesis, indicates "depressive-like" changes of 5-HT receptors in GC rats. Thus, the changes in the three monoaminergic (i.e. 5HT, norepinephrine and dopamine) brain systems observed in GC rats are in accordance with the hypothesis suggesting the involvement of these systems in depression pathogenesis.

Overall, numerous behavioral, endocrine and neurochemical changes observed in GC as compared to Wistar rats are a result of a long-term breeding for a vital adaptive character – defensive freezing reaction. The type and direction of these changes allow us to suggest GC rats as an animal model of depression-like disorders. This model meets all the three validity criteria and may therefore be regarded as a new promising model for the study of molecular and physiological mechanisms of endogenous depression and for the search for ways of its pharmacological correction.

Importantly, the fact that breeding of rats for an exaggerated fear-induced freezing reaction has resulted in development of a persistent depression-like state is not quite unexpected. Stupor is often observed at the peak of depression (Kraepelin, 1904, cited from Nuller, Mikhailenko, 1988; Weitbrecht, 1960; Leonhard, 1980). Besides, classical antidepressants and anxiolytics are known to attenuate fear-induced freezing (Ishida-Tokuda et al., 1996; Hashimoto et al., 1997) and neuroleptic-induced catalepsy (Khisti et al., 1997; Al-Khatib et al., 1989; Worms et al., 1987).

Table 1. Comparison between GC and FSL rat strains

Characteristics	GC	FSL
Behavioral traits		
Catalepsy	↑ [Barykina et al., 1983]	nd
Anhedonia	nd	↑ [Overstreet,1993]
Locomotions	↓ [Barykina et al., 1983]	↓ [Overstreet,1993]
Forced swim immobility	↑ [Nikulina et al.,1987]	↑ [Overstreet,1993]
Foot shock aggression	↑ [Nikulina et al.,1987]	↑ [Overstreet,1993]
Delta-sleep	↓ [Oganesian et al.,1990]	0 [Overstreet,1993]
REM-sleep	0 [Oganesian et al.,1990]	↑ [Overstreet,1993]
Serum hormone levels		
Corticosterone	↓ [Amstislavsky et al.,2000]	0 [Overstreet,1993]
Testosterone	↓ [Shul'ga et al.,1997]	nd
Thyroxine	↓ [Barykina et al.,2002]	nd
Chronic imipramine treatment		
Catalepsy	↓ [Kulikov et al.,2004]	nd
Forced swim immobility	nd	↓ [Zangen et al.,1997]
Brain monoamines		
Dopamine	↓ [Alekhina et al., 1994]	↑ [Zangen et al.,1999]
Norepinephrine	↓ [Alekhina et al., 1994]	↑ [Zangen et al.,1999]
Serotonin and 5-HIAA	↓ [Kolpakov et al.,2001]	↑ [Zangen et al.,1997]
5-HT_{2A} receptors	↓ [Kulikov et al.,1995]	↓ [Osterlund et al.,1999]

↑ - increased, ↓ - decreased, 0 – unchanged, nd – no data, up – unpublished data

Finally, it remains to compare the GC rats with other currently existing models of depression. Among various genetic animal models of depression, the FSL rat strain bred for a high sensitivity to the anti-acetylcholineesterase agent diisopropyl fluorophosphate meets the largest number of criteria established for animal models of depression (Table 1). The FSL rats are characterized by anhedonia, long time of immobility in the forced swimming test (Overstreet, 1993), an increased serotonin and 5-HIAA in hypothalamus, hippocampus, cortex and n. accumbens, compared to the control strain FRL (Zangen et al., 1997). Notably, all these changes disappeared after a chronic desipramine administration (Overstreet, 1993; Zangen et al., 1997), showing sensitivity of these rats to antidepressant drugs.

Overall, the behavioral changes observed in GC rats are in general similar to those in FSL rats (Table 1). Catalepsy of GC rats, like immobility in the forced swim test in FSL rats, reacts only to chronic imipramine administration. However, the direction of changes in dopamine, norepinephrine and serotonin levels in the brain of GC rats differ from those in FSL rats. We do not, nevertheless, see in this discrepancy any contradiction to the ideas of discussed earlier. Quite the reverse, the proposed new model supplements the body of models of depression, making it possible to study different aspects of this manifold pathology. Taken together, we suggest that GC rats represent a biological model of the processes taking place in endogenous depression complicated with hypothyroidism.

References

[1] Abrams R., Taylor M.A., Coleman-Stolurow K. Catatonia and mania: patterns of cerebral dysfunction. *Biol. Psychiatry*, 1979, 14:111-117.

[2] Alekhina T., Gilinsky M., Kolpakov V. Catecholamines level in the brain of rats with a genetic predisposition to catatonia. *Biog. Amin.*, 1994, 10:443-449.

[3] Al-Khatib I., Fujiwara M., Ueki S. Relative importance of the dopaminergic system in haloperidol-catalepsy and the anticataleptic effect of antidepressants and methamphetamine in rats. Pharmacol. *Biochem. Behav.*, 1989, 33:93-97

[4] Ammon G., Koppen U., Thome A. Sleep researches of bordeline patients compared with groups of patients with depression, schizophrenia and psychosomatic disease. *Dyn. Psychiatr.*, 1990, 23:120-129.

[5] Amstislavsky S., Buligina V., Maslova L., Alekhina T., Barykina N., Chuguy V., Popova N., Kolpakov V. Effect of cross-fostering on some physiological and behavioural features in Wistar and GC (genetically cataleptic) rat strains. *Russ. J. Physiol.*, 2000, 86:1630-1637.

[6] Anand A., Charney D., Norepinephrine dysfunction in depression. *J. Clin. Psychiatry*, 2000, 61 (Suppl.10):16-24.

[7] Arora R., Meltzer H. Serotonergic measures in the brains of suicide victims: 5-HT2 binding sites in the frontal cortex of suicide victims and control subjects. *Am. J. Psychiatry*, 1989, 146:730-736.

[8] Barykina N., Chepkasov I., Alekhina T., Kolpakov V. Breeding of Wistar rats for predisposition to catalepsy. *Genetika,* 1983, 19:2014-2021.

[9] Barykina N., Chuguy V., Alekhina T., Kolpakov V., Maksiutova A., Kulikov A. Effects of thyroid hormone deficiency on behavior in rat strains with different predisposition to catalepsy. *Physiol. Behav.*, 2002, 75:733-737.

[10] Bauer M., Whybrow P. Rapid-cycling bipolar affective disorder. II: Treatment of refractory rapid cycling with high-dose levothyroxine. A preliminary study. *Arch. Gen. Psychiatry*, 1990, 47:435-440.

[11] Baumann P., Bertschy G., Long-term treatment of depression: is there a use for depot antidepressants? *Int. Clin. Psychopharmacol.*, 1997, 12:77-80

[12] Blier P., de Montigny C. Current advances and trends in the treatment depresion. *Tr. Pharm. Sci.*, 1994, 15:220-226.

[13] Bondy B., Ackenheil M., Mueller-Spahn F., Hippius H. Biologische Marker endogener Psychosen. *Nervenarzt*, 1988, 59:565-572.

[14] Borsini F. Balance between cortical 5-HT_{1A} and 5-HT_2 receptor function: hypothesis for a faster antidepressant action. *Pharmacol. Res.*, 1994, 30:1-11.

[15] Burnet P., Michelson D., Smith M., Gold P., Sternberg E. The effect of chronic imipramine administration on the densities of 5-HT_{1A} and 5-HT_2 receptors and the abundances of 5-HT receptor and transporter mRNA in the cortex, hippocampus and dorsal raphe of three strains of rat. *Brain Res.*, 1994, 638:311-324.

[16] Carroll B., Curtis G., Mendels J. Neuroendocrine regulation in depression. I: Limbic system-adrenocortical dysfunction. *Arch. Gen. Psychiatry*, 1976, 33:1039-1044.

[17] Charney D., Deutch A., Krystal J., Southwick S., Davis M. Psychobiological mechanisms of posttraumatic stres disorder. *Arch. Gen. Psychiatry*, 1993, 50:294-307.

[18] Charney D., Bremner J., Redmond D. Noradrenergic neural substrates for anxiety and fear. Clinical asotiation based on preclinical research. In: Psychopharmacology:. The Fourth Generation of Progress. Bloom F. and Kupfer D. (eds) Raven Press. Ltd., New York, 1995, p.387-395.

[19] Clear A., McGregor A., O'Keane V. Neuroendocrine evidence for an association between hypothyroidism, reduced central 5-HT activity and depression. *Clin. Endocrinol.*, 1995, 43:713-719.

[20] Clear A., McGregor A., Chambers S., Dawling S., O'Keane V. Thyroxine replacement increases central 5-hydroxytryptamine activity and reduces depressive symptoms in hypothyroidism. *Neuroendocrinol.,* 1996, 64:65-69.

[21] Davidkova G., Zhou L., Morabito M., Zhang S., Weiss B. D2 dopamine antisense RNA expression vector, unlike haloperidol, produce long-term inhibition of D2 dopamine-mediated behaviors without causing Up-regulation of D2 dopamine receptors. J. *Pharmacol. Exp. Ther.* 1998, 85:1187-1196

[22] DeBattista C., Pasener J., Kalehzan B., Schatzberg A. Acute antidepressant effects of intravenous hydrocortisone and CRH in depressed patients: a double-blind, placebo-controlled study. *Am. J. Psychiatry,* 2000, 157:1334-1337.

[23] Duman R., Heninger G., Nestler E. A molecular and cellular theory of depression. *Arch. Gen. Psychiatry*, 1997, 54:597-606.

[24] Duval F., Mokrani M., Bailey P., Correa H., Diep T., Crocq M., Macher J. Thyroid axis activity and serotonin function in major depressive episode. *Psychoneuroendocrinol.,* 1999, 24:695-712.

[25] Frazer A Norepinephrine involvement in antidepressant action. *J. Clin. Psychiatry*, 2000, 61(Suppl.10):25-30.

[26] Frye M., Denicoff K., Bryan A., Smith-Jackson E., Ali S., Luckenbaugh D., Laverich G., Post R. Association between lower serum free T4 and greater mood instability and depression in lithium-maintained bipolar patients. *Am. J. Psychiatry*, 1999, 156:1909-1914.

[27] Fundaro A. Pinch-induced catalepsy in mice: a useful model to investigate antidepressant or anxiolytic drugs. Prog. Neuropsychopharmacol. *Biol. Psychiatry*, 1998, 22:147-158.

[28] Gershon E., Berettini W., Nurnberger J., Goldin L. Genetcs of affective illness. In: Psychopharmacology: The Third Generation of Progress. Meltzer H. (ed.), Raven Press, New York, 1987, p.481-492.

[29] Geyer M., Markou A. Animal models of psychiatric disorders. In: Psychopharmacolgy:. The Fourth Generation of Progress. Bloom F. and Kupfer D. (eds) Raven Press. Ltd., New York, 1995, p.787-798.

[30] Green A., Heal D. The effects of drugs on serotonin-mediated behavioural models. In: Green A. (Ed.) Neuropharmacology of Serotonin. Oxford University, Oxford, 1985, p.326-365.

[31] Greenway S., Pack A., Greenway F. Treatment of depression with cyproheptadine. *Pharmacotherap.,* 1995, 15:357-360.

[32] Grof P., Joffe R., Kennedy S., Persad E., Syrotiuk J., Bradford D. An open study of oral flesinoxan, a 5-HT1A receptor agonist, in treatment-resistant depression. *Int. Clin. Psychopharmacol.*, 1993, 8:167-172.

[33] Haggerty J., Stern R., Mason G., Beckwith J., Morey C., Prange A. Subclinical hypothyroidism: A modifiable risk factor for depression? *Am. J. Psychiatry*, 1993, 150:508-510.

[34] Howland R. Thyroid dysfunction in refractory depression: Implication for pathophysiology and treatment. *J. Clin. Psychiatry*, 1993, 54:47-54.

[35] Harro J., Oreland L. Depresion as a spreading neuronal adjustment disorder. *Eur. Neuropsychopharmacol.*, 1996,6:207-223.

[36] Hashimoto S., Inoue T., Koyama T. Effects of the co-administration of 5-HT1A receptor antagonists with an SSRI in conditioned fear stress-induced freezing behavior. *Pharmacol. Biochem. Behav.*, 1997, 58:471-475.

[37] Hrdina P., Demeter E., Vu T., Sotonyi P., Palkovits M. 5-HT uptake sites and 5-HT2 receptors in brain of antidepressant-free suicide victims/depressives: increase in 5-HT2 sites in cortex and amygdala. *Brain Res.*, 1993, 614:37-44.

[38] Ishida-Tokuda K., Ohno Y., Sakamoto H., Ishibashi T., Wakabayashi J., Tojima R., Nakamura M. Evaluation of perospirone (SM-9018), a novel serotonin-2 and dopamine-2 receptor antagonist, and other antipsychotics in the condutioned fear stress-induced freezing behavior model in rats. Jpn. J. Pharmacol., 1996, 72:119-126.

[39] Joffe R., Sokolov S., Singer W. Thyroid hormone treatment of depression. Thyroid, 1995, 5:235-239.

[40] Kanes S., DainsK., Cipp L., Gatley J., Hitzemann B., Rasmussen E., Sanderson S., Silverman M., Hitzemann R. Mapping the genes for haloperidol-induced catalepsy. *J. Pharmacol. Exp. Therap.*, 1996, 277:1016-1025.

[41] Karmanova I., Oganesian H. Physiology and Pathology of Sleep-Wakefulness Cycle. Evolutionary Aspects. St. Petersburg, Nauka, 1994.

[42] Kellar K., Cascio C., Butler J., Kurtzke R. Differential effects of electroconvulsive shock and antidepressant drugs on serotonin$_2$ receptors in rat brain. *Eur. J. Pharmacol.*, 1981, 69:515-518.

[43] Khisti R., Mandhane S., Chopde C. Haloperidol-induced catalepsy: a model for screening antidepressants effective in treatment of depression with Parkinson's disease. Indian. *J. Exp. Biol.* 1997, 35:1297-1301.

[44] Klemm W. Drug effects on active immobility responses: What they tell us about neurotransmitter systems and motor functions. *Prog. Neurobiol.*, 1989, 32:403-422.

[45] Klein D.E., Gittelman R., Quitkin F. Diagnosis and Drug Treatment of Psychiatric Disorders, 1980, 2nd ed., Williamsand Wilkins, Baltimore.

[46] Kolpakov V., Alekhina T., Amstislavskaya T., Chuguy V., Barykina N., Amstislavsky S. Influence of cross-fostering on manifestation of catalepsy and brain monoamine contents in cataleptic and control strains'of rats. *Russ. J. Physiol.*, 2001, 87:918-925.

[47] Kolpakov V., Barykina N., Alekhina T., Ponomarev I. Some Genetic Animal Models for Comparative Psychology and Biological Psychiatry. Novosibirsk, 1996.

[48] Kolpakov V., Barykina N., Chugui V., Alekhina T. Relationship between certain forms of catalepsy in rats. An attempt at genetic analysis. Genetika, 1999, 35:807-810.

[49] Kolpakov V., Nikulina E., Alekhina T., Gevorgian M. Effects of neuroleptics on different types of catatonia in rats with hereditary predisposition to catatonic reactions. Zh. VND im. I.P. Pavlova, 1995, 45:388-394.

[50] Kulikov A., Avgustinovich D., Kolpakov V., Maslova G., Popova N 5-HT2A serotonin receptors in the brain of rats and mice hereditary predisposed to catalepsy. *Pharmacol. Biochem. Behav.* 1995, 50:383-387.

[51] Kulikov A., Barykina N., Tikhonova M., Chuguy V., Kolpakov V., Popova N. Effect of chronic thyroxine treatment on catalepsy in rats. Neurosci. Lett., 2002a, 330:207-209.

[52] Kulikov A., Jeanningro R.The effects of hypothyroidism on 5-HT1A and 5-HT2A receptors and the serotonin transporter protein in the rat brain. *Neurosci. Behav. Physiol.*, 2001, 31:445-449.

[53] Kulikov A., Kolpakov V., Maslova G., Kozintsev I., Popova N. Effect of selective 5-HT_{1A} agonists and 5-HT_2 antagonists on inherited catalepsy in rats. *Psychoparmacol.*, 1994, 114:172-174.

[54] Kulikov A., Tikhonova M., Barykina N., Alekhina T., Chuguy V., Kolpakov V., Popova N. Effect of chronic imipramine administration on mRNA of 5-HT_{2A} receptors in brain frontal cortex in rat strains differing in predisposition to catalepsy. *Bull. Exp. Biol. Med.*, 2002b,134:194-196.

[55] Kulikov A., Tikhonova M., Chuguy V., Alekhina T., Kolpakov V., Popova N. Chronic administration of imipramine decreases freezing time in rats genetically predisposed to catalepsy. *Bull. Exp. Biol. Med.*, 2004,138:401-403.

[56] Kupfer D., Frank E., Ehler C. EEG sleep in young depressives:first and second night effects. *Biol. Psychiatry*, 1989, 25:87-97.

[57] Lafaille F., Welner S., Suranyi-Cadotte B. Regulation of serotonin type 2 (5-HT2) and adrenergic receptors in rat cerebral cortex following nowel clasic antidepressant treatment. *J. Psychiatr. Neurosci.*, 1991, 16:209-214.

[58] Lambert G., Johansson M., Agre H., Fribeg P. Reduced brain norepinephrine and dopamine release in treatment-refractory depressive illness: Evidence in support of the catecholimine hypothesis of mood disorders. *Arch. Gen. Psychiatry*, 2000, 57:787-793.

[59] Leonhard K. Aufteilung der endogenen Psychosen. Berlin, Akademie Verlag, 1980.

[60] Maes M., Meltzer H. The serotonin hypothesis of major depresion. In: Psychopharmacolgy:. The Fourth Generation of Progress. Bloom F. and Kupfer D. (eds) Raven Press, New York, 1995, p.933-944.

[61] Mendlewicz J., Sevy S., Mendelbaum K. Molecular genetics in affective illness. Minireview. *Life Sci.,* 1992, 52:231-242.

[62] Michael A., Jenaway A., Paykel E., Herbert J. Altered salivary dehydroepiandrosterone levels in major depression in adults. *Biol. Psychiatry*, 2000, 48:989-995.

[63] Musselman D., Nemeroff C. Depresion and endocrine disorders: Focus on the thyroid and adrenal system. *Br. J. Psychiat.*, 1996, 168 (Suppl.30):123-128.

[64] Nikulina E., Popova N., Kolpakov V., Alekhina T. Brain dopaminergic system in rats with a genetic predisposition to catalepsy. *Biog. Amin.,* 1987, 4:399-406.

[65] Nuller U., Mykhalenko I. Affective Psychoses. Mediisina, Leningrad, 1988.

[66] Oganesian H., Khomutetskaya O., Bogoslovsky M., Karmanova I., Kolpakov V., Barykina N. Wakefulness-sleep cycle in rats with genetic predisposition to catalepsy. *Zh. Evol. Biohim. Fiziol.*, 1990, 26:376-382.

[67] Onodera K. Effects of antidepressants and antihistaminics on catalepsy induced by intracerebroventricular administration of histamine in mice. Methods. *Find. Exp. Clin. Pharmacol.*, 1991, 13:397-403

[68] Osterlund M., Overstreet D., Hurd Y. The flinders sensitive line rats, a genetic model of depression, show abnormal serotonin receptor mRNA expression in the brain that is reversed by 17beta-estradiol. *Mol. Brain Res.*, 1999, 74:158-166.

[69] Overstreet D. Genetic models of endogenous depression. In: Genetically-defined Animal Models of Neurobehavioral Dysfunction. Driscoll P. (ed.), Birkhauser, Boston, 1992, p.253-275.

[70] Overstreet D. The Flinders Sensitive line rats: A genetic animal model of depression. *Neurosci. Biobehav. Rev.*, 1993, 17:51-58.

[71] Pare W.P. The performance of WKY rats on three tests of emotional behavior. *Physiol. Behav.*, 1992, 51:1051-1056.

[72] Pare W.P. Passive-avoidance behavior in Wistar-Kyoto (WKY), Wistar, and Fisher-344 rat. *Physiol. Behav.*, 1993, 54:845-852.

[73] Patel N., Hitzemann R. Detection and mapping of quantitative trait loci for haloperidol-induced catalepsy in a C57BL/6J x DBA/2J F2 intercross. Behav. Genet., 1999, 29:303-310.

[74] Petrova E. Change of congenital and acquired forms of behavior in rats with genetic catalepsy. Zh. VND im. I.P. Pavlova, 1990, 40:475-480.

[75] Popova N., Avgustinovich D., Kolpakov V., Plyusnina I. Specific 3H.8-OH-DPAT binding in brain regions of rats genetically predisposed to various defense behavior strategies. *Pharmacol. Biochem. Behav.*, 1998, 59:793-797.

[76] Popova N., Barykina N., Plyusnina T., Alekhina T., Kolpakov V. Expression of the startle reaction in rats genetically predisposed towards different types of defensive behavior. Neurosci. *Behav. Physiol.*, 2000, 30:321-325.

[77] Popova N., Kulikov A. On the role of brain serotonin in expression of genetic predisposition to catalepsy in animal models. *Am. J. Med. Genet.*, 1995, 60:214-220.

[78] Popova N., Kulikov A., Kolpakov V., Barykina N., Alekhina T. Changes in brain serotonin system of rats genetically predisposed to catalepsy. Zh. VND im. I.P. Pavlova, 1985a, 35:742-746.

[79] Popova N., Kulikov A., Pak D. Correlation between the number of serotonin type 2 receptors in the frontal cortex and intensity of serotonin-induced head twitches in mice. *Bull. Exp. Biol. Med*, 1985b, 100:322-324.

[80] Porsolt R., Le Pichon M., Jalfre M. Depression: a new animal model sensitive to antidepressant treatment. Nature, 1977, 266:730-732.

[81] Prange A. Novel uses of thyroid hormones in patients with affective disorders. Thyroid, 1996, 6:537-543.

[82] Qin Z., Zhou L., Zhang S., Wang Y., Weiss B. D_2 dopamine receptor antisense oligodeoxynucleotide inhibits the synthesis of a functional pool of D2 dopamine receptors. *Mol. Pharmacol.* 1995, 48:730-737

[83] Sampson D., Willner P., Muscat R. Reversal of antidepressant action by dopamine antagonists in an animal model of depression. *Psychopharmacol.,* 1991,104:491-495.

[84] Sanberg P., Bunsey M., Giordano M., Norman A. The catalepsy test: Its ups and downs. *Behav. Neurosci.*, 1988, 102:748-759.

[85] Schweiger U., Deuschle M., Weber B., Korner A., Lammers C., Schmider J., Gotthardt U., Heuser I. Testosterone, gonadotropin and cortisol secretion in male patients with major depression. *Psychosom. Med.,* 1999, 61:292-296.

[86] Sher L., Rosenthal N., Wehr T. Free thyroxine and thyroid-stimulating hormone levels in patients with seasonal affective disorder and matched control. *J. Affect. Dis.*, 1999, 56:195-199.

[87] Shtilman N., Alekhina T., Barykina N., Kolpakov V., Shtark M. Learning ability and protein metabolism in various brain structures of rats with genetic predisposition to catalepsy. Bull. Sib. Br. AS USSR, 1988, 20:86-92.

[88] Shul'ga V., Alekhina T., Kolpakov V. Adrenal cortex hormones and the testicles in emotional stress in rats with a genetic predisposition to cataleptic responses. *Neurosci. Behav. Physiol.,*1997,27:692-694.

[89] Spurlock G., Buckland P., O'Donovan M., McGuffin P. Lack of effect of antidepressant drugs on the levels of mRNAs encoding serotonergic receptors, synthetic enzymes and 5HT transporter. *Neuropharmacol.*, 1994, 33:433-440.

[90] Van Delft A., Sitsen J., Ruigt G. Antidepressant drugs can be differentiated by their effects on slow wave sleep in the rat. *Psychopharmacol.,* 1988, 96 (Suppl.):149.

[91] Van Praag H. Neurotransmitters and depression. Part A and B. In: Handbook of Psychiatry and Endocrinology. Beumont P., Burrows G (eds), Amsterdam, 1982, p.267-303.

[92] Weitbrecht H. Depressive und manische endogene Psychosen. In: Psychiatrie der Gegenwart. Berlin, Springer Verlag, 1960, 2:83-140.

[93] Willner P. Dopamine and depression: A review of recent evidence. *Brain Res. Rev.*, 1983, 6:211-246.

[94] Willner P. The validity of animal models of depression. *Psychopharmacol.,* 1984, 83:1-16.

[95] Willner P. Animal models as simulations of depression. *Tr. Neurosci.*, 1991, 12:131-136.

[96] Willner P. Animal models of depression: an overview. *Pharm. Ther.*, 1990, 45:425-455.

[97] Willner P. Dopaminergic mechanisms in depression and mania. In: Psychopharmacology: The Fourth Generation of Progress. Bloom F. and Kupfer D. (eds) Raven Press. Ltd., New York, 1995, p.921-931.

[98] Willner P., Golembiowska, Klimek V., Muscat R. Changes in mesolimbic dopamine may elplain stress-induced anhedonia. *Psychobiol.,* 1991,19:79-84.

[99] Worms P., Kan J., Wermuth C., Roncucci R., Biziere K. SR 95191, a selective inhibitor of type A monoamine oxidase with dopaminergic properties. I. Psychopharmacological profile in rodents. *J. Pharmacol. Exp. Ther.,* 1987, 240:241-50

[100] Zangen A., Overstreet D., Yadid G. High serotonin and 5-hydroxyindolacetic acid levels in limbic brain regions in a rat model of depresion: normalization by chronic antidepressant treatment. *J. Neurochem.*, 1997, 69:2477-2483.

[101] Zangen A., Overstreet D., Yadid G. Increased catecholamine levels in specific brain regions of a rat model of depression: normalization by chronic antidepressant treatment. *Brain Res.*, 1999, 824:243-250.

[102] Zhang M., Creeze I. Antisense oligodeoxynucleotide reduces brain dopamine D2 receptors: behavioral correlates. *Neurosci. Lett.* 1993, 161:223-226.

In: Animal Models in Biological Psychiatry
Editor: Allan V. Kalueff, pp. 75-95
ISBN 1-59454-814-5

Chapter 5

Experimental Study of Neurophysiological Basis for Hereditary Predisposition to the Development of Depression: Review

Natalia N. Kudryavtseva, Damira F. Avgustinovich, Irina V. Bakshtanovskaya, Luydmila A. Koryakina, Olga V. Alekseyenko, Tatiana V. Lipina and Natalia P. Bondar
Institute of Cytology and Genetics SD RAS, Novosibirsk, Russia

I. Introduction

It is well known that heredity plays the main role in the etiology of many psychoses, including depression and schizophrenia (Ehrman, Parsons, 1981; Zerbin-Rudin, 1987; Mackinnon, Mitchell, 1994; Sham, 1996; Bassett et al., 2002). This notion has been supported by numerous studies on twins or families suffering from these diseases. If one identical twin has depression, other twin with 70% probability will develop depression too. Children, parents, and siblings of depressed person (including non-identical twins) have about 15% chance of developing depression. However, according to many theories (Rosenthal, 1971; Gottesman, Shields, 1973), it is not the disease that is inherited, but a predisposition to it. It has long been recognised that environmental factors, often of psychogenic nature, determine the probability of development of psychopathology and form a provoking background. Stress situations induce the development of disease in persons predisposed to it.

It has been suggested that the action of genes, controlling development of depression or any other hereditary defined psychopathologies, must be characterized by threshold effect, which is determined by environment (Comings, 1979). The key questions are: what is the nature of genetic predisposition to the development of certain mental disease and what specific neurophysiological and psychosomatic features may predisposed persons have? These questions are out of interests of most specialists in medical genetics and psychiatrists because of numerous limitations associated with techniques for examining of brain functions in humans. Furthermore, as a rule, people come to their psychiatrists when symptoms of depression have already been developed, and only family analysis (if it may be carried out) might testify the genetic nature of this disease.

Traditionally, genetic approaches toward behavioral studies in animals have been focused on pre-existing, "natural" genetic variability amongst laboratory inbred strains (Trullas, Skolnik 1993; reviews, Crawley et al., 1997; Jones, Mormede 1999). Numerous studies demonstrate the interstrain differences in learned helplessness, fear and anxiety-related behavior in inbred mice and rats (reviews, Crawley et al., 1997; Zhukov, Vinogradova, 2002). Moreover, some inbred strains of rats are considered as a good genetic model for understanding depression mechanisms (review, Willner, Mitchell, 2002). For example, Wistar-Kyoto (WKY) rat strain is considered as an animal genetic model of depressive behavior (Tejani-Butt et al., 1994; Pare, Tejani-Butt, 1996; Pare, 2000) because these animals demonstrate motor retardation (Pare, 1993), significant decrease in the exploratory activity towards a female intruder (anhedonia) in stressed individuals (Pare, 2000), hyper-responsiveness to stress stimulation, higher restraint stress-induced ulceration (Pare, 1992), low level of activity and high level of immobility in the forced swimming test as compared to either normal inbred strains (Lahmame et al., 1997). Flinders Sensitive Line (FSL) of rats was established by genetically selecting (breeding) Sprague-Dawley rats for a behavioral trait, supersensitivity to cholinergic agents and was supposed as model of depression (Overstreet, Russell, 1982; Overstreet, 1986; Overstreet et al., 1986; Yadid et al., 2000).

Recently, Overstreet et al. (1996) have selectively bred two lines of rats with high and low sensitivities (HDS and LDS, accordingly) to the hypothermic effects of the 5-HT_{1A} receptor agonist, 8-OH-DPAT. HDS rats showed greater immobility in the forced swimming test, than either the LDS line or the randomly bred control group, suggesting that these rats may provide a useful genetic model of depression (Overstreet et al., 1996; Gonzalez et al., 1998; Knapp et al., 2000). WAG/Rij rats have also been considered as an genetic model of depression (Sarkisova, Kulikov, 2000) showing higher levels of fear and depressiveness (Bazian et al., 2001). Koltushi high avoidance rats (KHA) with active coping style were selected from Wistar rats using divergent performances in avoidance conditioning. They have been shown to be susceptible to learned helplessness following inescapable stress (oppositely to Koltushi low avoidance (KLA) rats) and suggested as a model of depressive-like state (review, Zhukov, Vinogradova, 2002). Notably, the specific behavioral strategy in stressful conditions of all these strains was considered as the key criterion of predisposition to depression in all these studies.

It has long been known that in most cases the disease does not arise suddenly. Indeed, there is period of development from the recipient stages to the deep ones, and similar negative social environments may produce different psychopathologies in individuals in dependence on their genetic predisposition. Knowledge of neurobiological basis of genetic predisposition to possible development of depression under influence of psychopathogenic factors is very important for pharmacological or psychological prevention of this disease.

Here we will discuss a feasible experimental approach to investigate such problem. As has been shown previously (Kudryavtseva et al., 1991a; reviews, Kudryavtseva et al., 1995; Kudryavtseva, Avgustinovich, 1998), social defeat repeatedly experienced in agonistic confrontations leads to dramatic changes in social and individual behaviors, as well as in welfare of submissive male mice (losers) of C57BL/6J (C57) strain. The etiology, response to treatment, and symptomatology of these changes are analogous to those of human depression. A severe behavioral deficit developed in male mice: after experiencing social defeat for 20 days, they could only demonstrate a passive defense and immobile postures, whilst in the beginning they preferred active defense and withdrawal. These social losers displayed reduced ambulation in the open-field, increased immobility time in the Porsolt's test and demonstrated no aggression in any, no matter how provoking situation. Clear-cut anxiety has been revealed in the plus-maze test and disturbed social communicative behavior in the partition test (Kudryavtseva, 1994; Avgustinovich et al., 1997). A loss of weight, decreased plasma testosterone levels (Kudryavtseva et al., 1995), immune responsiveness (Devoino et al., 1993; Popova et al., 1996; Gryazeva et al., 2001), and low stress reactivity (Kudryavtseva et al., 1991a) have also been demonstrated.

Repeated treatment with the antidepressants imipramine (Kudryavtseva et al., 1991a) or tianeptine (Kudryavtseva et al., 1995) decreased depressiveness (immobility in the Porsolt's test). Chronic ethanol consumption (Kudryavtseva et al., 1991b) and chronic treatment with ipsapirone and buspirone (Avgustinovich et al., 1999a, 2003) reduced the level of anxiety but did not prevent depression. Treatment with citalopram for three weeks lowered anxiety in the light-dark test in the chronically defeated losers (Keeney, Hogg, 1999).

Interestingly, many symptoms demonstrated by the losers were similar to the core and some additional symptoms of depressive patients (Table 1). The majors are vegetable symptoms, anxiety, total behavioral deficit in individual and social behaviors, sensitivity to anxiolytics and antidepressants. Chronic unavoidable social emotional stress is believed to be a pathogenic factor that leads to a mixed anxiety/depression state in C57 mice (Kudryavtseva, Avgustinovich, 1998; Borodin et al., 2002).

In parallel with these experiments, we studied mice of CBA/Lac (CBA) strain. Almost all behaviors in intact CBA mice differ from those in C57 mice (Kudryavtseva, 1987; Kudryavtseva, Sitnikov, 1988). Moreover, CBA mice are characterized by the highest susceptibility to catatonic (Kudryavtseva, Bakshtanovskaya, 1989; Kudryavtseva et al., 1989) or cataleptic (Kulikov et al., 1989, 1995) states in different tests among all mouse strains studied. Freezing or active defense prevailed in submissive behavior of CBA losers at the moment of the aggressor's attack (Bakshtanovskaya, Kudryavtseva, 1991). Long experience of defeats was not the provoking factor for the increasing of immobility time in the Porsolt's test. However, CBA losers after 20 days of repeated defeats demonstrated very strange forms of behavior that they had never shown in the first confrontations - cataleptic or catatonic postures (Kudryavtseva, Bakshtanovskaya, 1989), which C57 losers never displayed. It was supposed that chronic social stress provokes a cataleptic-like state in CBA losers because this strain has a hereditary predisposition to it. Thus, a similar psychogenic factor - long-term negative emotional stress - produced different psychopathologies in mice of different strains. It has been concluded that C57 mice have a genetic predisposition to the development of depression under the influence of pathogenic factors of an emotional nature. In contrast, CBA mice are non-depressive, but are genetically predisposed to catalepsy.

The aim of this study was to: 1) perform a comparative analysis of behaviors in different situations and brain serotonin function in male mice of "depressive" and "cataleptic" (non-depressive) genotypes, and 2) determine the most probable features that could be used to characterize the genetic predisposition to the development of depression.

Table 1. Parallels in depressive symptoms in patients (Hamilton, 1967) and C57 losers (adapted from Kudryavtseva, Avgustinovich, 1998; references in the text)

Depressed patients	Depressive mice-losers
Vegetative symptoms	
Somatic symptoms	Decreased testosterone level; higher corticosterone level; loss of weight; increased gastric mucosa damage; immune deficiency.
Eating disturbances	Loss of weight; increased ethanol consumption; gastric mucosa damage.
Motor retardation, decreased energy, rare movements	Total behavioral deficit: prevailing passive defense; appearance of postures of "waiting" "depression"; decreased ambulation and exploratory activity; increased immobility time in Porsolt's test.
Muscular tension	Increased time of rigid immobility in the reflex immobility reaction test.
Disturbances in mood	
depressed mood, loss of interest, indifference	Negative emotional state as a result of social defeats, high depressiveness in Porsolt's test, disturbances in social behavior: avoidance of social contacts and decreased communicative behavior, loss of interest to the partner, disappearance of natural aggressiveness.
Disturbed cognitions	
derealization, feeling of helplessness	Decreased exploration, high level of behavioral helplessness.
Anxiety, phobias	
avoidance-withdrawal	Increased level of anxiety; avoidance of social contacts, disappearance of natural aggressiveness, increased voluntary ethanol consumption.
Therapeutic effect of antidepressants and anxiolytics	Sensitivity to antidepressants and anxiolytics: chronic imipramine and tianeptine treatment (decreased depressiveness in the Porsolt's test); chronic ipsapirone and buspirone treatment (anxiolytic effect in the plus-maze test); chronic ethanol consumption (improved communication in the partition test)

Sensory contact model (Kudryavtseva, 1991a) for generation of aggressive and submissive behaviors in male mice was used in all our studies. Briefly, pairs of animals were placed in cages divided in two compartments by a perforated transparent partition allowing the animals to see, hear and smell their neighbor, but not to contact them physically. Every afternoon the partition was removed for 10 min to enable agonistic interactions. The procedure yielded equal numbers of males with an opposite social experience of aggression, evidenced by victories (aggressors, winners), and experience of social defeats (defeated mice, losers) in daily agonistic confrontations. The losers and winners were investigated in different periods of repeated defeat or victory experience in daily agonistic confrontations.

II. Behaviors of Mice of "Depressive" C57 and "Cataleptic" CBA Strains

Features of Submissive Behavior

During winners' attacks in the first agonistic confrontations, C57 losers escaped or defended themselves actively, demonstrating upright or sideways postures (Kudryavtseva et al., 1991a). After ten days (T10 losers) of agonistic interactions the losers tried to escape the attacks by running away or by falling down on the back. Sometimes this behavior resembled a strong panic reaction. Sometimes the flight ends up with a fainting-fit. This syncope lasts sometimes more than 3 min (during this period the winners do not interfere). Repeated social defeats during 20 days (T20 losers) of agonistic confrontations induced novel immobile postures (that the losers never showed in the first agonistic confrontations) – nose-to-corner or into the litter on the cage floor. These behaviors were interpreted as major symptoms of human depression - motor retardation, behavioral deficit, complete indifference and loss of interest even toward the threatening social factor - aggressors. In contrast, CBA losers showed a markedly different behavioral strategy in these conditions. Active defense, or mainly immobile postures – freezing - prevailed in the losers in any periods of confrontations. It was supposed that CBA mice demonstrated more adaptive behavior that decreased aggression in the winners during confrontations (Bakshtanovskaya, Kudryavtseva, 1991).

Open Field, Exploratory Activity and Porsolt's Test

In the open field test, CBA mice demonstrated high emotionality: the latency to the first movement of the central square and defecation scores were significantly larger and the number of crossed squares was significantly lower in CBA vs. C57 intact male mice (Kudryavtseva, 1991b; Avgustinovich et al., 2000). 20-day experience of defeats equally reduced motor activity (as assessed by crossed squares in the open-field test and a number of nose-pocking in the exploratory activity test) in the mice of both strains (Kudryavtseva, 1991b; Kudryavtseva, Bakshtanovskaya, 1988). However, the main parameters of emotionality, such as the number of fecal boli (defecation) and the latency to the first movement from center were changed only in the highly "emotional" group of CBA losers. Importantly, the immobility time in Porsolt's test was significantly increased in T20 C57 (but not CBA) losers (Fig. 1). We shall stress that this parameter is sensitive to antidepressants (Porsolt et al., 1977), and may therefore reflect the development of depression state (Kudryavtseva et al., 1991a).

Animal behavior in novel conditions may be interpreted also in terms of behavioral strategy. In these terms, C57 mice display high activity in the open field and may therefore be characterized by a preference for active avoidance of novel situations. The behavioral strategy of CBA mice was passive, especially in the open field: it was typical for them to freeze. This interpretation fits previous observations on C57 losers showing active defense or withdrawal when attacked by a stronger aggressive partner. In contrast, CBA losers predominantly freeze in this situation (Bakshtanovskaya, Kudryavtseva, 1991). Thus, C57 animals demonstrated active strategy of defensive behavior and CBA mice showed passive defensive strategy in novel experimental situations. It may also be assumed that active strategy in C57 mice is produced by panic reaction developing in stressful conditions.

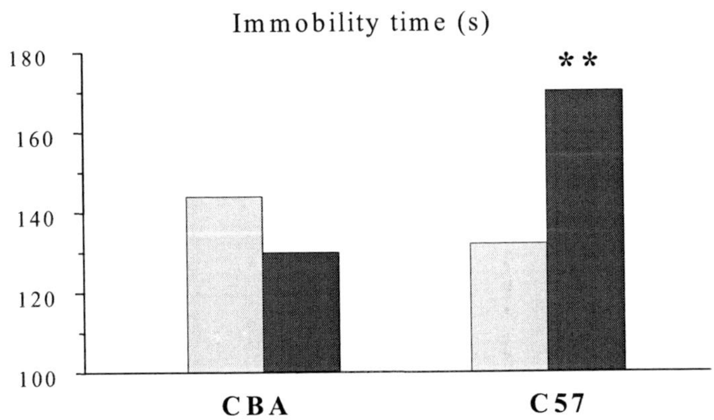

Fig. 1. Time of immobility in the control (gray) and T20 losers (black) male CBA and C57 mice in the Porsolt's test. ** P<0.01 vs the respective controls (adapted from Kudryavtseva et al., 1995).

Features of Anxiety-Related Behavior in C57 and CBA Mice

During an in-depth ethological analysis of our data, all behavioral phenotypes of these mouse strains in the above-mentioned tests were reconsidered (see further, also see: Avgustinovich et al., 1999c; Avgustinovich et al., 2000) in terms of state and trait anxiety (Lister, 1990; File, 1991; File, 1995).

State anxiety is defined as the emotion displayed by an individual when confronted with a stressful stimulus in unfamiliar environments, whereas trait anxiety is an enduring feature of the subject, that is, a stable characteristic (Belzung, Berton, 1997). It is assumed that state anxiety is environmentally determined, whereas trait anxiety is considered to be influenced mostly by genetic components (File, 1991). The elevated plus-maze, open field, light/dark choice tests were proposed to measure state anxiety (Belzung, Berton, 1997; review, Ramos, Mormede, 1998). Griebel et al. (1993) developed a test for measuring trait anxiety in mice under familiar unstressed conditions. Indices of emotionality such as decreased ambulation and increased defecation in a brightly lit open field were considered as those of anxiety (reviews, Crawley et al., 1997; Ramos, Mormede, 1998). In these terms, CBA mice may be more "state-anxious" in the open field than C57 animals. Indeed, crossed squares were significantly lower and defecation was higher in CBA than in C57 mice (Table 2).

Table 2. Comparison of intact C57 and CBA mice in behavioral tests

Parameters	**C57**		**CBA**	
BEHAVIOR OF MICE IN THE NOVELTY (STATE ANXIETY)				
OPEN FIELD TEST				
Crossed squares	119.3 ± 11.7		75.9 ± 11.1 *	
Latency to leave centre, s	6.6 ± 0.8		50.4 ± 23.4	
Rearing time, s	15.2 ± 3.1		17.9 ± 3.9	
Number of rearings	12.1 ± 2.0		11.8 ± 2.5	
Defecation	1.1 ± 0.6		4.0 ± 0.7 **	
ELEVATED PLUS-MAZE TEST				
Open arm time, %	2.8 ± 1.7		7.8 ± 2.8	
Central platform time, %	13.8 ± 2.0		40.7 ± 5.9 ***	
Enclosed arm time, %	83.4 ± 3.0		51.5 ± 6.6 ***	
Open arm entries, %	7.2 ± 1.9		12.5 ± 2.0	
Central platform entries, %	46.4 ± 1.0		49.8 ± 0.5 **	
Enclosed arm entries, %	46.5 ± 2.5		37.6 ± 2.1 **	
Total entries	15.4 ± 2.1		17.7 ± 1.6	
Head-dips	3.5 ± 0.8		5.5 ± 1.0	
BEHAVIOR OF MICE IN THE HOME CAGE (TRAIT ANXIETY)				
CUBIC BOX TEST				
Latency to approach, s	56.3 ± 12.3		49.3 ± 12.0	
Total number of approaches	9.3 ± 1.6		11.2 ± 1.8	
Total exploration time, s	12.8 ± 2.9		53.2 ± 17.8 *	
PARTITION TEST				
	Familiar neighbour	Unfamiliar neighbour	Familiar neighbour	Unfamiliar neighbour
Approaches to the partition	7.5 ± 1.2	4.9 ± 1.0	9.3 ± 0.9	10.2 ± 0.8
Time near the partition, s	40.4± 8.8	33.7 ± 8.1	76.7 ± 7.5 *	104.4 ± 10.1 •
Average time, s	4.6 ± 0.5	5.7 ± 0.8	7.9 ± 0.7 *	11.1 ± 1.3 •

One-way ANOVA test. *P<0.05; **P<0.01; ***P<0.001 - vs C57; • P<0.05 - vs familiar neighbor (for CBA; adapted from Avgustinovich et al., 2000).

However, plus-maze data (increased enclosed arm time and entries and decreased center platform time and entries) suggest that C57 mice are more anxious than CBA mice. These observations are in a good agreement with other works (review, Crawley et al., 1997) and may be interpreted as an attempt to avoid danger in any experimental situations demonstrated by C57 mice (Avgustinovich et al., 1999c; Avgustinovich et al., 2000). In contrast, CBA mice demonstrated a clear-cut passive behavioral strategy including long freezing episodes in the central platform of the elevated plus-maze.

Study of trait anxiety in a familiar environment as a response to unfamiliar stimuli in the home cage revealed a higher level of trait anxiety in C57 mice than in CBA mice. While C57 mice clearly avoided the novel cubic box placed into home cage or run away no sooner than approach it, their CBA counterparts willingly explored the novelty (Table 2) (Avgustinovich et al., 2000). A similar behavior was observed in the partition test (Kudryavtseva, 1994), measuring the level of communicative behavior as a reaction to the partner behind the perforated transparent partition in home cage. C57 mice demonstrated less reaction to the familiar partner in the neighboring compartment than did CBA mice. Replacement of the familiar partner by an unfamiliar animal increased significantly the level of the behavioral activity of CBA mice near the partition as response to other partner. In contrast, C57 mice avoided the partition and did not demonstrate curiosity. If these test situations, as suggested in (Avgustinovich et al., 2000), reveal trait anxiety, which is a permanent attribute of individual (Belzung, Berton, 1997; review, Ramos, Mormede, 1998), then C57 mice demonstrated higher level of trait anxiety in comparison with non-depressive strain. Since the trait anxiety is considered to be genotype-depended feature (File, 1991), it becomes clear that C57 mice demonstrated higher genetically defined trait anxiety. In these terms, it may be assumed that level of trait anxiety in CBA mice is lower than in C57 mice. As shown earlier, the repeated experience of defeat in 10 daily agonistic confrontations led to the development of pronounced anxiety in the plus-maze and partition tests (Avgustinovich et al., 1997; Kudryavtseva, Avgustinovich, 1998) in high trait anxious C57 (but not in CBA) losers.

The data presented here allow to suggest that "depressive" genotype (C57 mice) may also show panic-like avoidance in any novel dangerous (or not) situations and pronounced trait anxiety provoking generalized anxiety under influence of chronic social defeats. Indeed, in all behavioral tests used here (the open-field, the plus-maze, the partition tests, etc.) C57 losers demonstrated severe anxiety (Avgustinovich et al., 1997; Borodin et al., 2002).

Voluntary Ethanol Consumption

It has long been known that many depressive patients suffer from alcohol or drug abuse. Depressive symptoms are very common in alcoholics ranging from 28 to 98% (Keeler et al., 1979; Weissman, Myers, 1980; Brown, Schuckit, 1988). It has been shown that C57 mice highly prefer alcohol under the free choice conditions, while CBA mice are a low-preferring alcohol strain (Khodorova et al., 1984). In our experiments, consecutive defeat experience elevated (by 20%) voluntary ethanol consumption in the C57 losers, which was most robust on the second week of testing (Fig. 2). Notably, this phenomenon was not observed in CBA losers. Taken together, these data suggest (Kudryavtseva et al., 1995) that depression and alcoholism have a common genetic background and neurobiological basis. The provoking factor for development of both disorders may be chronic negative emotional stress stimulating ethanol consumption which attenuated anxiety.

Reflex Immobility Reaction

A slight pinch of the skin in the mouse scruff produces the reflex immobility reaction, accompanied by rigid muscular tension alternating by indirect body and tail movements (paroxysms). This test (Kudryavtseva et al., 1989) was intent for quantitative estimation of genetic predisposition to catatonic reactions in mice. It has been shown that CBA mice spent significantly more time immobile in this test than did C57 mice and mice of other strains (Kudryavtseva, Bakshtanovskaya, 1989). In other tests measuring cataleptic reactions (Ornstein, Amir, 1981) CBA mice also demonstrated the most robust catalepsy (Kulikov et al., 1989; Kulikov et al., 1993; Kulikov et al., 1995). It was concluded that CBA mice is genetically predisposed to catalepsy. Long experience of defeats in daily agonistic confrontations was found to induce development of expressed cataleptic reaction in free behavior in T20 CBA losers (but not in T20 C57 losers). Some of them froze near the wall for a long time in uncomfortable postures, sometimes lasting more than 3 min. When approached by other males, they froze deeply so that the conspecifics could turn them over as logs. In general, freezing and immobility behaviors in the wild nature represent typical adaptive mimicric reactions (review, Kolpakov, 1990). In these terms, it may be concluded that C57 mice demonstrate less adaptive reaction under unavoidable stressful conditions.

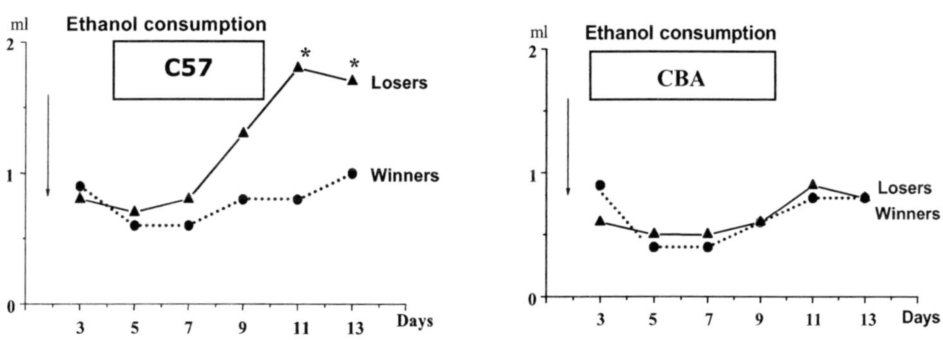

Fig. 2. Voluntary ethanol consumption in C57 and CBA losers and winners. Explanations are given in the text. Arrows show placing of water and 20% ethanol bottles to the winners and losers after 7 days of agonistic confrontations (adapted from Kudryavtseva et al., 1991b).

III. Behavior of C57 and CBA Social Winners

Obviously, genetic features of the nervous system may be realized and reflected in different forms of the social behavior. The consideration of interstrain differences in aggressive behavior among the victorious mice allowed us to reveal other features of the nervous system, to characterize the depressive genotype. For example, it has been shown that the latency to the first attack and the total attacking time were longer in C57 than in CBA victorious mice (Kudryavtseva, Popova, 1988). Noteworthy, the total attacking time and the number of attacks did not change significantly in these experimental situations and were considered as stable parameters reflecting nervous excitation in male mice: a long-lasting aggressive excitation in C57 mice and a short-lasting aggressive excitation in CBA mice in provoking conditions. After the partition was lowered to stop agonistic interactions, both winners and losers of CBA strain became quiet very quickly. The total time spent near the partition as response to the partners in the neighboring compartment was reduced to zero (Kudryavtseva, 1987), with all mice sitting in their nests and/or sleeping.

In contrast, C57 winners were still active near the partition for an hour. These data indirectly confirm those reported above. In C57 mice, the threshold of aggressive reaction (long latency of the first attack) is high. However, once arising, aggressive excitation lasts long, possibly because the inhibiting mechanisms act weakly. By contrast, CBA mice demonstrated a low threshold (short latency to aggression), and a short-lasting nervous excitation (evoking aggressive behavior). Using anthropomorphic terms, one may say that C57 individuals fall down into the emotional (positive or negative) state and stay longer time in this state, whereas CBA mice quickly "forget" emotional state developed under their social experience.

IV. Serotonergic System: Inter-Strain Differences

The key role of the serotonergic system in depression is supported by an enormous amount of clinical and preclinical data (for review, see: Kostowski et al., 1989). However, in spite of years of investigations, the role of serotonin (5-HT) in depressive psychopathology is not yet clear (Curzon, 1988; Kostowski et al., 1989; Yadid et al., 2000). The existing data do not allow unambiguous conclusions about the serotonergic regulation to be made, because the data and following hypothesis are often contradictory. Although, originally, the serotonin hypothesis of depression proposed a hypofunction of this system, subsequent researches made it unclear whether the 5-HT dysfunction in depression was related to hypofunction or hyperfunction of this system (review, Brown et al., 1994). Some authors link the mechanisms of depression to a functional deficit of brain serotonin (Lapin, Oxenkrug, 1969; Van Praag, 1984). Most but not all investigators have found decreased 5-hydroxyindoleacetic acid (5-HIAA) accumulation in cerebrospinal fluid (CSF) of depressed patients compared to normal persons (Bowers, 1974; Goodwin et al., 1977; Van Praag et al., 1970, 1973a,b; Asberg et al., 1984), suggesting decreased 5-HT metabolism in the brain.

However, in other studies, normal (Roy et al., 1985) or even higher (Reddy et al., 1992) levels of 5-HIAA were observed in the CSF of depressed patients. Several postmortem brain studies of suicide victims have demonstrated increased bindings of 5-HT_2 receptors in frontal cortex (Stanley, Mann, 1983; Mann et al., 1986; Arango et al., 1992) and in blood-platelets (Arora, Meltzer, 1989). A decrease in the uptake of 5-HT and an alteration in postsynaptic 5-HT receptors in depressed individuals were considered to be indicators of a compensatory mechanism for a generally low serotonergic activity (Meltzer, Lowy, 1987). Higher levels of 5-HT$_{1A}$ receptors have been reported in the prefrontal cortex of nonviolent depressed suicide victims than in the brain of violent suicidents and normal postmortem brains (Matsubara et al., 1991).

In other studies, the decreased sensitivity of 5-HT$_{1A}$ receptors in the hippocampus and amygdala of suicide victims were revealed (Cheetham et al., 1990). The density and affinity of 5-HT$_{1A}$ receptors in some brain regions were shown to be similar for suicide victims who took no drugs and for normal postmortem samples (Cheetham et al., 1990; Arranz et al., 1994). Similarly, the disturbances in the serotonergic-catecholaminergic balance is supposed to be the cause of depressive illness (Reinchard et al., 1983; Ressler, Nemeroff, 2000). One of explanations for these conflicting data in depressed patients in these studies may be due to the fact that serotonergic mechanisms of depression were investigated on different stages of pathogenesis.

Our preliminary data on 5-HT and 5-HIAA levels in various brain areas of C57 losers over different time periods of "depression" development allowed us to put forward a hypothesis of dynamic changes in the 5-HT turnover during the development of depression, depending on the duration and the depth of the disorder (Kudryavtseva, Bakshtanovskaya, 1988; Kudryavtseva et al., 1992). Numerous changes in 5-HT and/or 5-HIAA levels were revealed in the hippocampus, olfactory bulbs, amygdala and midbrain of T10 losers in comparison with the controls (Kudryavtseva et al., 1995). There were no significant differences in 5-HT and 5-HIAA levels in these areas after 20 and 30 days of agonistic confrontations in the losers compared to the controls. 5-HT level in hypothalamus was increased after 20 tests in losers, decreasing after 30 days of agonistic confrontations (Kudryavtseva et al., 1995). Also 5-HIAA level in this area was significantly decreased in T30 losers.

Collectively, these data strongly support the dynamic changes in serotonergic activity, involving changes in serotonin metabolism during the development of experimental depression (Avgustinovich et al., 2004). The incipient stage of depression has been speculated (Kudryavtseva, Bakshtanovskaya, 1988; Kudryavtseva et al., 1995) to be accompanied by activation of serotonin function in some brain areas, and the later stages by its exhaustion. As response to changes in serotonin metabolism in different brain areas, dynamic changes in 5-HT$_{1A}$ receptors have been shown by radioligand binding assay (Avgustinovich et al., 1999b; 2001a) in male mice during development of depression. It has been found that B_{max} of 5-HT$_{1A}$ receptor was lower in the frontal cortex and amygdala of T10 losers than in the control (Avgustinovich et al., 1999b). However increased B_{max} and K_d were found in amygdala of T20 losers in comparison with the controls and T10 losers (Avgustinovich et al., 2001a).

Pharmacological method revealed lesser behavioral reactivity to agonist 5-HT$_{1A}$ receptors flesinoxan in T10 losers compared to their intact counterparts (Kudryavtseva et al., 1996; Avgustinovich et al., 1998a). This suggests that chronic stress may cause desensitization of 5HT$_{1A}$ receptors, accompanying by increased serotonergic activity. Interestingly, in similar model based on the sensory contact paradigm, repeated defeat stress also produced dynamic changes in 5-HT$_{1A}$ receptors binding in some brain areas in three shrews (Flugge, 1995). We suggest that assessment of male mice genetically predisposed to the development of depression or catalepsy may be helpful to reveal some features of brain serotonergic function of depressive genotype.

Serotonin Metabolism in Brain Areas of C57 and CBA Mice

Mice of "depressive" and "cataleptic" strains have been found to differ in many parameters of their central serotonergic activity (Fig 3). The most obvious fact was different activity of tryptophan hydroxylase (TPH) - a key limiting enzyme of serotonin synthesis. TPH activity was lower in all brain areas of C57 mice. Compared to CBA mice, 5-HT and 5-HIAA levels were higher in the midbrain and nucleus accumbens and lower in hypothalamus of C57 mice, while 5-HT levels in amygdala and 5-HIAA levels in hippocampus were also reduced (Avgustinovich et al., 1998a).

Consecutive experience of defeats in daily agonistic confrontations produced different dynamic changes in brain serotonergic function in dependence on duration of agonistic confrontations as well as on strain of mice (Lipina et al., 1997; Avgustinovich et al., 2001b). Increase of serotonin level in the midbrain and nucleus accumbens and its decrease in hypothalamus and amygdala were shown in CBA losers compared to the control group in response to a short 3-day social stress. The most parameters of serotonergic metabolism in brain areas were recovered to the control level in CBA T10 losers. In C57 losers, the opposite changes in serotonin function were shown: decreased 5-HT level in midbrain and hypothalamus and increased in amygdala after 3 tests as compared to the control (Avgustinovich et al., 2001b). 5-HT and 5-HIAA levels in most brain areas were not recovered to 10th day of defeated stress. Higher serotonin level was maintained in hypothalamus of C57 T10 losers compared to control level.

Since activation of serotonergic system accompanies the stress reaction in animals (Chaouloff, 1993; Malyszko et al., 1994; Kawahara et al., 1995), high serotonin level in hypothalamus may indicate strong stress in C57 T3 and T10 losers. Collectively, we suggest that weak feedback (compensatory) mechanisms may lead to renewal of serotonergic metabolic processes under repeated stress in C57 mice (Avgustinovich et al., 2001b).

Serotonergic Receptors

Inter-strain differences in the central serotonergic function were confirmed pharmacologically in behavioral experiments. In C57 intact mice, $5HT_{1A}$ receptor agonist ipsapirone with anxiotropic properties (Griebel, 1995) produced anxiogenic effect, decreasing the percentage of open arm time and in open arm entries, as well as the number of open arm end exploration and the number of head-dips in the plus-maze test (Avgustinovich, Koryakina, 2000). In CBA mice, ipsapirone predominantly decreased ambulation. Agonist of $5\text{-}HT_{1A}$ receptors flesinoxan produced decrease in communicative behavior in the partition test in intact mice of both strains and CBA T10 losers and was ineffective in C57 T10 losers (Kudryavtseva et al., 1996). Desensitization of $5\text{-}HT_{1A}$ receptors resulted from long-term activation of serotonergic system under chronic social stress was supposed in C57 losers

(Kudryavtseva et al., 1996). In CBA losers pharmacological sensitivity to flesinoxan did not differ from the controls. This indirectly confirms our hypothesis that serotonergic metabolism quickly restores after stress in CBA losers.

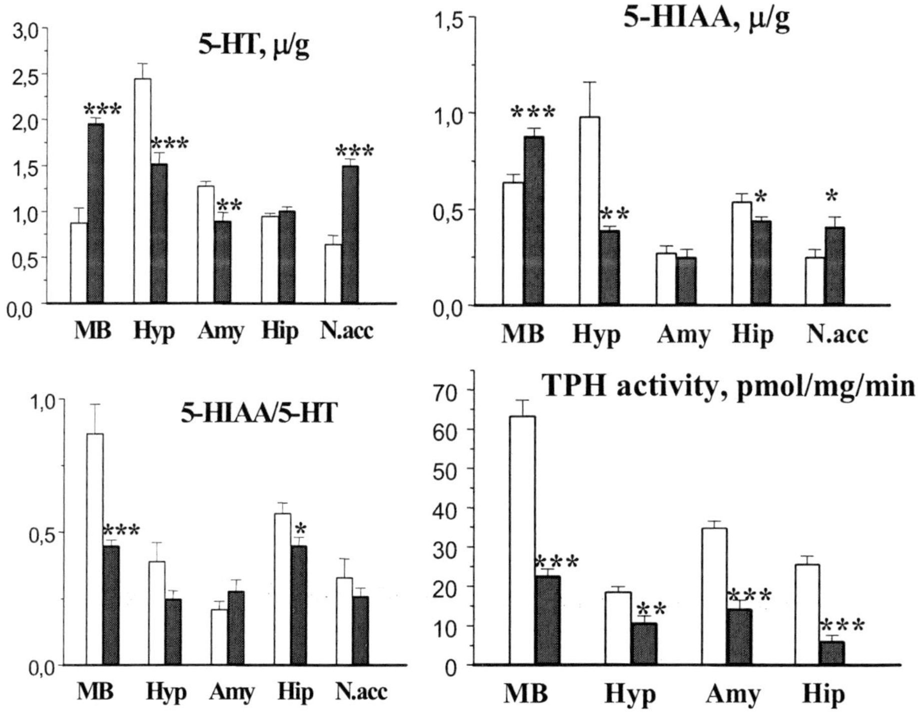

Fig. 3. Brain serotonergic activity in intact CBA (white) and C57 (black) mice. MB – midbrain; Hyp – hypothalamus; Amy – amygdala; Hip – hippocampus; N.acc. – nucleus accumbens. * $P<0.05$; ** $P<0.01$; *** $P<0.001$ – vs. CBA mice (adapted from Avgustinovich et al., 2001b)

Thus, the question arises as for which specific processes may underlie brain serotonin function genetic predisposition to the experimental depression evoked by pathogenic psychoemotional factors? In general, it may be suggested that depressive genotype is characterized by weak feedback mechanisms of autoreceptors and progressive dysregulation of normally adaptive relationships between serotonin synthesis, catabolism and receptors. As a result, dysfunctional alterations and incapability of serotonergic metabolism to be recovered after daily social stress and exhaustion of serotonin function (at least in hypothalamus) produce development of depression. In CBA mice, high TPH activity may provide rapid compensation of serotonergic function changed under stress.

Noteworthy, cataleptic genotype was described earlier at this Institute by V.Kolpakov for rats of GC-strain (Genetic Catatonics) that had been bred for more than 20 years from Wistar rats (reviews, Kolpakov, 1990; Kolpakov et al., 1996). The selective sign in these rats was catatonic reaction - an immobile vertical posture in stressful conditions. Dr. Kolpakov proposed these rats as a model of schizophrenia. Notably, high brain TPH activity in striatum, passive avoidance, freezing, immobility behaviors in GC rats (Kolpakov et al., 1996) and in CBA mice with genetic predisposition for catalepsy are remarkably similar.

V. Concluding Remarks

There is no doubt that it is necessary to add hereditary predisposition to the criteria (similarity of symptoms, biochemistry and sensitivity to antidepressants) of homology of animal models to human depression, as formulated by McKinney and Bunney (1969), for which the C57BL/6J mouse strain represents a good model meeting all these criteria. Moreover, it is known that stressful stimuli and events are the most potent environmental factors that may trigger or induce depressive episodes (Blanchard et al., 1998; Kalueff, 1998; Yadid et al., 2000). Consequently, animal models that involve a social context seem to be more appropriate (Koolhaas et al., 1995; Blanchard et al., 1998; Martinez et al., 1998) because they represent situations that individuals meet in their everyday lives. In this context, social defeat, negative emotions, permanent anxiety produced by fear over being attacked, threatened under the sensory contact model, and, in general, unavoidable psychoemotional social stress produced mainly by anticipation of negative events, may be considered as the relevant psychopathogenic etiologic factors in the development of experimental depression under sensory contact model.

A detailed data analysis showed that inclination to panic reaction in stressful conditions, pronounced trait anxiety, high alcohol consumption may be the markers for genetic predisposition to depression. Incapability of serotonergic metabolic processes to be recovered during long time after stress may be crucial for individuals genetically predisposed to depression. High brain TPH activity and passive avoidance, freezing, immobility behavior, high level of state anxiety in stressful situations may characterize mouse strain predisposed to catalepsy.

References

[1] Arango V, Underwood MD, Mann JJ. Alteration in monoamine receptors in the brain of suicide victims. *J. Clin. Psychopharmacol.* 1992. 12:8S-12S.

[2] Arora RC. Meltzer HY. Increased serotonin2 (5-HT_2) receptor binding as measured by ^{3}H-lysergic acid diethylamide (^{3}H-LSD) in the blood platelets of depressed patients. *Life Sci.* 1989. 44:725-734.

[3] Arranz B, Eriksson A, Mellerup E, Plenge P, Marcusson J. Brain 5-HT_{1A}, 5-HT_{1D}, and 5-HT_2 receptors in suicide victims. *Biol. Psychiat.* 1994. 35:457-463.

[4] Asberg M, Bertilsson L, Martensson B, Scalia-Tomba GP, Thoren P, Traskman-Bendz L. CSF monoamine metabolites in melancholia. *Acta Psychiat. Scand.* 1984. 69:201-219.

[5] Avgustinovich DF, Gorbach OV, Kudryavtseva NN. Comparative analysis of anxiety-like behavior in partition and plus-maze tests after agonistic interaction in mice. *Physiol. Behav.* 1997. 61:37-43.

[6] Avgustinovich DF, Lipina TV, Alekseyenko OV, Amstislavskaya TG, Kudryavtseva NN. Peculiarities of brain serotonergic system activity in natural and pathological anxiety in mice: strain differences. Zhurn. VND im. I.P. Pavlova. 1998a. 48:331-341.

[7] Avgustinovich DF, Lipina TV, Molodtsova GF, Alekseyenko OV. Koryakina LA, Amstislavskaya TG, Kudryavtseva NN. Changes in the activity of tryptophan hydroxylase and monoamine oxidase A during development of experimental depression induced by social confrontations. *Dokl. Biol. Sci.* 1998b. 363(3):523-525.

[8] Avgustinovich DF, Alekseyenko OV, Koryakina LA. Chronic treatment with ipsapirone affects anxiety, but not depression in mice. Eur. *Neuropsychopharmacol.* 1999a. 9 (Suppl 5): S301.

[9] Avgustinovich DF, Lipina TV, Alekseyenko OV, Kudryavtseva NN. Changes in brain serotonergic activity in anxious losers. *Biog. Amines.* 1999b. 15:4:395-404

[10] Avgustinovich DF, Lipina TV, Bondar NP, Kudryavtseva NN. Manifestations of genetically defined anxiety in male C57BL/6J and CBA/Lac mice. Zhurn. VND im. I.P. Pavlova. 1999c. 49:1008-1017.

[11] Avgustinovich DF, Lipina TV, Bondar NP, Alekseyenko OV, Kudryavtseva NN. Features of the genetically defined anxiety in mice. *Behav. Genet.* 2000. 30: 101-109.

[12] Avgustinovich DF, Koryakina LA. Revealing anxiety in mice of C57BL/6J, CBA/Lac, and BALB/c strains after ipsapirone injection. Zhurn. VND im. I.P. Pavlova. 2000. 50:95-102.

[13] Avgustinovich DF, Lipina TV, Kudryavtseva NN. Features of the brain serotonergic system reactivity to the social stress of different duration in mice of C57BL/6J and CBA/Lac strains. *Ross. Fiziol. Zhurn.* 2001b. 87(4):532-542.

[14] Avgustinovich DF, Alekseyenko OV, Tenditnik MV. Fighting among C57Bl/6J mice and its implications for (3H)8-hydroxy-N,N-dipropyl-2-aminotetralin binding in various brain regions. *Neurosci. Lett.* 2001a. 305:189-192.

[15] Avgustinovich DF, Alekseyenko OV, Koryakina LA. Effects of chronic treatment with ipsapirone and buspirone on the C57BL/6J strain mice under social stress. *Life Sci.* 2003. 72, 1437-1444.

[16] Avgustinovich DF, Alekseyenko OV, Bakshtanovskaya IV, Koryakina LA, Lipina TV, Tenditnik MV, Bondar NP, Kovalenko IL, Kudryavtseva NN. Dynamic changes of brain serotonergic and dopaminergic activities during development of anxious depression: Experimental Study. *Usp. Fiziol. Nauk.* 2004. 35(4):19-40.

[17] Bakshtanovskaya IV, Kudryavtseva NN. Strategy of submissive behavior of male mice: Influence of genotype and preliminary experience of agonistic confrontations. *Biol. Sci.* 1991. 11:73-79.

[18] Bassett AS, Chow EW, Weksberg R, Brzustowicz L. Schizophrenia and genetics: new insights. *Curr. Psychiat. Rep.* 2002. Aug;4(4):307-14.

[19] Bazian AS, Midzianovskaia IS, Kuznetsova GD, Sarkisova KIu, Getsova VM, Orlova NV, Lushkin AA. Possible mechanisms for forming typological features of behavior of WAG/Rij line rats. Zhurn. VND im. I.P. Pavlova. 2001. 51:709-716.

[20] Belzung C, Berton F. Further pharmacological validation of the BALB/c neophobia in the free exploratory paradigm as an animal model of trait anxiety. *Behav. Pharmacol.* 1997. 18 (6):541-548.

[21] Blanchard RJ, Hebert M, Sakai RR, McKittrick C., Henrie A., Yudko E., McEwen BS., Blanchard DC. Chronic social stress: changes in behavioural and physiological indices of emotion. *Aggress. Behav.* 1998. 24:307-321.

[22] Borodin JuI, Kudryavtseva NN, Tenditnik MV, Rachkovskaya LN, Shurlygina AV, Trufakin VA. Behavioural effects of novel enterosorbent Noolit on mice with mixed depression/anxiety-like state. *Pharm. Biochem. Behav.* 2002. 72:131-141.

[23] Bowers MB. Lumbar Csf 5-hydroxyindoleacetic acid and homovanillic acid in affective syndromes. *J. Nerv. Ment. Dis.* 1974. 158(5):325-330.

[24] Brown SA, Schuckit MA. Changes in depression among abstinent alcoholics. *J. Stud. Alcohol.* 1988. 49: 412-417.

[25] Brown S-L, Steinberg RL, van Praag HM. The Pathogenesis of Depression: Reconsideration of Neurotransmitter Data. In: den JA Boer, JM Sitsen (eds). Handbook of Depression and Anxiety. New York:Marcel Dekker Inc. 1994. p. 317-347.

[26] Chaouloff F. Psychopharmacological interaction between stress hormones and central serotonergic systems. *Brain Res. Rev.* 1993. 18:1-32.

[27] Cheetham SC, Crompton MR, Katona CL, Horton RW. Brain 5-HT1 binding sites in depressed suicides. *Psychopharmacol.* 1990. 102:544-548.

[28] Comings DC. Pc1 Duarte, a common polymorphism of a human brain protein and its relationship to depressive disease and multiple sclerosis. Nature. 1979.277:28-32.

[29] Crawley JN, Belknap JK, Collins A, Crabbe JC, Frankel W, Henderson N, Hitzemann RJ, Maxson SC, Miner LL, Silva AJ, Wehner JM, Wynshaw-Boris A, Paylor R. Behavioral phenotypes of inbred mouse strains: implications and recommendations for molecular studies. *Psychopharmacol.* 1997. 132:107-124.

[30] Curzon G. Serotonergic mechanism of depression. Clin. Neuropharmacol. 1988. 11:S11-S20.

[31] Devoino LV, Alperina EL, Kudryavtseva NN, Popova NK. Immune responses in male mice with aggressive and submissive behavior patterns: Strain differences. Brain *Behav. Immun.* 1993. 7:91-96.

[32] Ehrman L, Parsons PA. Behavior Genetics and Evolution. New York: McGraw-Hill Book Company. 1981.

[33] File SE. The biological basis of anxiety. In: HY Meltzer, D Nerozzi (eds). Current practices and future developments in the pharmacotherapy of mental disorders. Amsterdam: Elsevier. 1991. p. 159-165.

[34] File SE. Animal models of different anxiety states. In: G Biggic, E Sanna, E Costa (eds). GABAA receptors and anxiety, from neurobiology to treatment. New York: Raven Press. 1995. p. 93-113.

[35] Flugge G. Dynamics of central nervous 5-HT$_{1A}$-receptors under psychosocial stress. *J. Neurosci.* 1995. 15(11):7132-7140.

[36] Gonzalez LE, File SE, Overstreet DH. Selectively bred lines of rats differ in social interaction and hippocampal 5-HT$_{1A}$ receptor function: a link between anxiety and depression. *Pharm. Biochem. Behav.* 1998. 59(4):787-792.

[37] Goodwin FK, Rubovits R, Jimerson D, Post RM. Serotonin and norepinephrine subgroups in depression. *Sci. Proc. Amer. Psychiat. Assoc.* 1977. 130:108

[38] Gottesman II, Shields J. Genetic theorizing and schizofrenia. *Brit. J. Psychiat.* 1973. 122(15):15-30.

[39] Griebel G, Belzung C, Misslin R, Vogel E. The free exploratory paradigm, an effective method for measuring neophobic behavior in mice and testing potential neophobia-reducing drugs. *Behav. Pharmacol.* 1993. 4:637-644.

[40] Griebel G. 5-hydroxytryptamine-interacting drugs in animal models of anxiety disorders: more than 30 years of research. In: BE Leonard (ed.). *Pharmacol. Ther.* 1995. 65:319-395.

[41] Gryazeva NI, Shurlygina AV, Verbitskaya LV, Mel'nikova EB, Kudryavtseva NN, Trufakin VA. Changes in various measures of immune status in mice subject to chronic social conflict. *Neurosci. Behav. Physiol.* 2001. 31(1):75-81.

[42] Hamilton MA. Development of a rating scale for primary depressive illness. *Brit. J. Soc. Clin. Psychol.* 1967. 6:278-296.

[43] Jones BC, Mormede P. Neurobehavioral Genetics. Methods and applications. 1999. Boca Raton-London-New York-Washington: CRC Press.

[44] Kalueff AV. Problems on the study of stress induced behavior. Kiev: CSF. 1998. 134 p.

[45] Kawahara H, Kawahara Y, Yoshida M, Yokoo H, Nishi M, Tanaka M. Serotonin release in the rat amygdala during exposure to emotional stress. In: A Takada, G Curzon (eds). Serotonin in the central nervous system and periphery. Elseiver Science B. 1995. p. 89-95

[46] Keeler MH, Taylor CI, Miller WC. Are all recently detoxified alcoholics depressed? *Amer. J. Psychiat.* 1979. 136:586-588.

[47] Keeney AJ, Hogg S. Behavioral consequences of repeated social defeat in the mouse: preliminary evaluation of a potential animal model of depression. *Behav. Pharmacol.* 1999. 10:753-764.

[48] Khodorova NA, Vlasova NN, Maisky AI. Comparative study of the level of brain biogenic amines and ethanol kinetics in blood of C57BL/6 and CBA mice. *Bull. Exper. Biol. Med.* 1984. 9:284-285.

[49] Knapp DJ, Sim-Selley LJ, Breese GR, Overstreet DH. Selective breeding of 5-HT_{1A} receptor-mediated responses: application to emotion and receptor action. *Pharmacol. Biochem. Behav.* 2000. 67:701-708.

[50] Kolpakov VG. Catatonia in animals: Genetics, Neurophysiology, Neurochemistry. Novosibirsk: Nauka. 1990. 168 p.

[51] Kolpakov VG, Barykina NN, Alekhina TA, Ponomarev IYu. Some genetic animal models for comparative psychology and biological psychiatry. Novosibirsk: Institute of Cytology and Genetics. 1996. 172 p.

[52] Koolhaas JM, Meerlo P, De Boer SF, Strubbe JH, Bohus B. Social stress in rats: An animal model of depression? *Acta. Neuropsychiat.* 1995. 7:27-29.

[53] Kostowski W, Plaznik A, Archer T. Possible implications of 5-HT function for the etiology and treatment of depression. New Trends Experiment. *Clin. Psychiat.* 1989. 5(2):91-116.

[54] Kudryavtseva NN. Peculiarities of forming of agonistic behavior in mice using sensory contact model. Review. Novosibirsk: Institute of Cytology and Genetics. 1987. 39 p.

[55] Kudryavtseva NN. The sensory contact model for the study of aggressive and submissive behaviors in male mice. *Aggress. Behav.* 1991a. 17(5):285-291.

[56] Kudryavtseva NN. Mechanisms of agonistic behavior. Dr. Sci. Dissertation. 1991b. Leningrad. 366 p.

[57] Kudryavtseva NN. Experience of defeats decreases the behavioral reactivity to conspecific in the partition test. Behav. Proc. 1994. 32:297-304.

[58] Kudryavtseva NN, Avgustinovich DF. Behavioural and physiological markers of experimental depression induced by social conflicts (DISC). *Aggress. Behav.* 1998. 24:271-286.

[59] Kudryavtseva NN, Bakshtanovskaya IV. The development of depression-like state in submissive male mice of C57BL/6J strain. Novosibirsk: Institute of Cytology and Genetics. 1988. 39 p.

[60] Kudryavtseva NN, Bakshtanovskaya IV. Experience of defeat increases the susceptibility to catatonic-like state in mice. *Behav. Proc.* 1989. 20:139-149.

[61] Kudryavtseva NN, Bakshtanovskaya IV, Avgustinovich DF, Koryakina LA, Serova LI, Wishnivetskaya GB, Kaledin VI, Popova NA, Ilnitskaya SI, Kolesnikova LA, Amstislavskaya TG, Gorbach IV, Lipina TV, Shigantsov SN, Madorskaya IA, Denisova T.P. Social defeats, depression and anxiety: an experimental model. Review, Novosibirsk: Institute of Cytology and Genetics, 1995. 48 p.

[62] Kudryavtseva NN, Bakshtanovskaya IV, Koryakina LA. Social model of depression in mice of C57BL/6J strain. *Pharmacol. Biochem. Behav.* 1991a. 38(2):215-300.

[63] Kudryavtseva NN, Bakshtanovskaya IV, Popova NK. Catatonia as an element of submissive behavior in intermale mouse agonistic confrontations. Zhurn. VND im. I.P. Pavlova. 1989. 39:128-136.

[64] Kudryavtseva NN, Lipina TV, Vishnivetskaya GB, Avgustinovich DF. Participation of 5-HT_{1A} and 5-HT_2 receptors in formation of different levels of anxiety under the influence of experience of social victories and defeats in male mice. Zhurn. VND im. I.P. Pavlova. 1996. 46:370-377.

[65] Kudryavtseva NN, Madorskaya IA, Bakshtanovskaya IV. Social success and voluntary ethanol consumption in mice of C57BL/6J and CBA/Lac strains. *Physiol. Behav.* 1991b. 50:143-146.

[66] Kudryavtseva NN, Madorskaya IA, Bakshtanovskaya IV, Popova NK, Marona-Levicka D, Vetulani J. Experimental model of depression: Neurochemical changes, effects of imipramine and citalopram. Zhurn. *Nevropatol. Psihiat.* 1992. 1:106-109.

[67] Kudryavtseva NN, Popova NK. Comparative characteristics of parameters of aggressive reaction of two genotypes mice. Zhurn. VND im. I.P. Pavlova. 1988. 38:889-895.

[68] Kudryavtseva NN, Sitnikov AP. Influence of the genotype on the formation of aggressive and submissive behavior in mice. *Neurosci. Behav. Physiol.* 1988. 18:38-43.

[69] Kulikov AV, Kozlachkova EYu, Kudryavtseva NN, Popova NK. Correlation between tryptophan hydroxylase activity in the brain and predisposition to pinch-induced catalepsy in mice. *Pharmacol. Biochem. Behav.* 1995. 50(3):431-435.

[70] Kulikov AV, Kozlachkova EYu, Maslova GB, Popova NK. Inheritance of Predisposition to Catalepsy in Mice. Behav. Genet. 1993. 23(4):379-484.

[71] Kulikov AV, Kozlachkova EYu, Popova NK. Genetic control of catalepsy in mice. Genetics. 1989. 25(8):1402-1408.

[72] Lahmame A, del Arco C, Pazos A, Yritia M, Armario A. Are Wistar-Kyoto rats a genetic animal model of depression resistant to antidepressants? *Eur. J. Pharmacol.* 1997. 337:115-123.

[73] Lapin IP, Oxenkrug GF. Intensification of the central serotonergic processes as a possible determinant of the thymoleptic effects. Lancet. 1969. 1:132-136.

[74] Lipina TV, Avgustinovich DF, Alekseyenko OV, Amstislavskaya TG, Kudryavtseva NN. Features of the brain serotonergic system in animals with genetic predisposition for the development of depressive state. *Behav. Pharmacol.* 1997. 8(6-7):653.

[75] Lister RG. Ethologically based animal models of anxiety disorders. *Pharmacol. Ther.* 1990. 46:321-340.

[76] Mackinnon A, Mitchell PB. The genetics of anxiety and depression. In: JA den Boer, JM Sitsen (eds). Handbook of Depression and Anxiety. Basel: Marcel Dekker Inc. 1994. p. 71-118.

[77] Malyszko J, Takada Y, Urano T, Serizawa K, Kosima Y, Yan D. Peripheral and central serotonergic systems in rats subjected to footshock or water-immersion restraint stress. *Biog. Amin.* 1994. 10(4):303-310.

[78] Mann JJ, Stanley M, McBride PA, McEwen BS. Increased serotonin-2 and beta-adrenergic receptor binding in the frontal cortices of suicide victims. *Arch. Gen. Psychiatry.* 1986. 43(10):954-959.

[79] Martinez M, Calvo-Torrent A, Pico-Alfonso MA. Social Defeat and Subordination as Models of Social Stress in Laboratory Rodents: a Review. *Aggress. Behav.* 1998. 24:241-256.

[80] Matsubara S, Arora RC, Meltzer HY. Serotonergic measures in suicide brain: 5-HT_{1A} binding sites in frontal cortex of suicide victims. *J. Neural. Transm. Gen. Sect.* 1991. 85:181-194.

[81] McKinney WT, Bunney WE. Animal model of depression: A review of evidences and implications for research. *Arch. Gen. Psychiat.* 1969. 21:240-248.

[82] Meltzer HY, Lowy MT. The serotonin hypothesis of depression. In: HY Meltzer, MT Lowy (eds). Psychopharmacology: The Third generation of Progress. 1987. New York: Raven Press. p. 513-526.

[83] Ornstein K, Amir S. Pinch-induced catalepsy in mice. *J. Comp. Physiol. Psychol.* 1981. 95(5):827-835.

[84] Overstreet DH. Selective breeding for increased cholinergic function: development of a new animal model of depression. *Biol. Psychiat.* 1986. 21:49-58.

[85] Overstreet DH, Janowsky DS, Gillin JC, Shiromani PJ, Sutin EL. Stress-induced immobility in rats with cholinergic supersensitivity. *Biol. Psychiat.* 1986. 21:657-664.

[86] Overstreet DH, Rezvani AH, Knapp DJ, Crews FT, Janowsky DS. Further selection of rat lines differing in 5-HT-1A receptor sensitivity: behavioural and functional correlates. *Psychiat. Genet.* 1996. 6:3107-3117.

[87] Overstreet DH, Russell RW. Selective breeding for diisopropyl fluorophosphate-sensitivity: behavioral effects of cholinergic agonists and antagonists. *Psychopharmacol.* 1982. 78:150-155.

[88] Pare WP. Learning behavior, escape behavior and depression in an ulcer susceptible rat strain. Integr. *Physiol. Behav.* 1992. 27:130-141.

[89] Pare WP. Passive-avoidance in Wistar Kyoto (WKY), Wistar and Fischer 344 rats. *Physiol. Behav.* 1993. 54:845-852.

[90] Pare WP. Investigatory behavior of a novel conspecific by Wistar Kyoto, Wistar and Sprague-Dawley rats. *Brain Res. Bull.* 2000. 53(6):759-765.

[91] Pare WP, Tejani-Butt S. Effect of stress on the behavior and 5-HT system in Sprague-Dawley and Wistar Kyoto rat strains. *Integr. Physiol. Behav. Sci.* 1996. 31:112-121.

[92] Popova NA, Ilnitskaya SI, Kolesnikova LA, Kaledin VI, Kudryavtseva NN. The influence of social conflicts on some parameters of non-specific immune resistance in mice. Ross. Fiziol. Zhurn. 1996. 82(12):14-19.

[93] Porsolt RD, Le Pichon M, Jalfre M. Depression: A new animal model sensitive to antidepressant treatment. Nature. 1977. 266:730-732.

[94] Ramos A, Mormede P. Stress and Emotionality: a multidimensional and genetic approach. *Neurosci. Biobehav. Rev.* 1998. 22(1):33-57.

[95] Reddy PL, Khanna S, Subhash MN. Channabasavanna SM, Rao BS. CSF amine metabolites in depression. *Biol. Psychiat.* 1992. 31:112-118.

[96] Reinchard JF, Galloway PP, Roth RH. Noradrenergic modulation of serotonin synthesis and metabolism. Stimulation by 3-isobutil-11-methylxanthine. *J. Pharmacol. Exp. Ther.* 1983. 226(3):764-769.

[97] Ressler KJ, Nemeroff CB. Role of serotonergic and noradrenergic systems in the pathophysiology of depression and anxiety disorders. *Depress. Anxiety.* 2000. 12:2-19.

[98] Rosenthal D. Genetics of Psychopathology. New York: McGraw-Hill. 1971.

[99] Roy A, Pickar D, Linnoila M, Doran AR, Ninan P, Paul SM. Cerebrospinal fluid monoamine and monoamine metabolite concentrations in melancholia. *Psychiat. Res.* 1985. 15:281-292.

[100] Sarkisova KYu, Kulikov MA. A new experimental model of depression: WAG/Rij rats genetically predisposed to absence epilepsy. *Dokl. Biol. Sci.* 2000. 374(1-6):462-465.

[101] Sham P. Genetic epidemiology. *Brit. Med. Bull.* 1996. 52(3):408-433.

[102] Stanley M, Mann JJ. Increased serotonin-2 binding sites in frontal cortex of suicide victims. Lancet. 1983. 1(8318):214-216.

[103] Tejani-Butt SM, Pare WP, Yang J. Effect of repeated novel stressors on depressive behavior and brain norepinephrine receptor system in Sprague-Dawley and Wistar-Kyoto (WKY) rats. Brit. Res. 1994. 649:27-35.

[104] Trullas R, Skolnik P. Differences in fear motivated behaviors among inbred mouse strains. *Psychopharmacol.* 1993. 111:323-331.

[105] Van Praag HM. Studies in the mechanism of action of serotonin precursor in depression. *Psychopharmacol. Bull.* 1984. 20:599-602.

[106] Van Praag HM, Flentge F, Korf J, Dols LC, Schut T. The influence of probenecid on the metabolism of serotonin, dopamine and their precursors in man. *Psychopharmacol.* 1973a. 33:141-151.

[107] Van Praag HM, Korf J, Schut T. Cerebral monoamines and depression. An investigation with the probenecid technique. *Arch. Gen. Psychiat.* 1973b. 28:827-831.

[108] Van Praag HM., Korf J, Puite J. 5-Hydroxyindoleacetic acid levels in the cerebrospinal fluid of depressive patients treated with probenecid. Nature. 1970. 225(239):1259-1260.

[109] Weissman MM, Myers JK. Clinical depression in alcoholism. *Amer. J. Psychiat.* 1980. 137:372-373.

[110] Willner P, Mitchell PL. The validity of animal models of predisposition to depression. *Behav. Pharmacol.* 2002. 13:169-188.

[111] Yadid G, Nakash R, Deri I., Tamar G, Kinor N, Gispan I, Zangen A. Elucidation of the neurobiology of depression: insights from a novel genetic animal model. *Prog. Neurobiol.* 2000. 62:353-378.

[112] Zerbin-Rudin E. Psychiatric genetics and psychiatric nosology. J. Psychiat. Res. 1987. 21(4):377-383.

[113] Zhukov DA, Vinogradova KP. Learned Helplessness or Learned Inactivity after Inescapable Stress? Interpretation Depends on Coping Styles. Integr. *Physiol. Behav. Sci.* 2002. 37(1):35-43.

In: Animal Models in Biological Psychiatry
Editor: Allan V. Kalueff, pp. 97-117
ISBN 1-59454-814-5

Chapter 6

Neurosteroid Vitamin D and Anxiety: Insights from Mutant Mice

Allan V. Kalueff and Pentti Tuohimaa
Medical School, University of Tampere, Tampere University Hospital, Tampere, Finland

I. Introduction

Vitamin D hormone is essential for growth and differentiation in a variety of organs, including the brain (Garcion et al., 2002; Carswell, 1997; Yoshizawa et al., 1997). Numerous data suggest that vitamin D plays an important role in the brain through induction of many CNS genes, modulation of neuroprotection, neurotrophins release and activity of key neurotransmitter metabolism enzymes (Garcion et al., 2002; Carswell, 1997; Altemus et al., 1987). The functions of vitamin D are mediated through nuclear vitamin D receptors (VDR, a member of the nuclear receptors superfamily of ligand-activated transcription factors), which are widely distributed through the nervous system (Garcion et al., 2002; Yoshizawa et al., 1997). VDR is a 50-60 kDa protein, consisting of several functional domains responsible for ligand and DNA binding, heterodimerization, nuclear localization and transcriptional activation (see Table 1 for details).

Evidence for the presence of vitamin D, the enzymes of its bioactivation and metabolism and functional VDR in the brain implies that this vitamin may have some function in the CNS as an autocrine or paracrine neurosteroid hormone (Garcion et al., 2002). VDR are found in key brain areas including the cortex, cerebellum and limbic system, all known to regulate behaviour (Prufer et al., 1999; Walbert et al., 2001; Langub et al., 2001). In humans, vitamin D deficiency has long been known to be accompanied by irritability, depression, psychoses and defects in mental development (Carswell, 1997). The psychotropic mood-elevating effects of vitamin D have also been well-documented in the literature (Gloth et al., 2001).

In animals, vitamin D deficiency produces behavioural alterations including decreased exploration and maze performance (Altemus et al., 1987; also see recent interesting behavioural data in: Burne et al. 2004). Collectively, this suggests that vitamin D could be an important factor controlling behaviour in animals and humans. As such, various vitamin D and VDR-related disorders may therefore be a risk factor for abnormal emotional behaviour in both animals and humans. In the present chapter, we will discuss data suggesting that genetic ablation of VDR in mice may strongly affect their behaviours, especially anxiety.

Table 1. Domain structure of the vitamin D nuclear receptor (VDR)

Domains	Structure	Functions
A/B (≈21 aa)	Hyper-variable amino-terminal domain unusually short compared to many other nuclear receptors	Lacks transactivation potential, but possibly determines the overall transactivation capacity of VDR
C (≈66 aa)	DNA-binding domain (similar to that of other nuclear receptors) with two zinc fingers interacting with specific DNA sequences on the target gene	DNA binding, also participates in nuclear localization and dimerization with the retinoic acid X receptor (RXR)
E, or E/F (≈310 aa)	Ligand-binding domain (similar to other nuclear receptors, especially RXR); organized in 13 α-helices and 3 β-sheets forming a hydrophobic pocket. Also includes the ligand-dependent activation function-2 (AF-2, ≈18 aa, a short amplipatic C-terminal α-helix)	A multifunctional globular domain mediating selective interactions of VDR with the hormone, other nuclear receptor partners (e.g., RXR) and co-modulatory proteins (CP)*. AF-2 is crucial for ligand-activated transcription
D (≈30 aa)	Highly flexible "hinge" region	Confers rotation flexibility between C and E domains to allow simultaneous VDR dimerization and DNA-binding

aa – Amino acids. * CP include SRC family, DRIP multiprotein complex, and several other proteins interacting with and modulating the VDR transactivation/transrepression (see: Ahonen, 2002; Sutton and MacDonald, 2003; Ylikomi et al., 2002 for details).

II. Increased Anxiety in VDR Null Mutant Mice: A Battery of Tests

Methods

In our pioneering studies (Kalueff et al., 2004a,b) we assessed the behavioural performance of VDR null mutant mice tested in several behavioural tests of anxiety and activity. Subjects were adult mice (aged 24-52 weeks) bred in the University of Tampere (Finland). VDR gene mutant mice were bred in Tampere from the line initially generated in the University of Tokyo (Japan). 129 mouse substrain was used as a genetic background for these mutant mice. Ten null mutants were compared to ten control wild type (+/+) 129 mice and eight heterozygous (+/-) mice. The mice were maintained in groups of two to three animals per cage in a virus/parasite-free facility (temperature 24$\pm$1°C, humidity 50$\pm$5%) and exposed to a 12-h light, 12-h dark cycle (lights on 7.00 h) with food and water ad libitum (except food finding experiments, when in order to increase hunger, animals were food deprived for 10 h prior to testing). All testing was conducted between 17.00 and 19.00 h. To normalize the blood mineral ion levels, VDR-ablated animals were fed a diet containing 2% calcium, 1.25% phosphorum, and 20% lactose supplemented with 2.2 IU vitamin D/g (Lactamin AB, Sweden).

On test days, animals were transported to the dimly lit laboratory and left undisturbed for 2 h prior to testing. General locomotor activity was measured for 5 min in a plastic actometer box (30 x 30 x 30 cm) with a floor divided into 4 squares (15 x 15 cm). Conventional measures were horizontal activity (the number of squares visited) and vertical activity (the number of times an animal stood erect on its hind-legs with forelegs in the air of against the wall). This experiment was the first exposure of the mice to the behavioural testing. 10 days later, the visual sensory abilities and motor coordination of the mice were analysed in a novel object-finding test. The animals were placed in a plastic box (50 cm x 50 cm x 50 cm; with a floor divided into nine squares of 15 cm x 15 cm) and after a 5-min acclimation time, the novel object (5-cm metal sphere) was introduced in the diagonally opposite corner of the box. The latency (s) of finding the sphere was used as a measure of the animals' visual abilities; the number of contacts (the number of times an animal stood on its hind-legs with forelegs placed on the sphere) was used as a measure of animal motor coordination/manipulatory activity. 10 days later, the animals' ability to keep their balance was assessed in the horizontal bar test. The horizontal bar (wooden bar 1 cm thick) was fixed to a platform that was elevated 30 cm from the floor. The mice were tested for 3 min and the time (s) the animals could keep their balance was measured.

10 days later, animal behaviour was assessed in a battery of anxiety tests including the open field, the holeboard, the elevated plus maze and the light-dark paradigms. Each test was performed following a 10-day recovery time. Behaviours were recorded for 5 min. in each test by an experienced observer. The open field and holeboard tests were a plastic box (45 x 45 x 45 cm) with a floor divided into 9 squares (15 x 15 cm each). The holeboard removable floor had 64 holes (1 cm in diameter). Conventional measures in these tests were horizontal activity, vertical activity, total time spent grooming (s), and the number of holes inspected.

The elevated plus maze was made from Plexiglas and consisted of two open arms (30x10 cm) and two enclosed arms (30x10x10 cm) extending from a common central region (10x10 cm) elevated to a height of 60 cm. Conventional measures were the initial latency (s) to leave the centre, the frequencies of open- and closed-arm entries (4-paw criterion), as well as vertical activity. The final test was the light-dark transition paradigm. The test was a Plexiglas box consisting of two exploratory units (transparent and black, 30 x 30 x 30 cm each), interconnected by a sliding door. Conventional measures were the initial latency (s) to move from the dark to the light compartment, the number of the light entries (4-paw criterion), total time spent in the light compartment (s), and vertical activity. Between subjects, each apparatus was thoroughly cleaned (wet and dry cloths).

Animal care and experimental procedures were conducted in accordance with the European legislation and the guidelines of the National Institute of Health. All animal experiments were approved by the Ethical Committee of the University of Tampere.

Statistics

All results are expressed as mean ± S.E.M. Behavioural data were analysed by the Kruskal-Wallis test followed by post-hoc Mann-Whitney U-test. In all tests, a probability of less than 0.05 was considered statistically significant.

Results

Since genetically modified animals often demonstrate motor and sensory abnormalities which may non-specifically affect behaviour (Crawley, 1999), we first tested the general locomotion and sensory abilities of VDR null mutant mice (Kalueff et al., 2004a). Assessment of locomotor activity in the actometer test revealed that VDR null mutant, heterozygous and the wild type mice had similar baseline levels of horizontal and vertical activity (horizontal activity: 37±4, 42±4 and 40±5, respectively; vertical activity: 30±3, 32±3 and 35±5, respectively). All three groups had unaltered major sensory (visual/olfactory) abilities as assessed on the food- and novel object-finding tests (the latency to find food: 14±3s, 16±3s and 17±3s, respectively; the latency to find novel object: 20±4s, 16±3s and 17±3s, respectively) and motor coordination (contacts with novel sphere, Kalueff et al., 2004b). In addition, all three groups had unaltered vestibular system as assessed on the horizontal bar test (bar retention time: 125+17s, 104±15s, and 120±21s, respectively).

However, as can be seen in Fig. 1, marked behavioural alterations in VDR null mutants were found when the mice were subjected to a battery of anxiety tests. In the holeboard test, VDR null mutants demonstrated decreased horizontal and vertical activity (43±5; $P<0.05$, U-test and 3±2; $P<0.05$, U-test), compared to the wild type (60±7 and 10±2, respectively) and heterozygous mice (62±8 and 9±2, respectively).

In the open field, compared to the wild type and heterozygous control groups, VDR null mutants demonstrated decreased horizontal (37±4 vs. 63±8 and 58±9, respectively; $P<0.05$, U-test) and vertical exploration (3±1 vs. 9±1 and 8±2, respectively; $P<0.05$, U-test) as well as increased duration of grooming (12±2s vs. 5±1s and 5±1s, respectively; $P<0.05$, U-test). In the elevated plus maze, compared to the wild type and heterozygous groups, VDR null mutant mice demonstrated a dramatic decrease in vertical activity (0.7±0.4 vs. 3±1 and 4±1, respectively; $P<0.01$, U-test) as well as longer latency to leave the central area (11±1s vs. 6±1s and 5±1s, respectively; $P<0.01$, U-test).

As can be seen in Fig. 1, in the light-dark transition test, VDR null mutant mice showed less exploration of the light compartment than did their littermates from both control groups (the time spent in the light compartment: 30±7s vs. 48±11s and 46±13s, respectively (a tendency); vertical activity in the light compartment: 1±0.6s vs. 5±1s and 4±1s, respectively; P<0.05, U-test), also showing fewer entries to the light compartment (Fig. 1).

Calcium Levels

Since vitamin D plays an important role in the regulation of Ca^{++} homeostasis, a key factor likely to affect motor performance in mutant mice can be dysregulation of Ca^{++} homeostasis, which is usually associated with vitamin D-related disorders (Carswell, 1997; Langub et al., 2001). To test this hypothesis, in a separate experiment we measured plasma Ca^{++} level in these mutant mice. Indeed, despite a special rich Ca^{++} diet, they mice had generally lower plasma Ca^{2+} (2.04 ± 0.08 mmol/l, $P < 0.05$; $n = 6$), compared to 2.28 ± 0.10 mmol/l in the wild-type ($n = 3$) and 2.27 ± 0.48 mmol/l in heterozygous ($n = 7$) mice (Kalueff et al., 2004b).

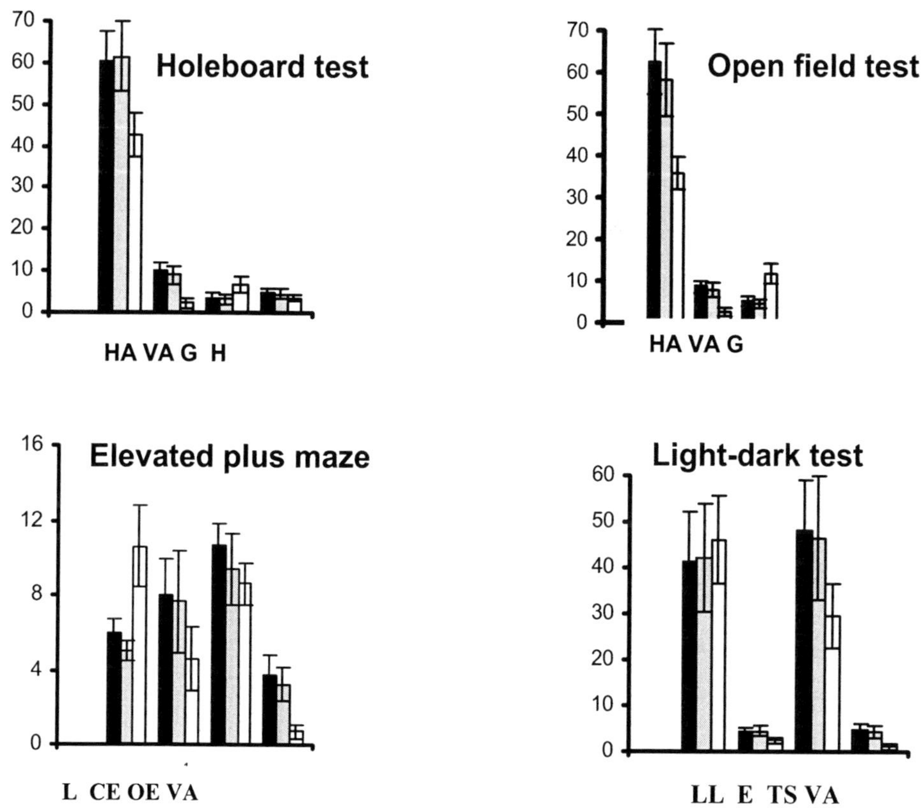

Fig. 1. Behaviours of VDR null mutant mice (-/-, white bars) compared to wild type (+/+; black bars) and heterozygous (+/-; grey bars) mice subjected to a battery of anxiety tests (adapted from Kalueff et al., 2004a) HA – horizontal activity, VA - vertical activity, G - grooming duration (s), H - holes inspected, L - latency to leave the centre (s), CE - closed entries, OE - open entries, LL - latency to enter the light area, E – entries to the light area, TS - time spent (s) in the light area (adapted from Kalueff et al., 2004a).

III. Anxiogenic Profile in the Protected Elevated Plus Maze

Methods

In a separate experiment, to further assess anxiety in VDR mutants, we subjected these mice to the protected elevated plus maze test. This modification of the regular elevated plus maze was made from plywood and consisted of two open arms with small side-walls (20 x 10 x 0.5 cm) and two enclosed arms (20 x 10 x 30 cm) extending from a common central region (10 x 10 cm) elevated to a height of 50 cm. The opposite walls of both enclosed arms were interconnected in the central region, forming two "doors" (7 x 7 cm each) leading to the open arms. Since this modification of the maze used smaller arms, lower height, opaque walls, interconnected walls of the closed arms, and special protective 0.5-cm walls in the open arms, this model generally utilizes less anxiogenic stimuli (compared to the transparent apparatus used in the previous experiments), and therefore was considered to be less stressful.

Since our previous experiments have shown 1) similar behavioural profiles of heterozygous and wild type animals in the behavioural tests including elevated plus maze (Fig. 1), 2) robust behavioural differences of both these groups from the VDR mutant mice, and 3) no sex differences between VDR mutant male and females (own unpublished observation), in this experiments we compared 10 VDR null mutant mice (6 males, 4 females) to 10 control mice (4 heterozygous and 1 wild type male, 3 heterozygous and 2 wild type female mice) tested in the protected elevated plus maze. The following behaviours were recorded for 5 min: head dipping from the open arms; the number of open, closed and total arm entries, vertical rears, vegetative behaviours (urination episodes + defecation boli), the number of grooming bouts and time spent grooming (s).

Results

In the protected elevated plus maze, the VDR null mutant mice demonstrated significantly lower exploration as assessed by head dipping behaviour, open entries and vertical activity (Fig. 2) compared to their controls. Overall, these behavioural responses are consistent with higher anxiety profile in the VDR null mutant animals. In addition, as can be seen in Fig. 2, these mutant mice showed fewer closed entries and total entries, unaltered defecation/urination scores and grooming bouts, and a tendency to more grooming duration ($P > 0.05$, U-test). Importantly, the ratio open:closed and open:total entries, although similar in both groups (1.02, controls; 0.84, VDR mutants; and 0.50, controls; 0.46, VDR mutants, respectively), showed a slight tendency to lower values (i.e., higher anxiety) in the mutant group.

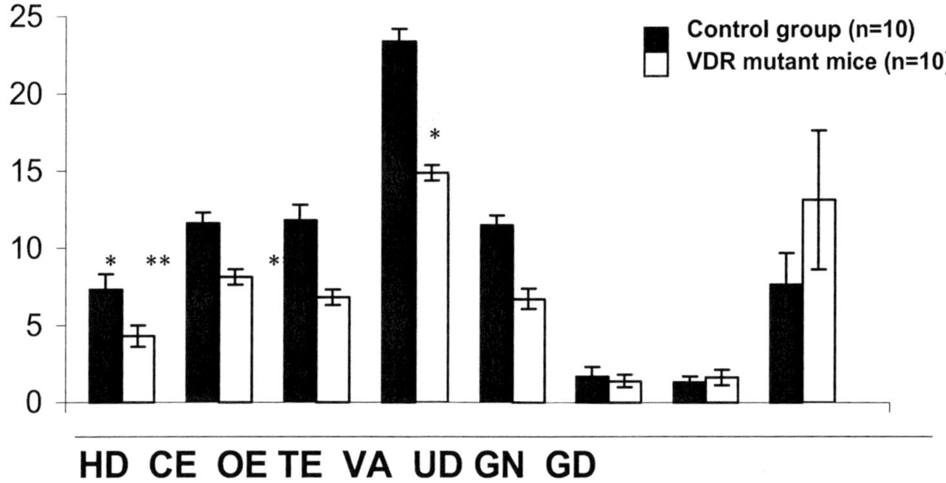

HD – head dips, CE – closed entries, OE – open entries, TE – total entries (CE + OE), VA – vertical activity (rears), UD – vegetative behaviours (urination spots/defecation boli), GN – grooming number (bouts), GD – grooming duration (s).

Fig. 2. Behavioural responses of VDR null mutant mice in the protected elevated plus maze compared to their wild type and heterozygous controls. * $P < 0.05$; ** $P < 005$ (U-test)

IV. Methodological Considerations

Can the elevated plus maze data be a key finding in behavioural phenotyping of VDR mutant mice? Our earlier studies using the regular version of this test (Fig. 1) failed to detect any behavioural response except a marked reduction in vertical exploration. The present experiment, using 'protected' version of the maze, partially reconfirms these findings showing a consistent reduction of vertical exploration in our mutant mice. In line with this, recent studies of another group (Burne et al., 2005) also showed reduced vertical activity of VDR null mutant mice in the regular (opaque acrylic plus maze with small 1-cm walls in the open arms), see Table 2 for details. Collectively, these data imply that reduced vertical exploration is the most robust behavioural response to stress in VDR null mutant mice, as has already been noted (Kalueff et al., 2004a).

Does the animal horizontal exploration change in the elevated plus maze novelty test? Our earlier experiments (Fig. 1, Kalueff et al., 2004a) failed to detect any difference between the mutant mice and both control groups in the regular transparent plexiglas plus maze with open arms without small side walls. Similar results were obtained by another group testing VDR mutant mice and their wild type controls in a slightly different plus maze apparatus (Burne et al., 2005). Inconsistent with traditional anxiety phenotype, these observations allowed this group to suggest that since the elevated plus maze is the most sensitive behavioural model of anxiety, the lack of open arms aversion in VRD mutants negates their anxiogenic profile.

However, the important question arises as for whether the elevated plus maze test can be feasible to assess anxiety in these mice. Several important factors have to be considered here in detail. First, although rich Ca^{++} diets used in both studies (Kalueff et al., 2004a, Burne et al., 2005) eliminate all major aberrant physiological features of these mice, this does not affect alopecia – a common diet-resistant phenotypic feature of all mice lacking VDR (Li et al., 1997; Yoshizawa et al., 1997). Thus, VDR null mutant mice have no or little body hair and have no whiskers by the age of 2.5-3 months, whereas both heterozygous and wild type groups have normal whiskers even at the age of 1-1.5 years (own systematic observations, 2003-2005).

Notably, tactile information obtained from whiskers is an important sensory input guiding novelty exploration behaviour in rodents (Staiger et al., 2000; Moore, 2004; Cardenas et al., 2001; Prchal et al., 2004). Since the whisker status of mice has been reported to affect their performance in the elevated plus maze, leading to unusually low aversion of the open arms (due to sensory impairment and inability to detect potential danger in the open arms; see Crawley, 1999 for details), the lack of whiskers in VDR mutant animals may be the main reason for their unusual responses in the elevated plus maze. Thus, the elevated plus maze may represent a particularly inappropriate model to study anxiety in VDR mutant mice. Therefore, it may be strongly recommended not to rely on one (even highly sensitive) behavioural model when analyzing behavioural phenotypes of mutant mice (Crawley, 1999; Kalueff and Tuohimaa, 2004a; also see previous neuroethological chapter in this book). Quite the opposite, only a detailed in-depth ethological analysis of their behaviours, using a wide range of different tests and behavioural indices, may represent the rational strategy in establishing behaviours of these mutant mice. Indeed, using a smaller and less aversive modification of the elevated plus maze, we were able to show anxiety-like response in these animals, manifest in consistent reduction of all forms of exploration (Fig. 2).

Another factor which theoretically may easily confound the plus maze data in our and other studies is the genetic background of these mice. Genetic background is known to affect anxiety-related behaviours in mutant mice, and has to be considered in all experiments (Gerlai, 1996). In our study, we used isogenic mutant mice and 129S1 mouse strain as the genetic background. In contrast, Burne et al. (2005) used mixed genetic background (129Sv x C57BL/6J) in their experiments. Since both groups employed a substantial portion of 129 genetic background, it is possible to assume that this common background factor may affect the behavioural profiles of mice tested in the elevated plus maze. Indeed, the fact that 129xC57 mice in many respects ethologically resemble their parental 129 strain, and differ from C57 mice (e.g., Voikar et al., 2001), further confirms this notion.

Notably, animals of the 129 mouse strain have long been known to perform "funny" in the elevated plus maze. For example, these highly anxious mice frequently display a robust "initial" anxiety when placed in the central part of the test, and spend more time in the center. In addition, 129 mice are known to show unusual center > open > closed arm preference in the plus maze. In line with this, (Burne et al., 2005) showed that wild type and mutant mice spent 53 and 59% test time in the center, respectively (also see similar phenomenon in the Y-maze in the same study). This observation clearly indicates robust "background" effect of their findings which, in our opinion, may "mask" all potential mutation-evoked behavioural alterations in these mice, and therefore shall not be interpreted as the lack of anxiety. The use of the protected elevated plus maze (where the visible central area is lacking due to the presence of walls interconnecting the opposite closed arms, thus representing a part of the closed arms area) allowed us to minimize the impact of the central area on mouse behaviours (Fig. 2) and obtain less confounded plus maze data. Indeed, as can be seen in Fig. 2, the robust reduction of arm exploration and head dips clearly supports the notion that VDR null mutant mice display high anxiety. Furthermore, while the control mice showed almost equal number of open and closed entries (most likely reflecting strong "background" effect), the VDR null mutants displayed a tendency to fewer open entries, lower open/closed and open/total entries, also consistent with their high anxiety phenotype reported previously (Kalueff et al., 2004a).

Another behavioural feature of all 129 mice is the robust tendency to avoid enclosed arms of the maze – the phenomenon which can be mistakenly interpreted as "anxiolysis". Taken together, this again indicates that the elevated plus maze may not be a valid model to study behaviours of VDR mutant mice, especially possessing portions of the 129 strain genome.

Similar conclusion may apply to the holeboard test – another highly sensitive behavioural paradigm widely used in behavioural neurogenetics (Crawley, 1999; Kalueff and Tuohimaa, 2004a). Both groups studying VDR mutant mice (Fig. 1, Burne et al., 2005) failed to detect any alteration in the specific anxiety-sensitive exploratory activity - nose poking. Inconsistent with traditional anxiety phenotype, this observation allowed Burne et al. (2005) to question the idea of high anxiety phenotype of these mice reported in our experiments. Again, this interpretation does not consider the important role of whiskers in nose-poking behaviours in rodents, and the fact that VDR mutant mice (but not their wild type counterparts) have no whiskers. Clearly, animals without whiskers will differ in the holeboard test, demonstrating altered nose-poking activity. In addition, specific behavioural features of "background" 129 mice (e.g., high initial anxiety, frequent freezing and general hypoactivity of this strain; see Kalueff and Tuohimaa, 2004b for details) may also dramatically affect their hole-poking activity, thus, making this well-validated behavioural paradigm inappropriate for the study of VDR mutant mice. Taken together, this suggests that the "lack" of anxiety response of VDR mutant mice tested in the holeboard test may be due to inability of this model to detect anxiety in these animals.

Overall, the importance of assessing general physiological status, locomotor, vestibular and sensory systems is widely recognized as a key part of behavioural analysis of mutant animals (Crawley et al., 1999). VDR deficiency in knockout mice has recently been reported to yield aberrant musculoskeletal development as well as rickets-like bone malformations (Yoshizawa et al., 1997; Endo et al., 2003). Using different behavioural tests we show that, despite these abnormalities, VDR null mutant mice exhibited unaltered baseline motor activity, movements coordination and sensory abilities. This observation is in line with previously published works showing no obvious motor and neurological abnormalities in VDR-deficient mice (Li et al., 1997; Yoshizawa et al., 1997). In addition, special Ca^{++}-rich diet used in our study (known to normalize all major physiological functions and reduce or eliminate muscular abnormalities in VDR mutants) also led to sufficient normalization of Ca^{++} plasma levels in mice tested in our behavioural experiments (Kalueff et al., 2004b).

In contrast, Burne et al. (2005) found aberrant motor functions in VDR null mutant mice, including poor rotaroid performance and a shorter stride length, suggesting that these mice may have severely impaired muscular and motor finctions rather than anxiety phenotype. We shall note, however, one principally important methodological difference between the two studies. While we used special Ca^{++}/Ph-rich diet with 20% lactose (Kalueff et al., 2004b), Burne et al. (2005) used water supplemented with 2mM Ca^{++}. Since lactose markedly increases Ca^{++} absorbtion from food, we may suggest that our diet was more effective to normalize mineral homeostasis in VDR mutant mice. Indeed, while our null mutant mice showed only moderate 11% hypocalcemia (2.04 vs 2.28 mmol/l in controls), the mice used by Burne et al. (2005) displayed markedly lower plasma Ca^{++} (1.7 vs. 2.5 mmol/l in controls). In our opinion, this 0.8-mmol/l difference in Ca^{++} levels between both genotypes may be considered as severe hypocalcemia (32%), representing a serious factor non-specifically impeding all behaviours in VDR null mutant mice. Therefore, motor impairments seen by Burne et al. (2005) may indeed be due to Ca^{++}-dependent imbalance in these mice, possibly due to insufficient Ca^{++} supplementation. However, these data to not contradict our findings. Indeed, the difference in plasma Ca^{++} between genotypes observed in our experiments (0.24 mmol/l) was almost 3-fold lower than in (Burne et al., 2005). We may suggest that this mild hypocalcemia may not lead to dramatic behavioural impairment in the VDR mutant group (Kalueff et al., 2004a), therefore enabling more specific assessment of behavioural phenotypes of these mutant mice. However, both cited studies support the notion that mineral homeostasis affected by VDR genetic ablation may strongly affect animal behavioural performance.

V. Additional Data Demonstrating High Anxiety in VDR Mutant Mice

Several additional behavioural phenomena further support our hypothesis linking ablated VDR to anxiety. First, although not statistically significant, lower head dipping scores have been reported for VDR null mutant mice in the elevated plus maze by Burne et al. (2005): 10.7 ± 3.4 compared to 14.3 ± 1.2 in the wild type group. In line with this, similar (but significant) reduction of this behaviour was found in our study in the VDR mutants tested in the protected elevated plus maze (Fig. 2). Second, since the marble burying test represents a traditional exploratory-based anxiety paradigm (Londei et al., 1998), lower burying activity in the VDR mutant group (Burne et al., 2005) may also indicate higher anxiety in these mice compared to their wild type counterparts. Third, a detailed ethological analysis of the mouse light-dark performance also supports their high anxiety phenotype. This test represents a traditional well-validated behavioural model of anxiety (Crawley, 1999; Kalueff and Tuohimaa, 2004a). As already mentioned, in our first study the VDR mutant mice showed significantly less exploration of the light compartment (entries, vertical rears, tendency to spend less time) than did their control littermates (Kalueff et al., 2004a).

Since the light-dark test provides a large number of ethologically-derived anxiety-sensitive behaviours (Kalueff and Tuohimaa, 2004a), and is generally less confounded by locomotor factors (than, for example, the open field or holeboard tests more reliant on horizontal activity scores), in a separate experiment we wanted to assess the mouse performance in this test in detail. For this, we used 10 VDR mutant and 10 control mice previously tested in the protected plus maze. Seven days later, the following behavioural parameters were assessed for 5 min in the light-dark apparatus used previously:

1. total number of light-dark transitions (dark-light and light-dark transitions, 4-paw criterion);
2. the number of dark-light entries ("unprotected" exploration, 4-paw criterion);
3. the number of dark-light exploratory looks ("abortive", protected exploration, attempted entries not meeting the 4-paw criterion);
4. total number of the light-directed exploration episodes (entries + looks);
5. the number of zones visited in the light compartment (zone 1: 0-15 cm, zone 2: 15-30 cm from the dark compartment; 4-paw criterion).

Overall, the VDR mutant group produced a tendency to fewer light-dark transitions (5.2 $\pm$ 1.1) and zones visited in the light compartment (3.8 $\pm$ 1.0) compared to the control group (8.5 $\pm$ 2.3 and 9.3 $\pm$ 2.7, respectively). This robust trend, however, was not statistically significant due to high variability of these behaviours. Interestingly, both groups produced similar number of exploratory episodes (VDR mutants: 9.0 $\pm$ 0.8, controls: 8.5 $\pm$ 1.3). However, while the control group displayed almost equal number of looks (4.2 $\pm$ 1.4, ≈51%) and entries (4.3 $\pm$ 1.2, ≈49%), the VDR mutant group showed slightly fewer "unprotected" entries (3.1 $\pm$ 0.6, ≈35%) but more "protected" looks (5.9 $\pm$ 1.0, ≈65%). Collectively, these data suggest that genetic ablation of VDR leads to lower exploratory motivation in these mutant mice, supporting their general anxiogenic profile (Kalueff et al., 2004a).

In a separate experiment using these two groups of mice, we tested them in the novel object finding test as described in (Kalueff et al., 2004b). Although both groups produced similar latency of finding the novel object (a 5-cm metal sphere), and the number of contacts with this object (sphere-leaning with forepaws), we also noted that he mutant group showed a dramatic reduction in the number of sniffing episodes (nose < 2 cm from the sphere) and time spent sniffing (4.8 $\pm$ 0.7 and 13.0 $\pm$ 2.1 s) compared to their controls (8.1 $\pm$ 0.8; $P < 0.01$, U-test; and 20.8 $\pm$ 2.8 s, $P < 0.05$, U-test; respectively). Since the latency of finding food was unaltered in the VDR null mutant mice (see above), suggesting their unimpaired olfactory functions, the latter observation may be interpreted as a robust neophobic response in these mice, generally consistent with higher anxiety phenotype.

Finally, assessing the VDR mutant mouse horizontal activity in different novelty arena tests, we noted that these mice differ markedly from their control counterparts (wild type or heterozygous mice) in their spatial strategies. Several behavioural observations have been made (own unpublished data, 2003-2005). First, we noted that the VDR mutant mice generally display longer latencies to leave the initial placement area (in the center of the novel arenas). For example, these mutant mice showed a tendency to a longer latency to leave the center in the holeboard (28 $\pm$ 6 vs. 24 $\pm$ 6) as well as significantly longer latency in the open field (37 $\pm$ 4 vs. 16 $\pm$ 3) tests, compared to the animals from the control group. Similar phenomenon was observed in the elevated plus maze (Kalueff et al., 2004a) where the mutant mice demonstrated almost twice longer latency to leave the central zone (Fig. 1) compared to both control groups.

Behavioural analyses of kinematics of leaving the initial placement area also show marked differences between the genotypes. While the control (wild type or heterozygous

129S1) mice moved to explore unfamiliar open field of holeboard arenas after a freezing episode, and generally did not demonstrate frequent withdrawals (moving backwards) once they "decided" to move, the VDR mutant mice showed frequent moving out (2 paws) followed by immediate withdrawals, also constantly changing the vector (direction) of their movements. Indeed, these mutant mice generally perform 3-9 such withdrawals (interpreted as fear-evoked behaviours) before finally leaving the center (Fig. 3). In addition, as can be seen in Fig. 3, during these novelty tests, VDR null mutants (but not their control counterparts) produced frequent stops accompanied by moving forward and backward and vector changes (possibly, due to general emotional excitation and higher levels of fear of novelty). Overall, we concluded that these behavioural observations are consistent with high anxiety phenotype reported for mice lacking VDR.

VI. Habituation in VDR Null Mutant Mice

In their recent comprehensive study, Burne et al. (2005) described the phenomenon of markedly impaired within-session habituation in VDR null mutant mice subjected to the open field novelty test. In contrast, the wild type controls demonstrated gradual reduction of their horizontal activity measures (distance traveled) over a 5-min test interval. Interestingly, these mutant mice also showed reduced habituation in the accoustic startle chambers, suggesting that VDR may be involved in the regulation of habituation (Burne et al., 2005).

Analyzing these interesting behavioural observations, we speculated that impaired open field habituation in VDR mutant mice are related to their altered exploratory strategies, and may be explained by underlying anxiety phenotype. Given our recent data showing altered spatial strategies of these mice (Fig. 3), this possibility seems indeed likely. For example, while unimpaired within-trial habituation implies relatively normal exploration strategies (commonly seen in various rodent species in the open field tests), poor habituation in this test (especially accompanied by lover exploratory activity, e.g., Burne et al., 2005), in our opinion, may reflect abnormal "anxious" novelty-coping strategy. Can this be the case for our VDR mutant mice? Indeed, it is possible to assume that VDR mutants do not reduce their exploration during the test because they are already highly anxious and do not want to fully explore the potentially dangerous environment. In contrast, they may prefer to use a highly conservative "cautious" strategy maintaining their exploration at a "safe" constantly low levels during the test.

In order to investigate this problem in detail, in a separate experiment we replicated the original Burne et al. (2005) habituation experiments, ethologically dissecting a wide spectrum of exploratory and non-exploratory open field behaviours in 10 VDR null mutant mice. We also chose to use a longer, 10-min observation time, allowing us to more fully assess the mouse habituation responses. The following behavioural measures (per min) were recorded for 10 min:

1. horizontal exploration (squares visited with 4 paws);
2. total vertical exploration (including "protected" and "unprotected" vertical rears);
3. "protected" vertical rears (wall-leanings with forepaws touching the walls);

4. "unprotected" vertical rears (with forepaws in the air);
5. stopping activity (the number of exploratory stops > 2 s);
6. grooming activity frequency (the number of grooming episodes); and
7. grooming duration (s).

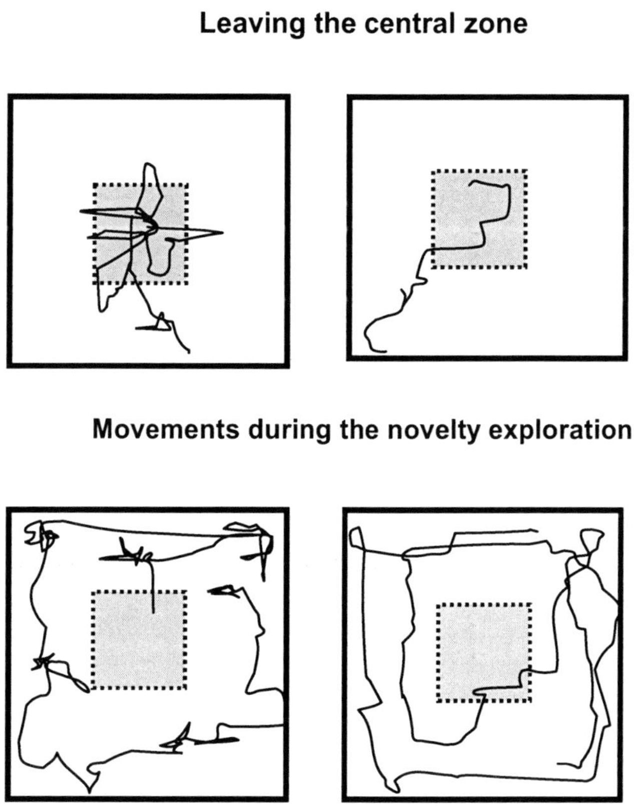

Fig. 3. Different spatial strategies used by the VDR mutant (left) and control mice (right) in the unfamiliar novel arena (adapted from Kalueff, 2005)

Overall, our experiments using a 10-min open field test confirm impaired habituation in the VDR null mutant mice previously described for horizontal activity in a shorter 5-min version of the test (Burne et al., 2005). As can be seen in Fig. 4, during the first 5 min and during the whole 10-min test, these mice maintained constant exploratory activity (13-15 squares/min, ≈9-12% of total activity scored). In addition, a strikingly constant (7-8 stops/min) level of stopping activity was observed in this group during the test (data not shown). Since stops represent an important exploratory behaviour in rodents, including mice (Golani et al., 1993; Drai et al., 2001) subjected to novel open arenas, the lack of their habituation in the VDR mutant mice may again support the idea of their abnormal exploratory strategy in the open field and other similar anxiety tests.

In contrast, total vertical activity of these mutant animals was very low at the beginning of the test (2-4 squares/min, ≈3-5%) but gradually increased with time reaching 9-14% (min

3-10). Similar effects were observed for other vertical activity measures (wall leanings, "unprotected" rears, Fig. 4). This suggests that the initial anxiety immediately after novelty exposure was very high (dramatically reducing vertical exploration of the VDR mutant group) but gradually decreased as the animals become more familiar with the environment.

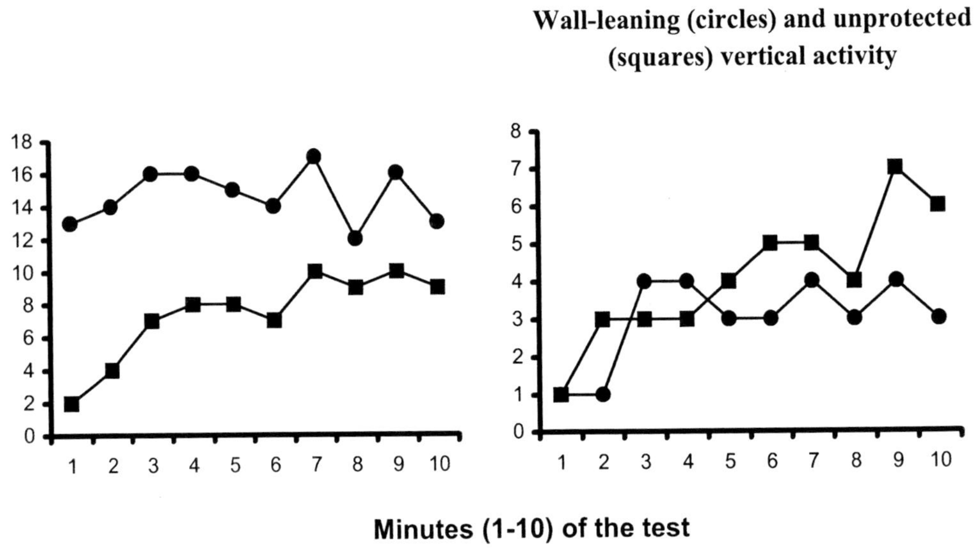

Fig. 4. Habituation in VDR null mutant mice tested in the open field test

On one hand, this observation further confirms our hypothesis that robust drop of vertical activity is the most specific pattern of emotional reactivity in the VDR mutant mice (Kalueff et al., 2004a). On the other hand, this clearly demonstrates that VDR mutant mice become more motivated to explore (and therefore less anxious) as they become more familiar with the environment. Interestingly, this phenomenon was most robust for "unprotected" vertical rears reflecting a typical exploratory activity particularly sensitive to anxiety. Indeed, this behaviour reached maximal levels (≈15-17%) by the end of the test (min 9-10), Fig. 4. Finally, grooming activity measures (frequency and duration) varied widely during the test, failing to reveal any behavioural tendency (data not shown). This observation is in line with our hypothesis (see further chapter in this book) that grooming in the VDR null mutant mice may represent a separate behavioural domain unlikely to reflect their anxiety (Kalueff et al., 2004c).

Taken together, these observations suggest that that within-trial habituation is impaired in the VDR null mutant mice, as assessed by their horizontal and stopping activity in the open field test. In contrast, vertical activity consistently increased with time, consistent with a gradual reduction of the initially high anxiety baseline. Collectively, these findings further support our earlier notion that VDR null mutant mice generally display high anxiety in various novelty-based anxiety tests (Kalueff et al., 2004a).

VII. General Discussion

In general, our study revealed that VDR mutant mice displayed consistent anxiety-like decreased exploration when subjected to anxiety tests (Fig. 1, 2). Notably, VDR null mutants react to stress by a robust decrease of vertical activity. Overall, these results indicate that VDR null mutant mice display a higher anxiety level compared to the wild type and heterozygous groups. Importantly, these findings are consistent with data from the literature showing that in rodents stress and anxiety are associated with decreased exploratory behaviours (Crawley, 1999; Prut and Belzung, 2003). Furthermore, since alterations in vertical activity reflect emotional components of rodent behaviour (Prut and Belzung, 2003; Thiel et al., 1999), our results are in line with earlier studies (Althemus et al., 1987) linking vitamin D deficiency to inhibition of open field vertical activity in rats.

Interestingly, the behavioural responses of heterozygous (+/-) mice were very similar to the wild type mice (Fig. 1). These behavioural observations are consistent with earlier data showing that heterozygous mice, possessing 50% of mutated VDR genes, show similar VDR gene mRNA expression, have no overt abnormalities and phenotypically are indistinguishable from the wild type animals (Yoshizawa et al., 1997; Li et al., 1997). This is also in line with our recent findings showing no behavioural differences between these two genotypes in self-grooming activity and some other behaviours (Kalueff et al., 2005). Together, our findings demonstrate that genetic ablation of VDR in mice is associated with increased anxiety-like behaviours, and that this effect can only be seen in VDR null mutant animals.

How can loss of VDR lead to increased anxiety? Vitamin D has been implicated in a number of physiological processes in the brain, including the modulation of brain neurotransmitters such as acetylcholine and catecholamines (review, Garcion et al., 2002; Carswell, 1997), mediators that have long been known to be involved in the regulation of emotional behaviours. The widespread VDR distribution in the brain suggests its functional properties in the CNS (Prufer et al., 1999; Walbert et al., 2001; Langub et al., 2001). Importantly, the highest brain VDR concentration has been found in the limbic system, the key emotiogenic brain structure, and its extensions in the brain (Walbert et al., 2001; Langub et al., 2001).

Given our findings in mutant mice, we can suggest that genetic ablation of VDR in the brain, especially in the emotiogenic limbic structures, may disrupt vitamin D-VDR signaling pathways which, associated with disturbed modulation of neurotransmitters in these regions, may cause the increased anxiety level seen in our experiments.

Our results directly link VDR deficiency to increased anxiety symptoms and indicate that the vitamin D-VDR system significantly affects emotional behaviour. Defects of this system may directly lead to emotional disorders, as has already been speculated (Garcion et al., 2002; Carswell, 1997; Gloth et al., 2001). Our studies allow us to introduce the vitamin D-related hypothesis of anxiety-related disorders, suggesting that anxiety may be a key disorder provoked by abnormal neuroendocrine vitamin D/VDR system (Kalueff et al., 2004a).

Notably, several recent studies from our (Kalueff et al., 2006a,b,c) and other (Buerne et al., 2006) groups have shown additional behavioural anomalies in these mutant mice, including increased sensitivity to seizures, reduced open field activity (but its unaltered temporal patterning), impaired swimming, as well as reduced barbering, aggressiveness and poorer maternal behaviours. Importantly, all these behaviours may, to some extent, be related to, underlie or contribute to, anxiety phenotype reported here.

Table 2. Comparison of the available published studies characterizing VDR mutant mice (adapted from Kalueff, 2005)

Behaviours and tests	Studies	
	Kalueff et al., 2004a,b,c	**Burne et al., 2005**
Vertical exploration		
open field	(-)	(-)
elevated plus maze	(-)	(-)
light-dark box	(-)	N/a
holeboard	(-)	(-)
Horizontal activity		
open field	Trend: (-)	(-)
elevated plus maze	0	(-)
light-dark box	0	
holeboard	(-)	(-)
Y-maze	N/a	(-)
Additional exploratory behaviours		
hole-poking (holeboard)	0	Trend: (-)
head-dips (plus maze)	N/a	0
open time (plus maze)	N/a	0
Y-maze arm alternation	N/a	(-)
Other anxiety-sensitive behaviours		
Urination	0*	(-)**
Defecation	0 ***	0**
Accoustic startle response	N/a	(-)
Marble burying	N/a	(-)
Other behaviours		
Memory in Y-maze	N/a	0
Digging (bedding test)	N/a	(-)
Open field habituation ****	N/a	(-)
Accoustic response habituation	N/a	(-)
Self-grooming ***	(+)	0 *****
Pre-pulse inhibition ******	N/a	(-)

N/a – not assessed. (+) – activation, (-) - reduction, 0 – no effects. * Unpublished data from (Kalueff et al., 2004a) study. ** Open field data. *** Open field, holeboard, plus maze, light-dark box data. **** Horizontal activity (distance traveled). ***** Holeboard test data. ****** To acoustic startle response (at long 256 ms, but not short 8-64 ms intervals).

Acknowledgements

This research was supported by research grants from CIMO, EVO, Tampere University and the Academy of Finland to PT. The authors are greatly indebted to Prof. S.Kato (University of Tokyo, Japan) for providing the knockout mice for our research. Authors also thank Dr. A. Galeeva (University of Tampere, Finland) for providing the protected elevated plus maze for our studies.

Inbox 1. Specific Motor Dysfunctions in VDR Null Mutant Mice

Since motor abnormalities have been reported for a number of mutant mice (Fortier at al., 1987; Fukamauchi et al., 1996; Costa et al., 1999; Lalonde et al., 1993), transgenic and knockout mice represent an increasingly popular tool to study the role of gene functions in motor behaviour. To examine the link between vitamin D-related disorders and motor activity, we studied VDR null mutant mice used in our previous study.

Motor Functions Test

The motor performance of 10 mutant, 10 wild type and 8 heterozygous mice (24-52 weeks) was assessed in the vertical screen test. Briefly, the mouse was placed on the centre of the screen consisting of a plastic frame (30 cm high and 15 cm wide, with 10-cm top and side walls) covered by a plastic net (2-mm mesh) elevated to a height of 60 cm from the floor. The screen was turned immediately to the vertical position with the mouse facing the upper end, and the retention time (the latency to fall off from the screen, s) was measured. To avoid any harm to the animals caused by falling from the screen, a thick cloth was placed under the screen. In addition, emotional reactivity was assessed by the number of defecation boli deposited during the first 5 min of the test.

The Swim Test

Animal motor performance was assessed in the swim test. In this experiment, 6 VDR null mutants were compared to 5 homozygous wild-type and 5 heterozygous controls. To rule out the impact of phenotypical difference in mice appearance (hairless VDR mutants vs. normal haired control groups), the hair of animals from both control groups was removed by shaving. Animals from all groups were anaesthetized with Hypnorm, and the shaving of the control mice was performed using small electric shears. Seven days later, behavioural testing was performed in a water tank consisting of a glass cylinder 50 cm tall and 30 cm in diameter filled with water (25 °C) to a height of 15 cm from the top. The mice were gently put onto the surface of the water, and their swimming behaviour was studied by an experienced investigator for a period of 3 min. The observer recorded the duration and number of immobility episodes (animal remaining motionless in the water with no limb movements except for small postural adjustments or minor head movements), the number of rotations (360° body turns), the number of defecation boli deposited and the number of sinking episodes (animal's nose going below the surface with the body in a vertical position head up). Behavioural data were analysed by the Kruskal–Wallis test followed by post-hoc Mann–Whitney test ($P < 0.05$).

In the vertical screen test, the mutant group demonstrated generally shorter retention time compared to both control groups, while no changes were seen in the number of defecation boli deposited. In the swim test, swimming patterns of the shaven wild-type and heterozygous mice were similar, including approximately equal number of immobility episodes and total immobility duration. In all three groups, no changes were seen in the number of defecation boli. However, we found severe impairment of swimming behaviour in the VDR null mutant mice, including swimming in a predominantly vertical body position, very short duration of immobility, frequent stereotypic rotations and specific catatonic-like upper limb spasms (seen most of the time except for short active swimming episodes). Another striking finding was that all the VDR null mutants demonstrated frequent sinking – an abnormal pattern not seen in the normal swimming of the control animals.

Our preliminary observations in this test showed that the mutant mice differ from the wild-type or heterozygous littermates, swimming in a predominantly vertical position, struggling throughout the test, and unable to remain immobile because they will sink as soon as stop moving. Although this is in line with the motor deficit we found in the vertical screen test, we noted that VDR mutant mice develop secondary alopecia and therefore differ phenotypically from both control groups. Thus, it was possible to assume that hair provides additional buoyancy, raising the possibility that poor swimming in VDR null mutant mice may be merely due to the lack of hair. To examine this possibility in the present study, we shaved all the control animals and compared their swimming patterns to those of VDR mutant mice. In line with our earlier observations, shaven mice from both control groups demonstrated normal swimming patterns similar to those of unshaven animals. In contrast, the VDR mutant group demonstrated abnormal swimming, which was markedly different from that of both control groups (Kalueff et al., 2004b). Overall, despite a dramatic reduction of immobility in an attempt to avoid sinking, these mice still could not perform proper swimming, demonstrating frequent rotation and sinking. Moreover, our recent study using less alopecic young animals (7-10 weeks), also showed their severely impaired swimming, despite retaining 50-70% of their body fur. Collectively, these experiments clearly indicate that specific motor impairment in mutant mice is not due to alopecia.

The apparent lack of any motor deficit in the mutants tested in the actometer and novel object-finding test (Kalueff et al., 2004a,b) suggests that their motor impairments do not appear in normal spontaneous behaviour, and can only be observed in more stressful situations requiring intense physical efforts (such as swimming or vertical screen retention). Together, our findings demonstrate that genetic ablation of VDR in mice is associated with specific impairments in motor performance in the vertical screen and swim tests, which are: (i) not accompanied by altered emotionality/activity; (ii) can only be seen if strong physical stressors are applied; and (iii) occur only in VDR null mutant (-/-) animals (Kalueff et al., 2004c).[7]

Given our findings in mutant mice, genetic ablation of VDR in the brain, especially in the structures involved in motor control, may disrupt brain vitamin D-VDR signalling pathways, which, associated with disturbed modulation of neurotransmitters in these regions, may cause the impaired motor performance reported in our experiments. As such, impairment of these functions in VDR mutant mice may be one of the reasons for the specific motor abnormalities, which we saw in our studies. In general, our data confirm that vitamin D and VDR are crucial for motor activity, and disorders related to them significantly impair animal motor functions. These findings may be important given the emerging problem of vitamin D-related neural disorders, especially since the growing number of motor disorders is being linked to deficit in vitamin D.

References

[1] Ahonen M. *Vitamin D in human ovarian and prostate cancer*. Acta Univer. Tamper. 2002; 885:1-215.

[2] Altemus KL, Finger S, Wolf C, Birge SJ. Behavioral correlates of vitamin D deficiency. *Physiol. Behav*. 1987; 39:435-440.

[3] Burne TH, Becker A, Brown J, Eyles D, Mackay-Sim A, McGrath JJ. Transient prenatal Vitamin D deficiency is associated with hyperlocomotion in adult rats. *Behav. Brain Res*. 2004; 154:549-555.

[4] Burne TH, McGrath JJ, Eyles D, Mackay-Sim A. Behavioural characterization of Vitamin D receptor knockout mice. *Behav. Brain Res*. 2005; 157:299-308.

[5] Burne TH, Johnston AN, McGrath JJ, Mackay-Sim A. Swimming behaviour and post-swimming activity in Vitamin D receptor knockout mice. *Brain Res. Bull*. 2006; 69: 74-78.

[6] Cardenas F, Lamprea MR, Morato S. Vibrissal sense is not the main sensory modality in rat exploratory behavior in the elevated plus-maze. *Behav. Brain Res*. 2001; 122:169-174.

[7] Carswell S. *Vitamin D in the nervous system: actions and therapeutic potential*. In Vitamin D. Feldman D, Glorieux FH, Pike JW (editors). San Diego: Academic Press; 1997. pp. 1197-1211.

[8] Costa ACS, Walsh K, Davisson MT. Motor dysfunction in a mouse model for Down syndrome. *Physiol. Behav*. 1999; 68:211–220.

[7] In line with this, Burne et al. (2006) have recently reported altered swimming patterns and increased fatigue in VDR -/- mice produced by forced swimming

[9] Crawley J. Behavioral phenotyping of transgenic and knockout mice: experimental design and evaluation of general health, sensory functions, motor abilities, and specific behavioral tests. *Brain Res.* 1999; 835:18-26.

[10] Drai D, Kafkafi N, Benjamini Y, Elmer G, Golani I. Rats and mice share common ethologically relevant parameters of exploratory behavior. *Behav. Brain Res.* 2001; 125:133-140.

[11] Endo I, Inoue D, Mitsui T, Umaki Y, Akaike M, Yoshizawa T, Kato S, Matsumoto T. Deletion of vitamin D receptor gene in mice results in abnormal skeletal muscle development with deregulated expression of myoregulatory transcription factors. *Endocrinol.* 2003; 144:5138-5144.

[12] Fortier PA, Smith AM, Rossignol S. Locomotor deficits in the mutant mouse, Lurcher. *Exp. Brain Res.* 1987; 66:271–286.

[13] Fukamauchi F, Mataga N, Wang YJ, Sato S, Yoshiki A, Kusakabe M. Abnormal behavior and neurotransmissions of tenascin gene knockout mouse. *Biochem. Biophys. Res. Comm.* 1996; 221: 151–156.

[14] Garcion E, Wion-Barbot N, Montero-Menei C, Berget F, Wion D. New clues about vitamin D functions in the nervous system. *Trends Endocrinol. Metabol.* 2002; 13:100-105.

[15] Gerlai R. Gene-targeting studies of mammalian behavior: is it the mutation or the background genotype? *Trends Neurosci.* 1996; 19:177-181.

[16] Gloth FM, Alam W, Hollis B. Vitamin D vs. broad spectrum phototherapy in the treatment of seasonal affective disorders. *J. Nutr. Health Aging* 2001; 3:5-7.

[17] Golani I, Benjamini Y, Eilam D. Stopping behavior: constraints on exploration in rats (Rattus norvegicus). *Behav. Brain Res.* 1993; 53:21-33.

[18] Kalueff AV, Lou Y-R, Laaksi I, Tuohimaa P. Increased anxiety in mice lacking Vitamin D receptor gene. Neuroreport. 2004a; 15:1271-1274.

[19] Kalueff AV, Lou Y-R, Laaksi I, Tuohimaa P. Impaired motor performance in mice lacking neurosteroid Vitamin D receptors. *Brain Res. Bull.* 2004b; 64:25-29.

[20] Kalueff AV, Lou Y-R, Laaksi I, Tuohimaa P. Increased grooming behavior in mice lacking Vitamin D receptors. *Physiol. Behav.* 2004c; 82:405-409.

[21] Kalueff A, Tuohimaa P. Experimental models of anxiety and depression. *Acta Neurobiol Experim.* 2004a; 64:439-448.

[22] Kalueff A, Tuohimaa P. Contrasting grooming phenotypes in C57BL/6 and 129S1/SvImJ mice. *Brain Res.* 2004b; 1028:75-81.

[23] Kalueff AV, Lou Y-R, Laaksi I, Tuohimaa P. Abnormal behavioural organization of grooming in mice lacking vitamin D receptor gene. *J. Neurogenet.* 2005; 67:169-77.

[24] Kalueff A. Behavioural anomalies in mice with partially deleted vitamin D receptor gene. Acta Univer. Tamper. 2005; 1105:1-79.

[25] Kalueff AV, Minasyan A, Keisala T, Kuuslahti M, Miettinen S, Tuohimaa P. Increased severity of chemically *induced seizures in mice with partially deleted Vitamin D receptor gene. Neurosci.* Lett. 2006a; 394:69-73.

[26] Kalueff AV, Keisala T, Minasyan A, Kuuslahti M, Miettinen S, Tuohimaa P. Behavioural anomalies in mice evoked by "Tokyo" disruption of the Vitamin D receptor gene. *Neurosci. Res.* 2006b; 54:254-260.

[27] Kalueff AV, Keisala T, Minasyan A, Kuuslahti M, Tuohimaa P. Temporal stability of novelty exploration in mice exposed to different open field tests. *Behav. Processes.* 2006c; 72:104-12.

[28] Kinuta K, Tanaka H, Moriwake T, Aya K, Kato S, Seino Y. Vitamin D is an important factor in estrogen biosynthesis of both female and male gonads. *Endocrinol.* 2000; 141:1317-1324.

[29] Lalonde R, Joyal CC, Cote C. Swimming activity in dystonia musculorum mutant mice. *Physiol. Behav.* 1993; 54:119–120.

[30] Langub MC, Herman JP, Malluche HH, Koszewski NJ. Evidence of functional vitamin D receptors in rat hippocampus. *Neuroscience.* 2001; 104:49-56.

[31] Li YC, Pirro AE, Amling M, Delling G, Baron R, Bronson R, Demay MB. Targeted ablation of the vitamin D receptor: an animal model of vitamin D-dependent rickets type II with alopecia. *Proc. Natl. Acad. Sci.* USA. 1997; 94:9831-9835.

[32] Londei T, Valentini AM, Leone VG. Investigative burying by laboratory mice may involve non-functional, compulsive, behaviour. *Behav. Brain Res.* 1998; 94:249-254.

[33] Moore CI. Frequency-dependent processing in the vibrissa sensory system. *J. Neurophysiol.* 2004; 91:2390-2399.

[34] Prchal A, Albarracin AL, Decima EE. Blockage of vibrissae afferents: I. Motor effects. *Arch. Ital. Biol.* 2004; 142:11-23.

[35] Prufer K, Veenstra TD, Jirikowski GF, Kumar R. Distribution of 1,25-dihydroxyvitamin D3 receptor immunoreactivity in the rat brain and spinal cord. *J. Chem. Immunol.* 1999; 16:135-145.

[36] Prut L, Belzung C. The open field as a paradigm to measure the effects of drugs on anxiety-like behaviors: a review. *Eur. J. Pharmacol.* 2003; 463:3-33.

[37] Staiger JF, Bisler S, Schleicher A, Gass P, Stehle JH, Zilles K. Exploration of a novel environment leads to the expression of inducible transcription factors in barrel-related columns. *Neuroscience.* 2000; 99:7-16.

[38] Sutton, ALM, MacDonald PN. Vitamin D: more than a “bone-a-fide” hormone. *Mol. Endocrinol.* 2003; 17:777-791.

[39] Thiel CM, Muller CP, Huston JP, Schwarting RK. High versus low reactivity to a novel environment: behavioural, pharmacological and neurochemical assessments. *Neuroscience.* 1999; 93:243-251.

[40] Voikar V, Koks S, Vasar E, Rauvala H. Strain and gender differences in the behavior of mouse lines commonly used in transgenic studies. *Physiol. Behav.* 2001; 72:271-281.

[41] Walbert T, Jirikowski GF, Prufer K. Distribution of 1,25-dihydroxyvitamin D3 receptor immunoreactivity in the limbic system. *Horm. Metab. Res.* 2001; 33:525-531.

[42] Ylikomi T, Laaksi I, Lou Y-R, Martikainen P, Miettinen S, Pennanen P, Purmonen S, Syvala H, Vienonen A, Tuohimaa P. Antiproliferative action of vitamin D. Vit. Horm. 2001; 64:357-405.

[43] Yoshizava T, Handa Y, Uematsu Y, Takeda S, Sekine K, Yoshihara Y et al. Mice lacking the vitamin D receptor exhibit impaired bone formation, uterine hypoplasia and growth retargation after weaning. *Nat. Genet.* 1997; 16:391-396.

In: Animal Models in Biological Psychiatry
Editor: Allan V. Kalueff, pp. 119-135
ISBN 1-59454-814-5

Chapter 7

Genetic Ablation of Vitamin D Receptor Gene Affects Grooming Activity and Sequencing in Mice

Allan V. Kaluef, and Pentti Tuohimaa
Medical School, University of Tampere, Tampere University Hospital, Tampere, Finland

I. Introduction

Neurosteroid vitamin D plays an important role in the nervous system including differentiation, regulation of Ca^{2+} homeostasis, modulation of neurotrophins release and activity of key brain genes and enzymes of neurotransmitter metabolism (Carswell, 1997; Garcion et al., 2002). The functions of vitamin D are mediated through the nuclear vitamin D receptor (VDR), a member of the nuclear receptors superfamily of ligand-activated transcriptor factors (Kato et al., 1999). VDR are widespread in the brain and the spinal cord including the areas involved in the regulation of motor activity and behavior (Prufer et al., 1999; Langub et al., 2001).

Several clinical and experimental studies outline the possible role of vitamin D and VDR in the regulation of various behaviours (Altemus et al., 1987; Carswell, 1997). Self-grooming is an ancient innate behaviour that is represented across most animal species and is a particularly important part of rodent behavioural repertoire (Sachs, 1988; Aldridge, Berridge, 1998; Greer, Capecci, 2003) sensitive to a number of endogenous and exogenous manipulations (van Erp et al., 1994; Kruk et al., 1998; Kalueff, 2000).

In rodents, a general pattern of self-grooming cephalocaudal progression is known to proceed as follows: paw licking, nose and face wash, head wash, body wash and fur licking, leg licking, tail/genitals licking and wash (Berridge et al., 1987; Sachs, 1988; Berridge, Whishaw, 1992). High concentrations of VDR were recently found in the basal ganglia, brainstem, hypothalamus and the limbic system (Veenstra et al., 1998; Prufer et al., 1999;

Langub et al., 2001; Walbert et al., 2001), the brain areas all reported to be involved in neural control of grooming and its sequencing (Grill, Norgen, 1978; Kruk et al., 1998; Strazielle, Lalonde, 1998; Meyer-Luehmann et al., 2002).

In addition, vitamin D has been reported to be involved in VDR-mediated modulation of brain neurotransmitters, including acetylcholine and dopamine (Carswell, 1997; Garcion et al., 2003), known to regulate grooming (Cromwell et al., 1998; Kalueff, 2002). Taken together, these data suggest that VDR may be important for the regulation of grooming behaviours and their patterning. Since genetically targeted animals provide a powerful tool extensively used in the field of neurobehavioral research (Flint et al., 1995; Crawley, 1999), several studies have focused on microstructure of grooming in different mutant mice (Coscia, Fentress, 1993; Bolivar et al., 1996; Cromwell et al., 1998; Strazielle, Lalonde, 1998; Greer, Capecci, 2003).

Mice with genetically impaired VDR are currently available for biomedical research focusing on the biological functions of vitamin D and VDR (Kallay et al., 2001; Song et al., 2003). Cloning and sequencing of the VDR gene (≈65 kb) has been carried out in some species including chickens, humans, rats and mice (Kamei et al., 1995). Structurally, the mouse VDR gene shows significant homology between these species: the most conserved fragments encode C (100% homology with rat and human VDR gene) and E domains (89-96% homology with human and rat VDR gene) of the receptor (Kamei et al., 1995). Several groups have independently generated VDR null mutant mice (NM) by targeted disruption of this gene. Yoshizawa et al. (1997) ablated exon 2 encoding the first zinc finger of the DNA-binding domain of the VRD gene, while Li et al. (1997) ablated a fragment spanning exons 3-5 and encoding the second zinc finger. In addition, Erben et al. (2002) have recently generated mice expressing non-functional VDR without the first zinc finger. Since the absence of functional VDR results in the target tissue insensitivity to vitamin D, the analysis of the behavior of these mutant mice seems to be an important tool to assess the role of the vitamin D/VDR system in the brain.

Our preliminary observations in the home cage showed that VDR null mutant mice appear to have similar motor activity levels but usually tend to spend more time grooming than do the wild-type animals. Our preliminary observations in several behavioural models have also shown that VDR null mutation in mice leads to abnormal grooming including increased grooming frequency and duration (Kalueff et al., 2004a) – the findings that further strengthen the link between vitamin D, VDR and grooming. However, various mutations have been reported to affect rodent grooming "activity" measures, sequencing of grooming or even both, implying different degrees of behavioural anomalies (Coscia, Fentress, 1993; Cromwell et al., 1998; Strazielle, Lalonde, 1998; Greer, Capecci, 2003). Therefore, it was important to assess in detail the role of VDR in the regulation of grooming by examining the impact of VDR genetic ablation on activity and sequencing of grooming in mice (Kalueff et al., 2005).

II. Methods

VDR gene mutant mice were bred in the University of Tampere from the line initially generated in the University of Tokyo (Kato et al., 1999). 10 homozygous (-/-) mutants were compared to 10 homozygous (+/+) wild type 129/S1 male mice. Mice of all genotypes were produced by heterozygous crosses. Adult mice aged 24-52 weeks were maintained in a virus/parasite-free facility and exposed to a 12-h light, 12-h dark cycle. Lights were turned off at 18.00h and on at 6.00h. The animals were experimentally naïve and housed in fours, with food and water freely available. All experiments were performed between 14.00 and 18.00.

In the present study, the animals were tested in a battery of behavioral tests including actimeter, open field, hole board, elevated plus maze, and horizontal rod tests (testing protocol was similar to those reported previously: Kalueff et al., 2004b). All testing was conducted between 1700 and 1900 h. During the testing sessions, the experimenter remained standing in front of (and 2 m away from) the testing boxes (Kalueff et al., 2005).

Three ethological measures of grooming activity were evaluated in all these tests:

1. frequency (the number of grooming bouts),
2. total time (s) spent grooming, and
3. average duration of a single grooming bout (s) calculated as total time spent grooming divided by the number of bouts.

In order to assess spontaneous novelty-induced grooming, the mice were placed individually in a clean plastic observation box (30 x 30 x 30 cm) and observed by an experienced investigator for a period of 10 min, timing the duration and number of grooming bouts. In order to asses "artificial" swim-induced grooming, the mice were placed individually in a water tank (30 cm glass cylinder 25 cm in diameter, filled with water (24 ± 1 ^{o}C) to a depth of 15 cm) for 30 sec. After a short swimming session, the mice were removed from the tank, placed individually in the observation box and observed by an experienced investigator for a period of 5 min, timing the duration and number of grooming bouts.

The following 6-point scaling system (Kalueff, Tuohimaa, 2004) was used in the present study:

- no grooming (0),
- paw licking (1),
- nose and face wash (2),
- head wash (3),
- body grooming (4),
- leg licking (5), and
- tail/genitals grooming (6).

Interruptions longer than 5 sec. determined separate grooming bouts. Grooming behavioural microstructure was assessed using the grooming analysis algorithm as described earlier (Kalueff, Tuohimaa, 2004). Briefly, "correct" transitions adhered to the cephalocaudal pattern as follows: (0-1), (1-2), (2-3), (3-4), (4-5), (5-6), and (6-0); "incorrect" transitions included all other possible transitions between grooming stages; a grooming bout was considered "interrupted" if at least one interruption was recorded within its transitions. Correct/incorrect grooming transitions and interrupted/uninterrupted grooming bouts were analyzed using the transition matrix (Kalueff, Tuohimaa, 2004), and the percentage of incorrect transitions and the percentage of interrupted grooming bouts were calculated for both genotypes. All animal experiments were approved by the Ethical Committee of the University of Tampere (Kalueff et al., 2005).

Statistics

All results are expressed as mean ± S.E.M. Behavioural data were analyzed by Mann-Whitney U-test for independent samples. A probability of less than 0.05 was considered statistically significant.

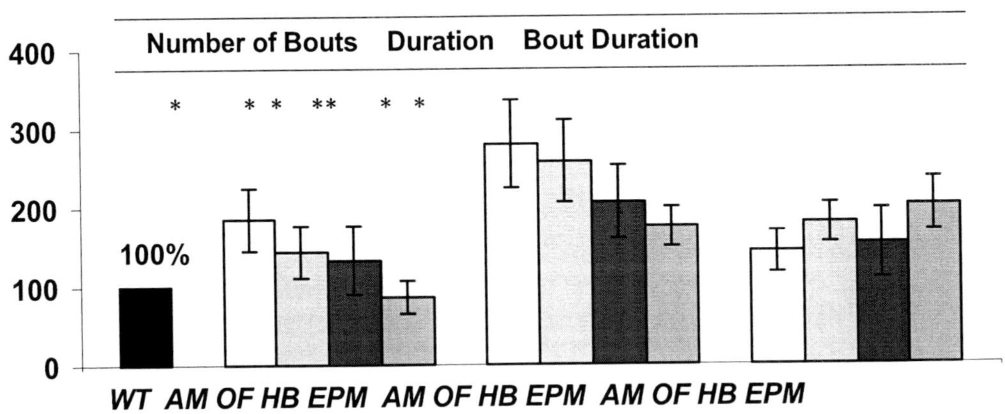

Fig. 1. Grooming behaviours in VDR null mutant mice in a battery of tests compared to their wild type (WT) controls (% of WT scores). Behavioural tests: AM – actimeter, OF – open field, HB – holeboard, EPM – elevated plus maze. Horizontal rod test results: WT mice: 0 (bouts, grooming duration, average bout duration); VDR mutant mice: 1.4 ± 0.3 bouts; 4.5 ± 0.9 grooming duration, 3.2 ± 0.4 average bout duration.

III. Results

Grooming Activity

The only marked behavioral difference found in the actimeter test, as can be seen in Fig. 1, was the increase in grooming activity (higher frequency, longer total time spent grooming, and a trend towards longer average duration of a single bout) in the VDR mutant mice compared to the wild type mice. In the open field test, the mutant mice again groomed more and longer than did their wild type counterparts, also showing significantly longer average duration of a single bout. In the holeboard test, the VDR null mutant animals showed a similar tendency for increased grooming activity (although this was not statistically significant; Fig. 1). In the elevated plus maze test, a significant increase in the VDR mutant group was found for the total time spent grooming and the duration of a single grooming bout (Fig. 1). Finally, as can be seen in Fig. 1 (legend), when placed on the horizontal rod, the mutant mice demonstrated grooming activity, which in this test was completely lacking in the wild type group.

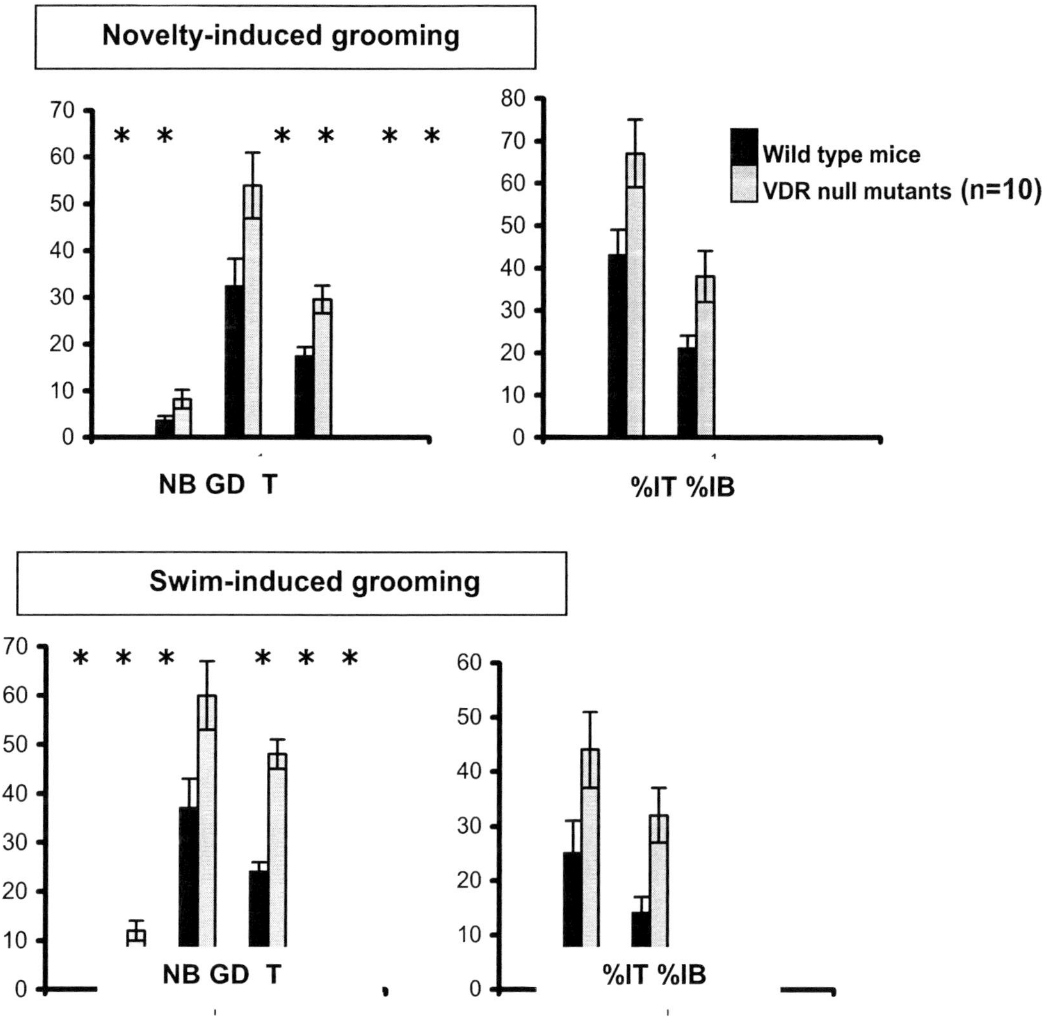

Fig. 2. Spontaneous (novelty-induced) and artificial (swim-induced) grooming in VDR null mutant mice compared to their wild type controls (n = 10). Data are expressed as mean ±S.E.M. NB – number of grooming bouts; GD – duration of grooming bouts (s); T – number of transitions between grooming stages; %IT – percentage of incorrect transitions (of T); %IB – percentage of interrupted bouts (of total NB).

Figure 2 shows spontaneous and artificial grooming of the wild type compared to the VDR null mutant mice. Overall, in line with our previous findings (Kalueff et al., 2004a), in both test situations the VDR null mutants spent more time on grooming, showing more bouts, and more transitions between stages, than did their wild type control littermates. In addition, our present study shows that not only grooming activity, but also its behavioural microstructure in these mice was significantly altered.

Grooming Patterning

A detailed ethological analysis using the grooming analysis algorithm (Kalueff, Tuohimaa, 2004) applied to both types of grooming activity reveals that mutant mice generally show a higher percentage of incorrect transitions and more interrupted bouts than their wild type counterparts (Fig. 2). Together, this proves that mice lacking functional VDR generally display abnormal grooming patterns, including altered sequencing and frequent interruptions.

IV. General Discussion

Explaining how the loss of VDR can lead to the phenomenon described here, we first suggested that genetic ablation of VDR may affect the brain neurophysiological mechanisms and pathways which control normal grooming and its sequencing (Aldridge, Berridge, 1998; Berridge, 1998). For example, vitamin D modulates several key brain neurotransmitters, including acetylcholine and dopamine (Garcion et al., 2003; Carswell, 1997), both known to regulate grooming (Kalueff, 2002). Given our findings in mutant mice, genetic ablation of VDR in the brain, especially in the structures involved in grooming motor control, may disrupt brain vitamin D-VDR signaling pathways which, associated with disturbed modulation of neurotransmitters in these regions, may cause the abnormal grooming behavior reported in our experiments (also see Inbox I for details of genetics of these behavioural anomalies).

Furthermore, genetic ablation of VDR, known to affect brain development (Eyles et al., 2003), may alter the formation of certain brain areas (such as basal ganglia and brainstem) involved in the control and regulation of grooming and its sequencing. This conjecture, if true, may also account for the abnormal grooming seen in VDR null mutants in the present study. Importantly, our recent studies have also shown that these mice seem to have unimpaired olfactory, visual and vestibular systems (Kalueff et al., 2004b,c), thus allowing us to eliminate sensory disturbances as a cause of the abnormal grooming patterning demonstrated by the VDR null mutant mice in the present study.

How specific is this behavioral abnormality in VDR mutant mice? Analyzing our data, we considered the possibility that the activation of grooming reported here may be due to possible difference in general motor activity levels between VDR mutants and the wild type mice. However, we found that the VDR mutant mice did not show any difference in motor activity levels in the actimeter test (Kalueff et al., 2004a). In line with this, behavioral measures reflecting the motor activity component in the elevated plus maze, such as closed arm and total arm entries, were unaltered in both groups (Kalueff et al., 2004a). Together, this allowed us to discount the "motor activity" factor while interpreting the results of our study.

Importantly, VDR null mutant mice have recently been shown to possess increased anxiety phenotype (Kalueff et al., 2004b). Since increased anxiety *per se* may produce alterations in rodent grooming, affecting both its activity measures and sequencing (Kalueff, 2000; 2002, Kalueff, Tuohimaa, 2004), it is possible to speculate that the abnormal grooming activity and sequencing reported in the present study may be associated with altered anxiety levels in these mice (also see previous Chapter on VDR mutant mice in this book). Indeed, since animal grooming, especially in rodents, is a robust stress-evoked "displacement" behavioural marker, it was possible to assume that the increased grooming activity in VDR mutant mice might be due to increased stress or anxiety. Although this possibility fits the idea of high anxiety phenotype reported previously for these mice (Kalueff et al., 2004b), our present study failed to demonstrate stress-dependent activation of grooming frequency or duration in a battery of behavioural tests (Fig. 1).

Since the degree of stress varies in the different test situations used in our study (actimeter < open field test < holeboard < elevated plus maze < horizontal rod test), we were also interested whether grooming increase might vary in different tests. However, our results clearly show that grooming activation did not follow "stress gradient" from low-stress actimeter test to high-stress elevated plus maze and horizontal rod tests. Quite the reverse, our data demonstrate a robust trend to lower grooming increase (vs. the respective wild type controls) in more stressful tests (Fig. 1) for both frequency and duration measures.

Inbox 1. The Character of Inheritance

Analyzing grooming behavior in these mice, we noted that impaired behavioural organization of grooming was only seen in VDR null mutant mice, whereas grooming patterns were unaltered in both heterozygous and wild type groups (Kalueff et al., 2005). This observation is in line with our previously published studies (Kalueff et al., 2004b,c) showing almost identical behavioural phenotypes of heterozygous and wild type mice in a number of anxiety and motor tests. Consistent with this, numerous observations show that heterozygous mice display similar VDR gene mRNA expression, have no overt anomalies, and phenotypically are indistinguishable from their wild type littermates (Yoshizawa et al., 1997; Kato et al., 1999). Moreover, all other mutant mice with non-functional VDR (Li et al., 1999; Erben et al., 2002) also reveal similar phenotypes in both these groups. Firstly, the fact that the heterozygous and wild type mice were physiologically and behaviorally normal, implies that only one wild type control group is necessary for behavioural analysis of VDR null mutant mice. Secondly, our results reveal the degree of dominance (i.e. harmful recessive) observed for behavioural phenotypes of these mutant mice. Thirdly, given recent data on reduced VDR level in heterozygous mice (Yoshizawa et al., 1997; Kallay et al., 2001), our findings raise the possibility that a limited number of functional VDR may be enough to maintain both normal physiological and behavioural phenotypes in mice. Importantly, numerous clinical data on hereditary vitamin D-resistant rickets (associated with various VDR gene mutations) parallel these data, showing normal phenotypes in heterozygous carriers (Malloy et al., 1997). Taken together, these findings support the notion that that physiological and behavioural anomalies induced by VDR impairment are inherited as a recessive in both mice and humans.

Furthermore, stress has long been known to synchronize grooming behavior by decreasing its individual variability (Van Erp et al., 1994). However, analysis of S.E.M. data (Kalueff et al., 2004a) indirectly reflecting grooming variability, has shown that in all tests used in the present study the VDR null mutant mice displayed equal or even higher variability of grooming activity measures compared to the wild type group (Fig. 3). This clearly contradicts the "synchronizing" effect of stress on grooming variability. Taken together, these observations seem to negate the idea that higher grooming activity in VDR null mutant mice is merely the result of their high emotional reactivity.

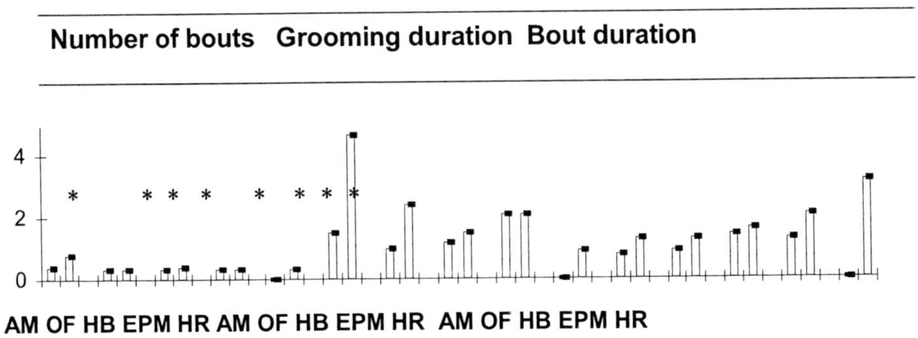

Fig. 3. Analysis of individual variability (only +S.E.M. values shown) of grooming scores in VDR null mutant (right bars) mice and their wild type controls (left bars) * $P < 0.05$ - significant behavioural differences (U-test, given for reference purpose) refer to the respective mean behavioural indices (Kalueff et al., 2004a). Behavioural tests: AM – actimeter, OF – open field, HB – holeboard, EPM – elevated plus maze, HR – horizontal rod test.

In general, our data suggest that activated grooming in these mice is not related to changes in their stress or emotionality, but rather represents a specific independent behavioural domain, in addition to their higher anxiety (Kalueff et al., 204b) and specific motor abnormalities (Kalueff et al., 2004c); Fig. 4. Although no correlation between anxiety and grooming frequency and duration was shown in our studies on these mice (Fig. 1, Kalueff et al., 2004a), some alterations of grooming sequencing were indeed reported in VDR null mutant mice subjected to different stressors (Kalueff, Tuohimaa, 2004), supporting the idea of the stress-related nature of abnormal grooming sequencing in these mice. Clearly, this interesting aspect of VDR null mutant mouse behavior needs further experimental investigation.

Since behavioural effects of genetic mutations may be affected by behavioural features of the animals' parental strains (Crawley, 1999), it was important to consider the role of genetic background in our experiments. The 129 mouse strain, used as genetic background in this study, generally displays callosal dysgenesis, hypoactivity and high anxiety (Crawley, 1999; also see the Mouse Phenome Database: http://www.jax.org). In addition, some of its sub-strains (including 129/S1 sub-strain used in our studies) are known to show generally low motor activity including grooming. We hypothesize that the background and the mutation-specific phenotypes may overlap, indirectly affecting grooming in the VDR mutant mice. For example, anxious phenotype of the 129 strain and "anxiogenic" VDR null mutation (Kalueff et al., 2004b) may cause additive effects on grooming, leading to its abnormal patterning reported here.

For example, this may explain frequent short, incomplete and interrupted bouts of mainly rostral ("anxiety-like") grooming seen in both genotypes in the present study. However, it is also possible that low-grooming background phenotype interacts with high-grooming phenotype of VDR null mutant mice (Kalueff et al., 2004a), collectively disorganizing their grooming patterning. Clearly, further studies are necessary to examine these possibilities in detail. For example, it may be necessary to further assess the strain differences in grooming activity of these mutant mice by comparing grooming and anxiety phenotypes of VDR null mutant mice generated on different genetic backgrounds (for example, C57, NMRI, BALB/c, etc). Nevertheless, marked differences in both the amount of grooming (Fig. 1, Kalueff et al., 2004a) and its behavioural organization (Fig. 2, Table 1, Kalueff et al. 2005) between the background (wild type) and VDR null mutant animals strongly support the crucial role of VDR genetic ablation in the abnormal grooming patterns reported here.

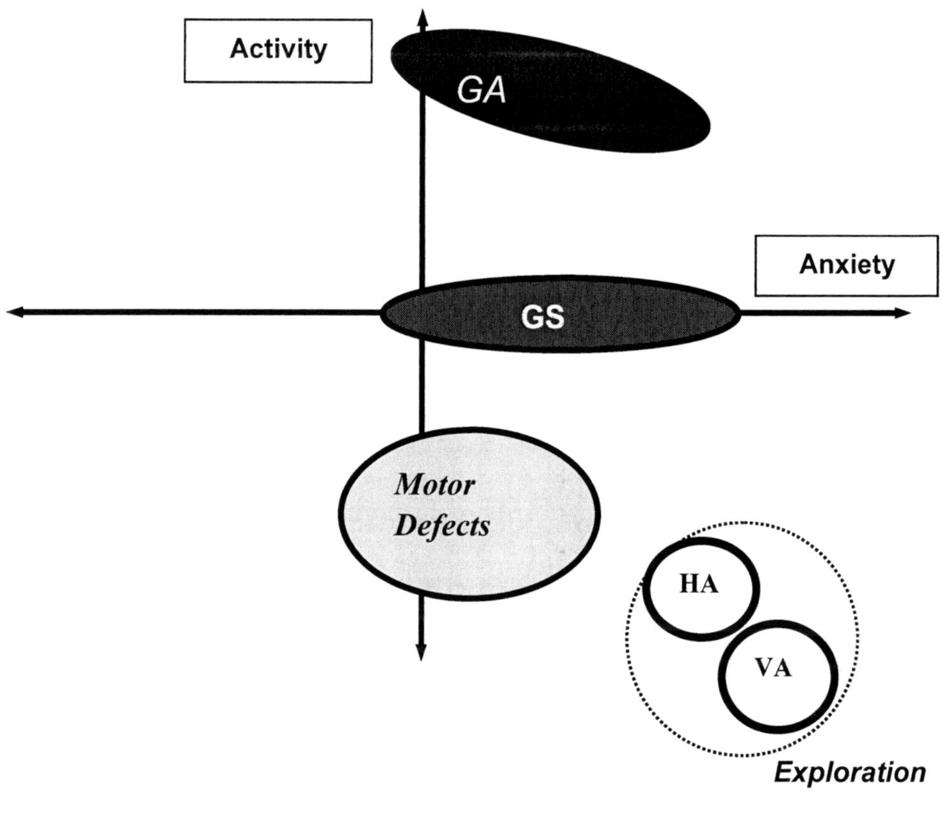

Fig. 4. Schematic presentation of behavioural domains in VDR null mutant mice, see (Kalueff et al., 2004a-c) for details. GA – grooming activity measures (frequency, duration), GS – grooming sequencing (behavioural microstructure), HA – horizontal activity, VA – vertical activity.

Since vitamin D plays an important role in the regulation of Ca^{2+} homeostasis (Garcion et al., 2003), another possible explanation for our findings in VDR null mutants may be disregulation of Ca^{2+} homeostasis, which is usually associated with vitamin D/VDR-related disorders (Carswell, 1997). A causal link between disturbances in Ca^{++} and various behavioral abnormalities in both animals and humans has been reported in the literature

(Altemus et al., 1987; Carswell, 1997). Since VDR mediate vitamin D regulation of plasma and brain Ca^{2+} (Garcion et al., 2003), behavioral abnormalities such as the abnormal patterning of grooming in VDR null mutant mice seen in our experiments, may be attributed to the disturbed Ca^{2+} homeostasis previously reported for these mice (Yoshizawa et al., 1997; Kalueff et al., 2004c).

Furthermore, since vitamin D is synthesized in the skin after sun exposure and was found in body grease and fur (Carpenter, Zhao, 1999), certain animal behaviors, such as outdoor activities and self-grooming, may represent important physiological adaptations of the organism in respect to regulation of the vitamin D system. For example, the evolutionary significant link between vitamin D and grooming behavior (Carpenter, Zhao, 1999) might lead to a very interesting hypothesis, requiring further testing, as to why abnormal grooming might be observed in animals with disturbed vitamin D/VDR system. For example, it is possible to speculate that disturbed vitamin D-VDR signalling in mice lacking VDR may be "interpreted" by the brain as the "lack" of vitamin D. Thus, increased grooming behaviour in these mice may represent a behavioural physiological adaptation aiming to "restore" the levels of vitamin D by extracting it from fur/body grease during grooming. Interestingly, the fact that hetero-grooming behaviour is also increased in VDR null mutant mice (own unpublished homecage observations) seems to indirectly support this hypothesis.

Moreover, it is known that several behavioral disorders in humans and animals are associated with vitamin D dysfunctions (Carswell, 1997). Stereotypic behaviors are repetitive inappropriate responses and represent a common symptom of many behavioral disorders. Since grooming is a common stereotypy in both animals and humans, it therefore seems possible that increased grooming activity may be some kind of behavioral stereotypy, typical for VDR mutant mice. Consistent with this, in all tests, prolonged time spent grooming was the most marked behavioral alteration in the VDR mutant group, which also demonstrated 1.5- to 2-fold increase in the average duration of a single grooming bout (Fig. 1). Moreover, in the horizontal rod test, where retaining their balance on the rod was crucial for mice, grooming was not seen in the wild type mice. However, as can be seen in Fig. 1, VDR mutants did demonstrate this "inappropriate" behavior while tested in this paradigm. Taken together, this lends indirect support to the hypothesis that in VDR mutant mice increased grooming might represent stereotypic behavior. This contention will certainly require further experimentation to be confirmed. For example, it would be of interest to explore if the behavioral characteristics of animals with vitamin D deficiency and/or impaired VDR might include some other (i.e., non-grooming) stereotypic behaviors. However, if true, this might explain the stereotypies frequently seen in patients with vitamin D-related disorders (Carswell, 1997) and, based on VDR ablation in mice, could lead to the development of several interesting animal models of vitamin D-related stereotypic behavioral disorders.

Another possible factor may be peripheral (cutaneous) effects of VDR genetic ablation, evoking different patterns of grooming activity. However, the significant portion of multiple-area grooming seen in these mice, with a clear cephalocaudal trend in both genotypes (Kalueff et al., 2005), is consistent with centrally-controlled, programmed grooming, rather than stimulus-driven grooming (Table 1). Indeed, if altered grooming in these mutant mice was merely a response to peripheral stimuli, one would not expect grooming patterns to sequence from one area to another (Ekstein and Hart, 2000). A clear displacement (stress-evoked) character of grooming observed in VDR null mutants tested on the horizontal rod (Kalueff et al., 2005) also negates the role of peripheral factors in abnormal grooming patterning observed in the present study.

Finally, the mice tested in the present study were approximately 6-12 month old, the age which can be classified as "adult-to-aged", according to the standard behavioural protocols (Crawley, 1999). Our general knowledge of the age-related progression of motor disorders indicates that this age-related aspect, although not directly tested in the present study, may be especially important to consider, since VDR null mutant mouse behaviour has not yet been fully examined in detail. For example, interesting data on rats (Kametani et al., 1984) show marked age-related alterations in grooming sequencing. Therefore, it is possible to assume that the abnormal sequencing of grooming found in the VDR null mutant mice can be age-dependent, and that the age of the mice used here did affect our findings accordingly. As such, sequencing of grooming in VDR null mutant mice, especially when tested at different ages, may provide a useful model to assess possible age-related motor/sequencing deficits associated with vitamin D/VDR-related disorders. Moreover, since abnormal sequencing may be seen not only for grooming behaviours, a detailed ethological analysis (especially focusing on patterning of other, non-grooming behaviors) would justify further studies on these mutant mice.

Table 1. Regional distribution of spontaneous (novelty-induced) and artificial (swim-induced) grooming activity in VDR null mutant mice (NM) compared to their wild type (WT) controls, assessed in the actimeter test for 5 min (Kalueff et al., 2005).

Grooming parameters	**Body areas**							
	Forepaws and head		**Body**		**Hind legs**		**Tail and genitals**	
	WT	*NM*	*WT*	*NM*	*WT*	*NM*	*WT*	*NM*
Novelty-induced grooming								
% patterns	50±5	72±4*	23±4	7±1*	15±2	21±3*	12±2	0*
% time grooming	48±6	65±7	32±4	16±1*	10±2	19±3*	10±1	0*
% interruptions	78±5	84±11	10±3	4±1	9±2	12±2	3±1	0
Water-induced grooming								
% patterns	63±5	73±7	22±5	12±3	12±2	15±2	3±0.5	0
% time grooming	54±7	81±6*	36±5	7±1*	5±1	12±1*	5±1	0*
% interruptions	83±7	72±8	12+4	8+2	5+1	20+6	0	0

- P<0.05, compared to the WT control group. Briefly, in order to assess the regional distribution of grooming in these mice, we analysed grooming activity directed to the following anatomic areas: forepaws and head, body, hind legs and tail/genitals. The percentage of grooming patterns, the percentage of time spent grooming, and the percentage of interruptions were calculated for each area. In the wild type group, novelty-induced grooming was directed most often to the forepaws and head. Other groomed areas, in rank order, were: body, hind legs and tail/genitals. Swim-induced grooming was distributed similarly to the novelty-induced grooming, showing, however, more gradual cephalocaudal progression. In contrast, the mutant group showed different regional distribution of novelty-induced grooming, including significantly higher frequency of forepaws and head grooming, a trend to more time spent grooming this area, significantly higher frequency and duration of hind legs grooming, and significantly lesser frequency and duration of body grooming. Interestingly, tail and genitals grooming was not observed in this group. Swim-induced grooming was organized similarly to the novelty-induced grooming, including significantly longer grooming of forepaws, head and hind legs, a trend to higher frequency of grooming directed to these areas, as well as significantly lesser body grooming frequency and duration ($P<0.05$, U-test). Tail and genitals grooming was also lacking in this group. Moreover, the regional distribution of interruptions failed to reveal any significant difference between both groups of mice, since interruptions were predominantly associated with forepaws and head grooming in all our experiments. The lack of tail/genitals grooming in the mutant mice resulted in 100% incomplete grooming bouts, compared to a slightly lesser percentage in the wild type group (88-97%).

- In addition, each grooming bout was categorised as being directed to (i) multiple regions or (ii) a single region. The percentage of grooming bouts and the percentage time spent grooming were calculated for both categories. Overall, the wild type mice dedicated $76\pm10\%$ of novelty-induced grooming bouts and $82\pm8\%$ of time spent grooming to multiple-body regions, compared to $55\pm7\%$ and $63\pm9\%$ in the VDR mutant group, respectively ($P<0.05$, U-test). For swim-induced grooming, the mutant group dedicated $35\pm8\%$ of grooming bouts and $57\pm11\%$ of time spent grooming to multiple-body regions, compared to $45\pm9\%$ and $67\pm11\%$ in the wild type group, respectively (although this difference did not reach significance).

Interestingly, in many species, genetics of complex patterned behaviours has numerous examples when mutations lead to excessive but functionally impaired behaviours. In fruit flies, *dsf* and *plt* mutations lead to vigorous courtship but impair copulation; *fru* mutation impairs copulation without disrupting courtship activity, while *fic* mutation evokes repetitive bouts of prematurely terminated copulation (Yamamoto, Nakano, 2003). Similar situation is commonly seen in mice. For example, *Hoxb8* mutation leads to higher grooming activity scores but shows abnormal regional distribution of grooming (Greer, Capecci, 2002), while *weaver* mutation (affecting both striatum and cerebellum) leads to a greater number of grooming bouts but produces smaller forelimb strokes and incomplete stereotypic sequences (Coscia, Fentress, 1993; Bolivar et al., 1996). To some extent, our present results coincide with these observations, allowing us to speculate that increased grooming activity in VDR mutant mice (Fig. 1) may be used to "compensate" their putative mutation-induced reduction of "functional effectiveness" of grooming due to its impaired sequencing (Fig. 2).

In summary, the main conclusion of our study is that mice with ablated VDR receptors display high self-grooming activity and abnormal sequencing of grooming, including increased percentages of incorrect transitions and interrupted bouts. What can be potential implications of these results?

A growing number of genetic anomalies have been found in human VDR gene, including missence and nonsence mutations, splice site mutations, and partial deletion of the VDR gene (Malloy et al., 1997, 2002). Such mutations, affecting DNA-binding, nuclear localization, ligand-binding, heterodimerization and other functions of the VDR, lead to partial or total hormone resistance and rickets (Malloy et al., 2002), with many behavioural anomalies (Carswell et al., 1997) sometimes associated with more severe psychiatric phenotypes (Ozer et al., 2004). For the development of effective treatments for such disorders, it is therefore necessary to increase our knowledge on the central function of the vitamin D/VDR system. Analysis of various behaviours (including grooming) in mutant mice with impaired VDR may be necessary to study various motor/sequencing and emotional deficits associated with vitamin D/VDR-related disorders (Kalueff et al., 2005).

In general, our data give support to the long-standing and continuously mounting evidence for the role of vitamin D in the brain (Carswell, 1997; Garcion et al., 2002) and contribute to the growing recognition of the importance of VDR in regulation of behavior (Kalueff et al., 2004a,b,c)[8]. We can suggest that the use of genetic animal models of vitamin

[8] In a recent study using VDR mutant mice on a mixed (C57-129) genetic background, Burne et al. (2006) replicated, with modifications, our initial experiments (Kalueff et al., 2004a, 2005) reported here. Using only 8 WT and 6 mutant mice, they found no significant difference in the baseline grooming activity in both groups of mice. Although the duration of grooming, in line with our studies, was predictably higher in the mutant group (25 s) vs. their WT controls (19 s), we believe that a small group size (surprisingly small for a behavioural study) might affect their findings, not allowing these authors to reach significance (also see similar predictable trend for a shorter grooming latency in VDR mutants: 79 s vs. 92 s in the WT group).

In contrast, post-swim "fatigue" grooming was dramatically impeded in the mutant group (Burne et al., 2006) – the finding which again needs some re-consideration. In our opinion, this result can indeed reflect higher fatigue in these mice, but do not allow to make conclusion about *reduced* grooming per se, due to apparent behavioral non-specificity in this study, and a global inhibition of all VDR mutant behaviors. We believe that different apploaches, using behavioral (rather than non-specific) ways to induce grooming, may assist in further analyses of grooming in these mice.

Finally, we view our own data (Kalueff et al., 2004a, 2005) in a more general sense - as an example how a mutation can lead to altered complex behavior. Clearly, grooming activity and patterning represent a good model for such studies. Robust alterations in grooming have also been reported in several mouse strains with spontaneously occurring mutations. For example, *Lurcher* mice display reduced grooming of forelimb, abdomen, back and hind limb, also showing less complex bouts (Strazielle and Lalonde, 1998). In contrast, *weaver* mice show a greater number, but shorter duration of grooming bouts, perform a higher proportion of smaller forelimb strokes and more incomplete grooming sequences (Coscia and Fentress, 1993; Bolivar et al., 1996). *Jimpy* mice (Bolivar and Brown, 1994) spend less time grooming, whereas s*taggerer* mice show less grooming but unaltered patterning (Fentress, 1999). With systematic data on aberrant grooming phenotypes in various transgenic and mutant mice already accumulating in the Mouse Genome Informatics Database, available for on-line search, new interesting studies analyzing grooming and its behavioral microstructure in various mice might be expected soon.

The existing mouse background strains phenotype databases (e.g., Mouse Phenome Database) may also benefit from including systematic grooming and barbering profiles of different mouse strains. Providing more comprehensive coverage of mouse behavioral phenotypes and offering clever ideas on how known

D/VDR-related behavioural disorders, such as those reported here, may be a useful tool for further studies focusing on the role of vitamin D and VDR in the brain.

Acknowledgements

This research was supported by grants from CIMO Finland, EVO and the Academy of Finland. We are greatly indebted to Professor Shigeaki Kato (University of Tokyo, Japan) for providing the initial VDR null mutant mice for our research.

References

[1] Aldridge, J.W., Berridge, K.C. 1998. Coding of serial order by neostriatal neurons: a "natural action" approach to movement sequence. *J. Neurosci.*, 18, 2777-2787.

[2] Altemus, K.L., Finger, S., Wolf, C., Birge, S.J. 1987. Behavioral correlates of vitamin D deficiency. *Physiol. Behav.*, 39, 435-440.

[3] Berridge, K.C. 1989. Progressive degradation of serial grooming chains by descending decerebration. *Behav. Brain Res.*, 33, 241-253.

[4] Berridge, K.C., Fentress, J.C., Parr, H. 1987. Natural syntax rules control action sequence of rats. *Behav. Brain Res.*, 23, 59-68.

[5] Berridge, K.C., Whishaw, I.Q. 1992. Cortex, striatum and cerebellum: control of serial order in a grooming sequence. *Exp. Brain Res.*, 90, 275-290.

[6] Bolivar, V.J., Danilchuk, W., Fentress, J.C. 1996. Separation of activation and pattern in grooming development of weaver mice. *Behav. Brain Res.*, 75, 49-58.

[7] Bolivar, V.J., Brown, R.E. 1994. The ontogeny of ultrasonic vocalizations and other behaviors in male jimpy (jp/Y) mice and their normal male littermates. Dev. *Psychobiol.,* 27, 101-110.

[8] Burne, T.H., Johnston, A.N., McGrath, J.J., Mackay-Sim, A. 2006. Swimming behaviour and post-swimming activity in Vitamin D receptor knockout mice. *Brain Res. Bull.,* 69, 74-78.

[9] Carpenter, K.J., Zhao, L. 1999. Forgotten mysteries in early history of vitamin D. J. Nutr., 129, 923–927

[10] Carswell, S. 1997. Vitamin D in the nervous system: actions and therapeutic potential. In: Feldman, D., Glorieux, F.H., Pike, J.W. (Eds) Vitamin D. Academic Press, San Diego, pp. 1197-1211.

[11] Coscia, E.M., Fentress, J.C. 1993. Neurological dysfunction expressed in the grooming behavior of developing weaver mutant mice. *Behav. Genet.*, 23, 533-541.

grooming peculiarities may affect other behaviors of different mouse strains, it will assist researchers in correct data interpretation and selecting appropriate mouse models for their tests.

USEFUL WEB-RESOURCES

MPD, Mouse Phenome Database	http://www.jax.org/phenome
MGI, Mouse Genome Informatics Database	http://www.informatics.jax.org/

[12] Crawley, J. 1999. Behavioral phenotyping of transgenic and knockout mice: experimental design and evaluation of general health, sensory functions, motor abilities, and specific behavioral tests. *Brain Res.*, 835, 18-26.

[13] Cromwell, H.C., Berridge, K.C., Drago, J., Levine, M.S. 1998. Action sequencing is impaired in D1A-deficient mutant mice. *Eur. J. Neurosci.,* 10, 2426-2432.

[14] Ekstein, R.A., Hart, B.L. 2003. The organization and control of grooming in cats. Appl *Animal Behav Sci.*, 68, 131-140.

[15] Endo, I., Inoue, D., Mitsui, T., Umaki, Y., Akaike, M., Yoshizawa, T., Kato, S., Matsumoto, T. 2003. Deletion of vitamin D receptor gene in mice results in abnormal skeletal muscle development with deregulated expression of myoregulatory transcription factors. *Endocrinol.* 144, 5138-5144.

[16] Erben, R.G., Soegiarto, D.W., Weber, K., Zeitz, U., Lieberherr, M., Gniadecki, R., Moller, G., Adamski, J., Balling, R. 2002. Deletion of deoxyribonucleic acid binding domain of the vitamin D receptor abrogates genomic and nongenomic functions of vitamin D. Mol. *Endocrinol.*, 16, 1524-1537.

[17] Eyles, D., Brown, J., Mackay-Sim, A., McGrath, J., Feron, F. 2003. Vitamin D3 and brain development. *Neurosci.,* 118, 641-653.

[18] Flint, J., Corley, R., DeFries, J.C., Fulker, W., Gray, J.A., Miller, S., Collins, A.C. 1995. A simple genetic basis for a complex psychological trait in laboratory mice. Science, 268, 1432–1435.

[19] Garcion, E., Wion-Barbot, N., Montero-Menei, C., Berget, F., Wion, D. 2002. New clues about vitamin D functions in the nervous system. *Tr. Endocrinol. Metab.*, 13, 100-105.

[20] Greer, J.M., Capecci, M.R. 2003. Hoxb8 is required for normal grooming behaviour in mice. Neuron, 33, 23-34.

[21] Grill, H.J., Norgren, R. 1978. Neurological tests and behavioral deficits in chronic thalamic and chronic decerebrate rats. *Brain Res.*, 143, 299-312.

[22] Kallay, E., Pietschmann, P., Toyokuni, S., Bajna, E., Hahn, P., Mazzucco, K., Bieglmayer, C., Kato, S., Cross, H.S. 2001. Characterization of a vitamin D receptor knockout mouse as a model of colorectal hyperproliferation and DNA damage. Carcinogenesis, 22, 1429-1435.

[23] Kalueff, A.V. 2000. Measuring grooming in stress and comfort. Proced. Measur. Behav. 3, 148-149.

[24] Kalueff, A.V. 2002. Grooming and stress, KSF, Kiev, 148 pp.

[25] Kalueff, A.V., Tuohimaa, P. 2004. Grooming analysis algorithm for neurobehavioural stress research. *Brain Res. Protocols*, 13, 151-158.

[26] Kalueff, A.V., Lou, Y.-R., Lakssi, I., Tuohimaa, P. 2004a. Increased grooming behavior in mice lacking Vitamin D receptors. *Physiol. Behav.*, 82, 405-409.

[27] Kalueff, A.V., Lou, Y.-R., Lakssi, I., Tuohimaa, P. 2004b. Increased anxiety in mice lacking Vitamin D receptor gene. *Neuroreport,* 15, 1271-1274.

[28] Kalueff, A.V., Lou, Y.-R., Lakssi, I., Tuohimaa, P. 2004c. Impaired motor performance in mice lacking neurosteroid Vitamin D receptors. *Brain Res. Bull.*, 64, 25-29.

[29] Kalueff, A.V., Lou, Y.-R., Lakssi, I., Tuohimaa, P. 2005. Abnormal behavioural organization of grooming in mice lacking Vitamin D receptor gene. *J. Neurogenet.*, 19, 1-24.

[30] Kamei, Y., Kawada, T., Fukuwatori, T., Ono, T., Kato, S., Sugimoto, E. 1995. Cloning and sequencing of the gene encoding the mouse vitamin D receptor. Gene, 152, 281-282.

[31] Kametani, H., Osada, H., Inoue, K. 1984. Increased novelty-induced grooming in aged rats: a preliminary observation. Behav. *Neural. Biol.*, 42, 73-80.

[32] Kato, S., Takeyama, K., Kitanaka, S., Murayama, A., Sekine, K., Yoshizawa, T. 1999. In vivo function of VDR in gene expression-VDR knock-out mice. J. Steroid Biochem. *Mol. Biol.*, 69, 247-251.

[33] Kruk, M.R., Westphal, K.G.C., Van Erp, A.M.M., Van Asperen, J, Cave, B.J., Slater, E., de Koning, J., Haller, J. 1998. The hypothalamus: cross-roads of endocrine and behavioral regulation of grooming and aggression. *Neurosci. Biobehav. Revs*, 23, 163-177.

[34] Langub, M.C., Herman, J.P., Malluche, H.H., Koszewski, N.J. 2001. Evidence of functional vitamin D receptors in rat hippocampus. *Neurosci.,* 104, 49-56.

[35] Li, Y.C., Pirro, A.E., Amling, M., Delling, G., Baron, R., Bronson, R., Demay, M.B. 1997. Targeted ablation of the vitamin D receptor: an animal model of vitamin D-dependent rickets type II with alopecia. *Proc. Natl. Acad. Sci.* USA, 94, 9831-9835.

[36] Malloy, P. J., Eccleshall, T. R., Gross, C., Van Maldergem, L., Bouillon, R., Feldman, D. 1997. Hereditary vitamin D resistant rickets caused by a novel mutation in the vitamin D receptor that results in decreased affinity for hormone and cellular hyporesponsiveness. *J. Clin. Invest.*, 99, 297-304.

[37] Malloy, P.J., Zhu, W., Bouillon, R., Feldman, D. 2002. A novel nonsense mutation in the ligand binding domain of the vitamin D receptor causes hereditary 1,25-dihydroxyvitamin D-resistant rickets. *Mol. Genet. Metab.*, 77, 314-318.

[38] Meyer-Luehmann, M., Thompson, J.F., Berridge, K.C., Aldridge, J.W. 2002. Substantia nigra pars reticulata neuron code initiation of a serial pattern: implications for natural action sequences and sequential disorders. *Eur. J. Neurosci.*, 16, 1599-1608.

[39] Ozer, S., Ulusahin, A., Ulusoy, S., Okur, H., Coskun, T., Tuncali, T., Gogus, A., Akarsu, A.N. 2004. Is vitamin D hypothesis for schizophrenia valid? Independent segregation of psychosis in a family with vitamin-D-dependent rickets type IIA. Progr. *Neuro-Psychopharm. Biol. Psych.*, 28, 255-266.

[40] Prufer, K., Veenstra, T.D., Jirikowski, G.F., Kumar, R. 1999. Distribution of 1,25-dihydroxyvitamin D3 receptor immunoreactivity in the rat brain and spinal cord. *J. Chem. Immunol.*, 16, 135-145.

[41] Sachs, B.D. 1988. The development of grooming and its expression in adult animals. *Ann. NY Acad. Sci.,* 525, 1-17.

[42] Strazielle, C., Lalonde, R. 1998. Grooming in Lurcher mutant mice. *Physiol. Behav.,* 64, 57-61.

[43] Van Erp, A.M., Kruk, M.R., Meelis, W., Willekens-Bramer, D.C. 1994. Effect of environmental stressors on time course, variability and form of self-grooming in the rat:

handling, social contact, defeat, novelty, restraint and fur moistening, *Behav. Brain Res.* 65, 47-55.

[44] Veenstra, T.D., Prufer, K., Koenigsberger, C., Brimijoin, S.W., Grande, J.P., Kumar, R. 1998. 1,25-Dihydrovitamin D_3 receptors in the central nervous system of the rat embryo. *Brain Res.*, 804, 193-205.

[45] Walbert, T., Jirikowski, G.F., Prufer, K. 2001. Distribution of 1,25-dihydroxyvitamin D3 receptor immunoreactivity in the limbic system. Horm. Metab. Res. 33, 525-531.

[46] Yamamoto, D., Nakano, Y. 1998. Genes for sexual behavior. *Biochem. Biophys. Res. Commun.,* 246, 1-6.

[47] Yoshizawa, T., Handa, Y., Uematsu, Y., Takeda, S., Sekine, K., Yoshihara, Y., Kawakami, T., Arioka, K., Sato, H., Uchiyama, Y., Masushige, S., Fukamizu, A., Matsumoto, T., Kato, S. 1997. Mice lacking the vitamin D receptor exibit impaired bone formation, uterine hypoplasia and growth retardation after weaning. *Nat. Genet.,* 16, 391-396.

In: Animal Models in Biological Psychiatry
Editor: Allan V. Kalueff, pp. 137-152
ISBN 1-59454-814-5

Chapter 8

Antibodies to S-100 Protein in Anxiety-Depressive Disorders in Experimental and Clinical Conditions

Tatiana A. Voronina, Svetlana A. Sergeeva, Andrey V. Martyushev-Poklad, Julia L. Dugina and Oleg I. Epstein
Materia Medica Holding, Research Department, Moscow, Russia

I. Introduction

Since the immune system actively interacts with the nervous and endocrine systems, substances with immunobiological profiles of action represent a new promising group of drugs. On one hand, the immune system's functions are under neuro-humoral control; on the other hand, antibodies to neuromediators, peptides and structural elements of brain exert influence upon the nervous system modulating functional characteristics of certain brain structures and cell ensembles contributing to pathogenesis (Ashmarin,1997; Kryzhanovskiy et al., 1997; Poletaev, 1995). Thus, antibodies should be regarded not only as a humoral component of the body's biological defense but also as important molecules of internal bioregulation.

Traumatic, inflammatory, psychic, neurological and somatic disorders, accompanied by impairment of the blood-brain barrier lead to appearance of circulating antibodies to neurospecific proteins, receptors and neuromediators. Interacting with their specific antigen targets, modifying or blocking them, these antibodies are capable of both impairing normal functioning of neurons (thus enhancing the existing disorders) or, quite the contrary, hinder the disease progression (Chekhonin et al., 2000; Asakura, Rodriguez, 1998). Therefore, appearance of high-affinity antibodies or elevation of their content in blood serum is regarded as diagnostic/prognostic markers of a number of diseases.

In the recent years, researchers have shown a growing interest in the family of brain-specific S100 proteins. This family comprises more than 20 members and is the largest subgroup of Ca^{2+}-binding proteins regulating functions of neuronal membranes, modulating intracellular processes, maintaining neurochemical balance and cerebral immune status (Heizmann, 2002).

Expression of S100 proteins changes with the onset of many diseases, such as neurodegenerative diseases, cancer, and cardiomyopathy. Therefore, S100 itself and specific antibodies to it are used as diagnostic markers in cardiac and brain hypoxia (Bottinger et al., 2001; Kiewitz et al., 2000; Missler et al., 1997), traumatic lesions of brain (Rommer et al., 2000), Alzheimer's disease and Down syndrome (Griffin et al., 1998; Yu, Frazer, 2001), epilepsy (Griffin et al., 1995), schizophrenia (Gattaz et al., 2000) and metastatic cancer (Platt-Higgins et al., 2000).

S100 proteins are important regulators of brain activity (Shtark, 1985; Barraclough, 1998) including generation and conduction of nerve impulse and synaptic transmission. Enhanced S100 expression in the brain results in hyperactivity as well as impaired hippocampal functions, learning and memory.

Some members of this family (e.g., S100B and S100A12) are secreted from cells and produce extracellular cytokine-like effect. These proteins trigger the cascade of signaling mechanisms via various routes including binding to recently discovered superficial RAGE receptors (receptor for advanced glycation end product) (Hofmann et al., 1999; Schmidt et al., 2000). Proproten consists of affinely purified antibodies (at ultra-low doses) to brain-specific protein S100 (Epstein et al., 1998). Since antibodies to pro-inflammatory cytokines, such as tumor necrosis factor (TNF)-α and γ-interferon, are efficient upon parenteral administration in the treatment of certain autoimmune disorders (e.g., rheumatoid arthritis, Crohn's disease, etc.), a similar same mechanism of action may be suggested for proproten.

However, ultra-low doses of antibodies to neuromediators, peptides and structural elements of the brain may have their own peculiar profiles of activity. Contrary to the classic immunological phenomena (antibody-induced suppression of the activity of endogenous regulators), the ultra-low doses of antibodies may specifically modulate and catalyze the activity of these molecules via modifying the system of natural antibodies to their particular regulators (Epstein, 1999). Thus, subtle targeted influences may be exerted via the immune system, targeting the impaired internal regulation of the pathological process. Thereupon it may be suggested that proproten produces restoring effect upon pathologically impaired functions of the S100 protein. Given the key role of S100 in the generation and conduction of nerve impulse, synaptic transmission and neurodegenerative processes, this study assessed the effect of proproten on stress-mediated functional disorders of the central nervous system, such as anxiety and depression.

II. Experimental Studies

Animals

Male outbred albino rats weighting 230-250 g (Stolbovaya Farm, RAMS, Moscow, Russia) were used in the experiments.

Preparations

Potentiated antibodies to the brain-specific protein S100 (Proproten, Materia Medica Holding, Russia) were administered at 2.5 ml/kg (0.25 ml/100 g body weight). Diazepam (2 mg/kg), amitriptyline (10 mg/kg) and mexidol (100 mg/kg) were used as reference drugs; control rats received distilled water. The substances were administered per os: a single dose 30 min. prior to testing or for 5 days (twice a day, at 9.00 and 18.00 h). In order to block gamma-aminobutyric acid (GABA) A-type receptors, a GABA-A receptor antagonist bicucullin (ICN Biomedicals Inc., USA; 1 mg/kg) was administered intraperitoneally (i.p.). To block Cl^-channel of GABA-benzodiazepine receptor complex, the channel blocker picrotoxin (ICN Biomedicals Inc., USA, 1 mg/kg i.p.) was used here.

Behavioural Tests

Conflict Test

The model (rev.: Voronina, Seredenin, 2000; Molodavkin, Voronina, 1995; Sanger, 1991; Triet, 1985; Vogel et al., 1971) is based on conflict between two motivations: drinking motivation and defense reaction, when each attempt of an animal to take water was punished by painful electric stimulation. For this, rats were water-deprived and a habit of taking water from a special bowl was developed. On Day 3, 10 sec after the first water intake, a continuous 0.2-mA current was put through the electrode floor of their chamber (punished water intake). The number of punished water intakes was registered for 10 min.

The elevated plus maze (Voronina, Seredenin, 2000; Dawson, Tricklebank, 1995; File, 1995; Pellow, File, 1986)

This is based on the fear of open space and height. The maze consists of 4 arms fixed at right angles. Two opposite arms are closed and the other two are open. The maze was elevated 50 cm off the floor. The animals were placed on the central section of the maze and their behavior was monitored for 3 min. Latency to the first entry into the open arms (open entry), the number of complete and incomplete entries and their duration, number of leanings over the edges of the open arms of the maze, the number of fecal boli and urination episodes were registered in this study.

Emotional stress in the open field test

This was induced by placing an animal into the center of an open brightly lit square arena (1 x 1m) for 3 min. The number of squares crossed (horizontal activity), vertical rears (vertical activity), entries into the center of the arena, hole exploration (exploratory activity) and grooming or combing episodes were registered. Animals' activity was monitored using a Pentium 200 MMX computer and special software.

Behavioral Despair/Helplessness (Porsolt et al., 1978).

A rat was placed into a cylinder-shaped tank 40-cm in diameter filled with water (25° C; 60 cm deep). The duration of immobility episodes for 10 min. reflected the severity of depression (antidepressants generally shorten this measure).

Forced SwimmingiIn a Tank with Freely Revolving Wheels

The Nomura's test, see (Molodavkin et al., 1994; Nomura et al., 1982) for details, consists of a tank 64 x 30 x 42 cm, subdivided into 4 equal compartments, in which the wheels were placed. The tank was filled with water (25°C) up to the middle of the wheels. The rats were placed into the tank (one into each compartment, snouts away from the wheel). The number of revolutions was registered using electromechanical counters for 10 min.

Statistical data analysis was performed using Mann-Whitney U- and Student's t-tests ($P < 0.05$).

Results

Anxiolytic Effect of Proproten on Punished Drinking in the Conflict Test

On the day of the experiment, a rat of the control group (when placed into the conflict test chamber) usually starts drinking from the bowls as it used to do before, but after an electric shock it jumps away from the water bowl and the number of its attempts to drink decreases dramatically. The average number of punished water intakes in control animals within 10 min. of observation was 303.7 (Table 1). Proproten (2.5 ml/kg) in the conflict test produced a marked anxiolytic effect, significantly increasing the number of punished water intakes compared to the control group (Fig.1). Diazepam at 2 mg/kg produced similar effects, markedly increasing the number of punished water intakes. Anxiolytic effect of a chronic (5-day) treatment with proproten was similar to the effect of diazepam.

Administration of bicucullin, a GABA-A receptor blocker, or picrotoxin, a Cl^- channel blocker, produced proconflict anxiogenic effect, reducing the number of punished responses (1.6 and 1.8-fold, respectively) vs. the control animals (Fig. 1). Combined administration of proproten and bicucullin inhibited anti-conflict effect of proproten, reducing the number of punished water intakes (1.76-fold) compared proproten alone. The effect of bicucullin on anxiolytic properties of diazepam and mexidol was similar, markedly reducing the number of punished water intakes in the conflict test. Finally, combined administration of picrotoxin with proproten, diazepam or mexidol also lowered the number of punished water intakes, clearly antagonizing anxiolytic properties of the drugs (Fig. 1).

Anxiolytic effect of proproten in the elevated plus maze

Overall, the behavior of control animals in the elevated plus maze was characterized by fewer open entries, shorter open time spent, and fewer leaning from the edges. In addition, high levels of the plus-maze anxiety in the control group was seen, as assessed by increased number of fecal boli and urinations.

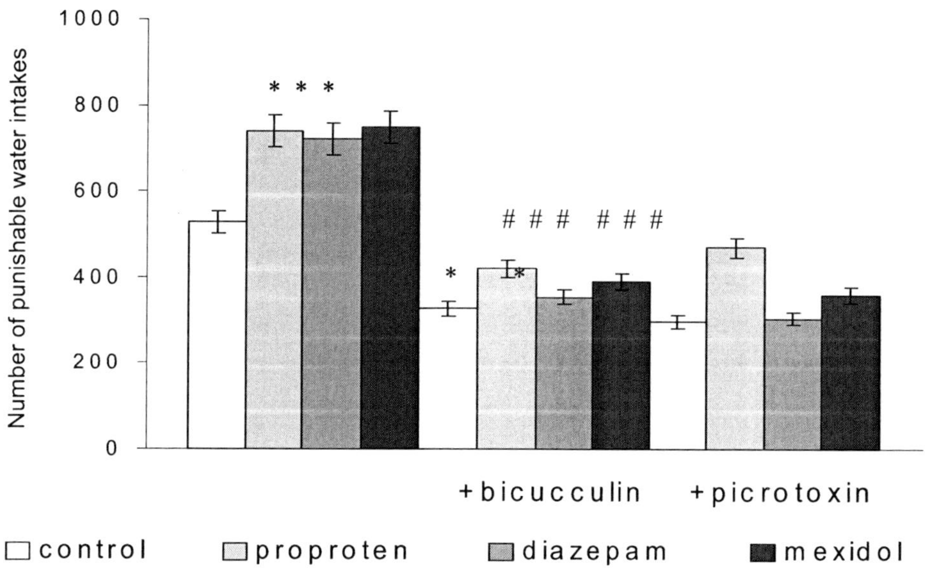

Figure 1. Effects of antagonists of the GABA-A-benzodiazepine receptor complex on anxiolytic effect of proproten, diazepam and mexidol. * P<0.5: vs. controls; # P < 0.05 vs. single proproten, diazepam or mexidol

Table 1. Anxiolytic effects of proproten in the elevated plus maze. * P <0.05 vs. controls

Indices of behavior	Control	Proproten 2.5 ml/kg	Diazepam 2 mg/kg
Number of open entries	1.1 ± 0.55	2.1 ± 0.42*	2.6 ± 0.8*
Time spent in the open arms	12.1 ± 3.15	65.41 ± 27.46*	85.25 ± 38.51*
Number of incomplete entries	0.7 ± 0.43	65.41 ± 27.46*	85.25 ± 38.51*
Number of leanings-over	0.5 ± 0.13	2.44 ± 0.95*	4.5 ± 1.12*
Number of closed entries	2.8 ± 0.65	2.3 ± 0.48	1.5 ±0.8
Number of fecal boli	5.2 ± 1.9	1.2 ± 0.8	1.4 ± 0.6
Number of urination episodes	3.7 ± 0.8	0.8 ± 0.5	1.1 ± 0.7

In contrast, following administration of proproten, the rats displayed more open entries (1.9-fold) and open time spent (5.4-fold) compared to their controls. As can be seen in Table 1, the proproten-treated rats also more frequently (4.8-fold) leaned from the edges of the open arms of the maze, and showed a significant decrease in the number of fecal boli and urinations. The effect of diazepam was similar to that of proproten but was more robust, increasing open entries 2.3-fold and open time spent 7-fold (Table 1).

Anxiolytic Effect of Proproten in the Open Field Test

Table 2 shows that proproten did not alter horizontal and vertical motor activity in the open field in all groups tested. At the same time, in contrast to the control group, migration of animals into the center of the lit arena was observed following proproten and diazepam treatment, indicating reduced anxiety of these animals. Moreover, diazepam but not proproten produced a distinct sedative effect as assessed by robust and significant decrease of horizontal activity (Table 2).

Table 2. Effect of proproten on behavior of rats in the open field test. * P <0.05 vs. controls

Substances	Doses	Horizontal activity	Vertical activity	Exploratory activity	Entries to the center
Control	-	18.2 ± 2.4	8.2 ± 3.3	11.1 ± 3.1	0 ± 0
Proproten	2.5 ml/kg	15.8 ± 2.1	5.8 ± 2.6	8.9 ± 1.6	2.4 ± 0.7 *
Diazepam	2 mg/kg	12.5 ± 1.8 *	6.2 ± 1.4	8.7 ± 1.5	1.8 ± 0.9 *

Antidepressant Effect of Proproten in Behavioral Despair/Helplessness Test

In this test, the control animals first make attempts to escape from the aversive situation, and later hang immobile in the water performing only small movements necessary to keep their snouts above the water. The onset of the immobility reflects the animals' helplessness (depressiveness) (Fig. 2).

Single administration of proproten (2.5 ml/kg) produced a distinct antidepressant effect in this test (Fig. 2), including statistically significant 1.6-fold shortening of the immobility (vs. control rats). Standard antidepressant amitriptyline at 10 mg/kg produced a similar effect, almost twice shortening the immobility duration (Fig. 2).

Repeated administration of proproten and amitriptyline for 5 days also resulted in a marked antidepressant effect in this test, significantly shortening the immobility duration.

However, amitriptyline, in contrast to proproten, produced a distinct sedative effect manifest in significant decrease of motor activity.

In another modification of this test (the Nomura's model), control rats, when placed in the tank with wheels, first try to get out of the water. However, as the wheels revolve freely, these attempts become unsuccessful, and the animals soon give up their efforts and hang in the water, indicating the onset of despair (depression). A single administration of proproten at 2.5 ml/kg reduced animal despair, enabling the animals to turn the wheels more energetically, almost twice increasing the number of the revolutions of the wheels. Amitriptyline at 10 mg/kg produced similar effects, enhancing the rats' activity in this test (Table 3).

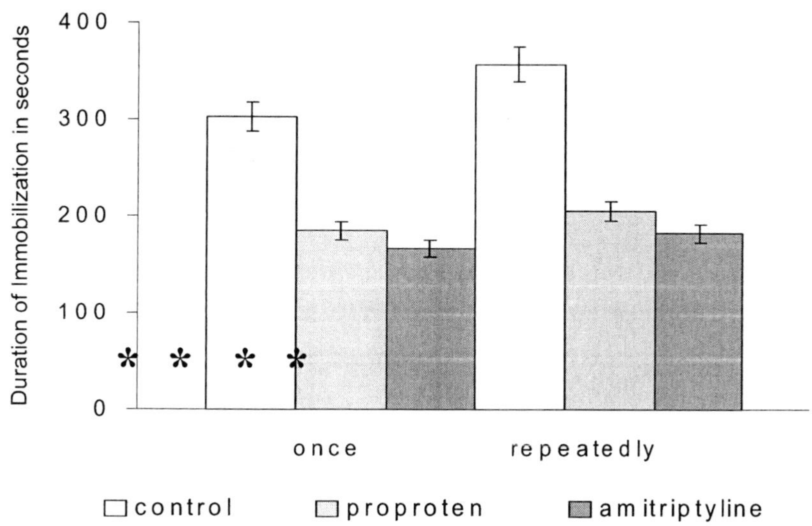

Figure 2. Effect of proproten (single and repeated administration) on duration of immobility in Porsolt's behavioral despair (helplessness) forced swimming test. * $P<0.05$

Table 3. Antidepressant effect of proproten in the Nomura's test. * $P<0.05$ vs. controls

Substance	Dose	Wheel revolutions per 10 min.		
Control	0 ml/kg	64.7	±	15.9 (100%)
Proproten	2.5 ml/kg	118.3	±	27.4 * (180%)
Amitriptyline	10 mg/kg	115.1	±	24.6 * (177%)

Antistress Effects of Proproten in Animals with Various Types of Individual Reaction to Stress

The experiment consisted of two phases. First, the type of individual reactivity was determined in the forced swimming test with freely revolving wheels. After this, the animals' behavior was assessed in the conflict test. In the present study, 24 animals (of 100) were found to be highly active at >80 wheel revolutions, whereas 28 animals showed low activity at <40 revolutions. 48 rats (40-80 revolutions) were regarded as moderately active in this study.

The second phase of the study investigated anxiolytic effects of proproten in high- and low-activity rat groups in the conflict test. Overall, control high-activity animals (selected in the Nomura's test by the number of wheel revolutions) also demonstrated higher activity in the conflict test. In contrast, low-activity rats were inactive in the conflict test. In control high-activity animals, the number of punished water intakes was 498.5, and in low-activity rats – 112.7.

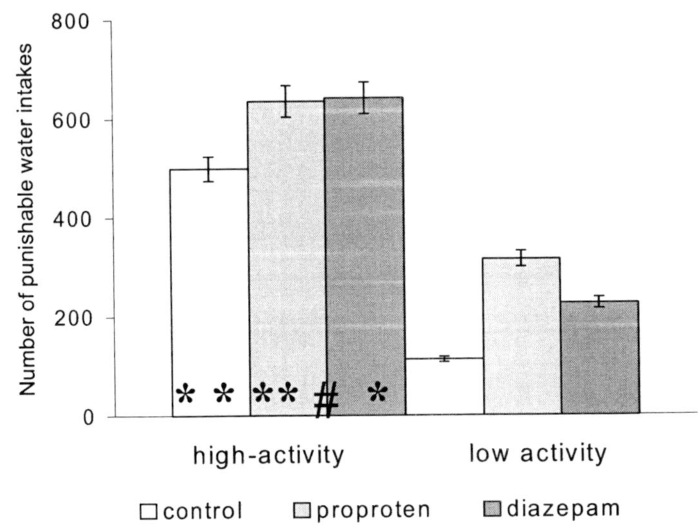

Figure 3. Anxiolytic effect of proproten in the high-activity and the low-activity rats in the conflict test: * $P < 0.05$ vs. controls; ** high- vs. low-activity groups; # proproten vs. diazepam

Our results show that anxiolytic effect of proproten in the low-activity rats was much more pronounced than in the high-activity animals. Indeed, the number of punished water intakes in low-activity proproten-treated rats increased 2.8-fold, showing only 1.3-fold increase in the high-activity group. Anxiolytic effect of diazepam was less pronounced in the low-activity group than that of proproten, producing only 2-fold increase in punished water intakes (Fig. 3).

Taken together, our findings show clear anxiolytic effects of proproten in various behavioural tests including conflict test, the elevated plus maze and the open field tests. Proproten was as effective as diazepam in all these tests. Bicucullin-induced blockage of GABA-A receptor and picrotoxin-induced blockage of the Cl- channel at GABA-A receptor significantly impeded anti-conflict effect of proproten and diazepam, suggesting that these subunits of GABA-benzodiazepine/Cl-ionophore receptor complex may be involved in anxiolytic effects of these drugs.

At the same time, some significant differences were observed between anxiolytic effects of proproten and diazepam, since in the low-activity rats (with aesthetic type of behavior)

proproten was highly effective, whereas diazepam had only mild effects. These results indicate that proproten possesses antiasthenic stimulating effect, compared to diazepam (whose anxiolytic effect is combined with sedation). Proproten, unlike diazepam, possesses neither muscle relaxant effect nor negative influence upon memory.

Anxiolytic and antiasthenic effect of proproten is combined with pronounced antidepressant effects in the behavioral despair and the revolving wheels tests. Notably, proproten shows antidepressant activity similar to the well-known reference antidepressant drug amitriptyline. However, the advantage of proproten over amitriptyline is its ability to preserve individual and adequate behavior patterns in animals in stressful situation and the lack of behavioural sedation.

III. Antidepressant and Anxiolytic Effects of Proproten

Proproten is used in clinical practice to treat alcohol withdrawal syndrome (AWS) and alcoholism. Clinical studies have demonstrated that this drug arrests the key somatovegetative and psychopathological disorders, suppresses pathological craving for alcohol, and can be used as a monotherapy. Moreover, in many patients proproten decreases anxiety, worries and stress (Alexandrova et al., 1999; Gofman et al., 2000, 2002, 2003).

A double blind placebo-controlled clinical study to assess the effects of proproten on AWS in patients with marked depressive and anxiety disorders has been carried out in parallel with open comparative clinical study of proproten, phenazepam and amitriptyline in AWS. The study was carried out on 256 patients (grade II of alcohol-dependence) suffering from AWS. The first (background) testing was performed prior to therapy. Subsequently, the patients were monitored daily during the whole period of AWS. For data standardization, the individual assessment cards were used to register the core symptoms of AWS according to the 3-point scale. Proproten or placebo was administered sublingually (1 tablet per intake). The first 5 doses were administered hourly, then every 2-3 h. After 5-6 h treatment, 87 patients responded to therapy and 85 failed to respond (corresponding exactly to the proproten and placebo groups of the study). Later on, the responsive patients continued to receive proproten monotherapy, whereas irresponsive patients received additional detoxication and general restorative therapy. From the second day of the study, irresponsive patients were regarded as the control group. Amitriptyline (75 mg) and phenazepam (2 mg) were administered daily. Both drugs were combined with standard detoxication therapy.

Pathological craving for alcohol, depressive and somato-vegetative symptoms, anxiety and insomnia subsided rapidly in the proproten-treated group. Comparison of the effects of proproten, phenazepam, amitriptyline, detoxication and general restorative therapy revealed their selective action on specific AWS symptoms (Table 4). All treatments arrested craving for alcohol faster compared to detoxication therapy. In the phenazepam- and proproten-treated groups, anxiety subsided faster than in the control group. Depressive and somato-vegetative disorders subsided faster in patients treated with proproten. Rapid normalization of sleep was observed in the patients treated with phenazepam ($P<0.001$). Improvement of sleep was also registered in the group of patients treated with proproten (P<0.05). In contrast, amitriptyline demonstrated rather low efficiency to affect AWS.

The results of our double-blind placebo-controlled clinical study revealed highly significant proproten-induced reduction in the number of patients craving, lowered anxiety and depression scores and somato-vegetative symptoms by the second day of the study. Among the patients with anxiety depression, the number of subjects responsive to proproten exceeded 50% on the second day of study, indicating a robust therapeutic effect.

Anxiolytic effects of proproten were also studied in patients with cardio-vascular disorders at the Cardiology Unit of Voronezh Regional Hospital (Volodina et al., 2002). 12 patients aged 24-65, suffering from cardio-vascular diseases (essential hypertension, ischemic heart disease or both) with excessive anxiety received proproten (1 tablet daily) in addition to conventional therapy for 2 weeks. 12 "control" patients were treated with conventional medications. Severity of anxiety manifestations was assessed (using a 5-point scale: 0-4) before and after 2-week therapy. In addition, Hamilton's scale (14 pp) was used in the present study. Initial score of anxiety in both groups of patients was 25.

Table 4. Average duration of psychopathologic and somatic and vegetative disorders in patients having alcoholic abstinence syndrome after treatment with proproten, amitriptyline and phenazepam. *P<0.05, **P<0.01 vs. placebo

Symptoms	Placebo	Proproten	Ami-triptyline	Phena-zepam
Craving for alcohol	2.7±0.12	1.9±0.09*	2.0±0.25*	2.1±0.29
Anxiety	2.4±0.15	1.9±0.11*	2.5±0.22	1.6±0.09*
Depression	3.5±0.17	1.9±0.14**	3.7±0.42	3.6±0.29
Sleep disorders	3.2±0.11	2.6±0.13*	3.1±0.35	1.4±0.09**
Somatic/vegetative disorders	3.4±0.13	2.9±0.17*	4.9±0.53	4.1±0.32
Total number of patients	85	87	34	50

Following proproten treatment, anxiety-like symptoms (anxious expectations, irritability, inability to concentrate, rigid muscles, hyperemia, paleness, weakness, etc.) subsided considerably. Sleep and sweat secretion returned to the normal levels, heart palpitation occurred less frequently, vision became less blurred, while mouth dryness, paresthesias and tinnitus disappeared. In the proproten-treated group, the average score of anxiety reduced 2.4-fold, reaching 10.5 pp (vs. 1.7-fold reduction, 14.4pp in the control group). In patients receiving background proproten treatment, anxiolytic effects were significantly more pronounced than in patients receiving only conventional therapy.

Thus, both a double blind placebo-controlled study and an open comparative clinical study of AWS patients demonstrated antidepressant, anxiolytic, hypnotic and vegetostabilizing effects of proproten. It has been found that antidepressant effect of proproten significantly (p<0.001) surpasses thymoleptic effect of amitriptyline, whereas anxiolytic effect of proproten does not yield to that of phenazepam. At the same time, proproten significantly reduces anxiety symptoms in patients with cardiovascular diseases as assessed by Hamilton's scale (anxious mood, feeling of strain, insomnia, somatic, sensory and vegetative disorders). In addition, no sedative or other side effects of proproten were registered in this study.

In 2005, a new drug based on anti-S100 antibodies - "Tenoten" - was approved in Russia as an anti-anxiety medication. Its efficacy and safety was studied in 2003-2004 in a multicenter open-label controlled randomised trial performed in 4 clinical centres in Moscow and St-Petersburg (Martyushev-Poklad et al., 2005). Patients meeting ICD-10 criteria for generalized anxiety disorder, mixed anxiety and depressive disorder, adjustment disorders with anxiety, or neurasthenia, and presenting with moderate to severe anxiety (total score of Hamilton anxiety scale, HAM-A, >=20) were randomised to receive tenoten (anti-S100 antibodies, ultra-low doses for oral use) – 10 orally disintegrating tablets/day (n=127), or diazepam – 15 mg/day (n=120) for 4 weeks. After 7, 14, and 28 days of treatment the patients were interviewed to assess the level of anxiety (by HAM-A and State-Trait Anxiety Inventory) and the safety (by structured scale of adverse events). Although diazepam provided more rapid and statistically significant reduction of anxiety (Table 5), the benefit/risk ratio for tenoten was undoubtedly superior. The new oral antibody drug neither caused sleepiness nor affected performance in any way, which is important for a daytime tranquilizer. Tenoten was completely equivalent to diazepam (with regard to efficacy) in the subgroups of patients with generalized anxiety disorder and with severe anxiety (baseline HAM-A >=30).

Table 5. Efficacy and safety of tenoten versus diazepam in 4-week treatment of anxiety

Endpoints	Diazepam 15 mg (n=120)	Tenoten (n=127)
Baseline total HAM-A score	28.6±0.5	27.4±0.5*
Total HAM-A score after week 4	11.0±0.6	12.1±0.5*
Proportion of patients with positive response at week 4 (>=50% improvement of total HAM-A)	78.3%	69.3%*
Proportion of patients with any adverse event	39.2%	5.6%*
Number of adverse events per 100 patients	299.2	20.4*

* - difference from diazepam group statistically significant at $p<0.05$

These findings suggest that the drug can become a good alternative for benzodiazepines in short-term treatment of anxiety. A long-term study is planned to assess the efficacy of tenoten in establishing remission in anxiety disorders.

Interestingly, the clinical anxiolytic and antidepressant effects of oral anti-S100 drugs agree very well with earlier experimental findings. Therefore, neuroprotective effects of anti-S100 revealed in animals (Romanova et al., 2005) can translate into drug's clinical efficacy in ischemic stroke, and positive experimental effects on cognition revealed in scopolamine-induced amnesia (Voronina T.A., unpublished data), may appear beneficial in the treatment of dementias.

IV. General Discussion

The results obtained here show that proproten may be an efficient neuropsychotropic medicine with antistress, anxiolytic, antiasthenic and antidepressant effects devoid of side-effects of conventional therapy. The unusual profile of psychotropic effects of proproten suggests its unique mechanism(s) of action.

For example, it is well known that conventional benzodiazepine and non-benzodiazepine tranquilizers target the limbic brain structures, hypothalamus and cortex, controlling impulse-mediated prolonged activation of neurons. Thus, excitability thresholds of the hippocampus and the amygdala are modified by tranquillizers (Alexandrovskiy, 2000; Voronina, Seredenin, 2002). It has been shown that proproten exerts marked influence on these brain structures. Proproten reduces the frequency of self-stimulation of lateral hypothalamus and inhibits neuronal activity of the limbic structures (Shtark et al., 2000; Epstein, 1999; Epstein et al., 1999b). Thus, it is possible to suggest that proproten may target the same brain structures affected by the conventional anxiolytic drugs.

Moreover, neurochemical mechanism of action of benzodiazepine tranquillizers (e.g., diazepam) is based on their ability to bind directly to benzodiazepine receptor and alter the conformation of GABA-A receptor. This increases the frequency and duration of chloride channel opening, which in turn lowers neuronal excitability and alters synaptic transmission (Alexandrovskiy, 2000; Voronina, Seredenin 2002). However, the effect of many novel anxiolytic drugs is not based on direct interaction with the receptor. For example, mexidol is a membrane modulator of the GABA-A-benzodiazepine receptor complex, exerting its targeted regulation via membrane-receptor interaction, and strengthening the bond of direct agonists with the receptors (Voronina 2001).

The ability of bicucullin and picrotoxin to reduce psychotropic effects of proproten suggests that GABA-benzodiazepine Cl^--ionophore complex is involved in the effects of proproten. However, it has been shown earlier that proproten possesses a distinct membranotropic effect. Experiments on giant neurons of snails have shown that proproten induces membrane depolarization, lowers the amplitude, suppresses generation of action potential and reduces maximal conductibility (Epstein et al. 1999c). Given these membranotropic properties, it is possible to hypothesize that proproten may affects membrane mechanisms related to GABA-A receptors.

Notably, proproten consists of ultra-low doses of antibodies to brain-specific protein S100, regulating key brain functions such as generation and conduction of nervous impulse (Heizmann et al., 2002; Barraclough, 1998). As a Ca^{++}-binding protein, S100 secures long-term potentiation (LTP), which is of critical importance for synaptic processes. It has been shown that proproten modifies inhibitory effects of native anti-S100 serum on LTP in hippocampal slices (Epstein, 1999; Epstein et al., 1999a), indicating the possibility of proproten's influence on synaptic processes.

It may also be suggested that actions or proptoten are based on subtle targeted influence on the functions of S100 protein via the immune system. For example, contrary to the classical antibody-induced suppression of activity of endogenous regulators, proproten (containing ultra-low doses of antibodies) may specifically modulate and catalyze the activity of such target molecules (such as S100 protein). This may occur via modifying the system of natural antibodies to this particular regulator. One of the evidences in favor of this mechanism is the effect of proproten on LTP. Indeed, as already mentioned, S100 proteins take part in LTP, native anti-S100 serum suppresses LTP in microscopic sections of hippocampus (Lewis, Teyler, 1986) and proproten clearly modifies this effect. Further experimental studies are necessary to analyze these interesting properties of proproten.

In conclusion, here we show that proproten may represent an efficient neuropsychotropic agent with anxiolytic and antidepressant effects devoid of side effects of conventional medications. Our data suggest that the mechanisms of its anxiolytic effects are associated with its ability to modify functional activity of brain-specific protein S100 and affect the synaptic transmission in the brain limbic structures via modulation of membrane-receptor interaction, especially targeting GABA-A receptor complex.

References

[1] Alexandrova N.V., Gofman A.G., Krylov Ye.N., Epstein O.I. (1999). Experience of using potentiated preparations for arresting the abstinence syndrome and opium anstinence syndrome. Bull. Sib. Branch RAMS, 1, 95-99.

[2] Alexandrovsky Yu.A. (2000). The border-line mental disorders, Med., Moscow, 345 p.

[3] Ashmarin I.P. (1997). Autoantibodies as regulators of biochemical and physiological processes in the healthy organism. *J. Evol. Biochem. Physiol.*, 33, 228-233.

[4] Borovikov V.P. (2001). Statistics: The art of analyzing data on computer for professional. - St. Petersburg, Piter, 241p.

[5] Voronina T.A., Seredenin S.B. (2000). Methodological guidelines on investigation of tranquilizing (anxiolytic) effect of pharmacological substances. A manual in experimental (pre-clinical) study of new pharmacological substances. Remedium, Moscow, 126-130.

[6] Voronina T.A., Seredenin S.B. (2002). Anxiolytics. Present-day situation and prospects for search. Problem article. *Exp. Clin. Farmacol.*, 65, 3-10.

[7] Voronina T.A. (2001). Antioxidant mexidol. Main neuropsychotropic effects and mechanism of action. *Psychopharmacol. Biol. Narcol.*, 1, 2-12.

[8] Gofman A.G., Krylov Ye.N., Grazhensky A.V. et al. (2000). Use of the preparation Proproten100 for arrest of alcoholic abstinence syndrome. Proc. 13th Conf. *Russ. Psych.*, 236.

[9] Gofman A.G., Krylov Ye.N., Grazhensky A.V. et al. (2002). The adequacy of using of the preparation Proproten-100 for arrest of alcoholic abstinence syndrome. *New drugs: Expr. Inform.*, 2, 53-58.

[10] Gofman A.G., Pyatnitskaya I.N., Valentik Y.V., Krylov E.N., Epstein O.I. (2003). Proproten-100 in the therapy of patients with the alcohol withdrawal syndrome. Bull. Exp. Biol. Med. 135, *Suppl 1,* 167-170.

[11] Kryzhanovsky G.N., Magayeva S.V., Makarov S.V. (1997). *Neuroimmunopathology,* Moscow, 283 p.

[12] Martyushev-Poklad A., Dugina J., Epstein O., Sergeeva S. (2005). A Novel antibody anxiolytic: Results of short controlled clinical trials. Proc. XIIIth *World Congr. Psychiatry*, Cairo, Egypt, 432.

[13] Molodavkin G.M., Voronina T.A., Mdzinarishvili A.L. (1994). Peculiarities of the effect of pharmacological substances of different classes on forced swimming in rats. *Exp. Clin. Farmacol.*, 57, 3-5.

[14] Molodavkin G.M., Voronina T.A. (1995). Multi-channel unit for search of tranquilizers and study of mechanisms of their action according to the method of conflict situation. *Exper. Clin. Farmacol.*, 58, 54-56.

[15] Poletayev A.B. (1995). Monoclonal antibodies in neurobiology (Eds: Shtark M.B., Starostina M.V.), *Novosibirsk*, p.36-45.

[16] Romanova G.A., Voronina T.A., Dugina Y.L., Martyushev-Poklad A.V., Sergeeva S.A., Epstein O.I., Barskov I.V. (2005). Neuroprotective activity of proproten in rats with experimental local photothrombosis of the prefrontal cortex. *Bull. Exp. Biol. Med.* 139(4), 404-407.

[17] Starostina M.V., Shtark M.B. et al., (2002). Effects of small doses of antibodies and synaptic plasticity. *Ibid.,* 30-41.

[18] Chekhonin V.P., Dmitriyeva T.B., Zhukov Yu.A. (2000). Immunochemical analysis of neurospecific antigens. Moscow, *Medicina*, 416 p.

[19] Shtark M.B. (1985) Brain-specific proteins (antigens) and functions of the neuron, *Novosibirsk*, 313 p.

[20] Shtark M.B., Beregovoy N.A., Starostina M.V. et al. (2000). Basic mechanisms of therapy of mental disorders with ultra-low doses of antibodies to the brain-specific Protein-100 (the preparation Proproten-100). *Proc. 13th Conf. Russ. Psych.*, 374.

[21] Shtark M.B., Epstein O.I., Komarov Ye.V. (2002). Ultra-low doses of antibodies to neurospecific substances as a new class of psychotropic preparations. In: Proproten-100. Moscow, *MSUL*, p.124 –127.

[22] Epstein O.I. (1999). Possible mechanisms of the effect of potentiated medicines and some problems of biological systems function. *Bull. Sib. Branch RAMS*, 1, 132-149.

[23] Epstein O.I., Beregovoy N.A., Sorokina N.S., Starostina M.V., Shtark M.B. (1999a). Effect of different dilutions of potentiated antibodies to the brain-specific protein S-100 on dynamics of post-tetanic potentiations in surviving hippocampus slices. *Bull. Exp. Biol. Med.*, 127, 317-320.

[24] Epstein O.I., Vorobyova T.V., Berchenko O.G., et al. (1999b). Effect of potentiated form of antibodies to the brain-specific protein S-100 on integrative activity of brain. *Bull. Exper. Biol. Med.*, 5, 547-549.

[25] Epstein O.I., Gainutdinov Kh.L., Shtark M.B. (1999c). Effect of homeopathic doses of antibodies to the antigen S-100 on electric characteristics of neuronal membranes. *Bull. Exp. Biol. Med.,* 4, 466-477.

[26] Epstein O.I., Voronina T.A., Molodavkin G.M., Sergeyeva S.A. (2002). Proc. 1st Int. Symp. Stress Extr. Cond., *Kara-Dag,* 90-91.

[27] Epstein O.I., Komarov Ye.V. (2000) Use of ultra-low doses of substances of endogenous origin in clinic in case of alcoholic dependence. IV Int. Conf. Act. Probl. New Med. *Prep. Nat. Orig.*, Veliky Novgorod, 254-258.

[28] Asakura R., Rodriguez M. (1998). A unique population of circulating autoantibodies promotes central nervous system remyelination. *Mult. Scler.* 4(3), 217-221.

[29] Barraclough R. (1998) Calcium-binding protein S-100A4 in health and disease. *Biochem. Biophys. Acta.*, 1448, 190-199.

[30] Bottinger B.W., Mobes S., Glatzer R. et al., (2001). Astroglial protein S100 is an early and sensitive marker of hypoxic brain damage and outcome aftter cardiac arrest in humans. *Circulation*, 103, 2694-2698.

[31] Dawson G.R., Tricklebank M.D. (1995). Use of the elevated plus-maze in the search for novel anxiolytic agents, *Tr. Pharmacol. Sci.*, 16, 33-36.

[32] File S.E. (1995). Animal models of different anxiety states., In: GABAa receptors and anxiety: from neurobiology to treatment., N.Y. *Raven Press*, p.93-113.

[33] Gattaz W.F., Lara D.R., Elkis H., et al. (2000) Decreased S100B protein in schizophrenia: preliminary evidens. *Schizophr. Res.*, 43, 91-95.

[34] Gofman A.G., Grazhenskiy A.V., Krylov E.N., et al. (2002) Proproten-100 in arresting alcohol abstinence syndrome. In: Proproten-100. Materia Medica Holding, Moscow, p.117-121.

[35] Griffin W.S.T., Stanley L.C., Ling C., et al. (1998) Brain interleukin 1 and S-100 immunoreactivity are elevated in Down syndrom and Alzheimer disease. *Proc. Natl. Acad. Sci.* USA, 86, 7611-7615.

[36] Griffin W.S.T., Yerelan O., Sheng F.A., et al. (1995). Overexpression of the neuritrophic cytokine S100B in human temporal lobe epilepsy. *J. Neurochem.,* 65, 228-233.

[37] Heizmann C.W., Fritz G., Schafer B.W. (2002). S100 proteins: structure, functions and pathology. *Frontiers Biosci.*, 7, 1356-1368.

[38] Hofmann M.A., Drury S., Fu C., et al. (1999). RAGE mediates a novel proinflammatory axis: a central cell surface receptor for S100/calgranulin polypeptides. *Cell*, 97, 889-901.

[39] Kiewitz R., Acklin C., Minder E., Huber P.R., et al. (2000). S100A1, a new marker for acute myocardial ischemia. *Biochem. Biophys. Res. Comm.*, 274, 865-871.

[40] Lewis D., Teyler T.J. (1986). Anti-S-100 serum blocks long-term potentiation in hippocampal slice. *Brain Res.*, 383, 159-164.

[41] Missler U., Weismann M., Fredericch C., Kaps M. (1997). S-100 Protein and neuron-specific enolase concentrations in blood as indicators of infarction volume and prognosis in acute ischemic stroke. *Stroke*, 28, 1956-1960.

[42] Nomura S., Shimizu J., Kinjo M. et al. (1982). A new behavioral test for antidepressant drugs. *Eur. J. Pharm.*, 83, 171-175.

[43] Pellow S. and File S.E. (1986). Anxiolytic and anxiogenic drugs effects on exploratory activity in an elevated plus-maze. A novel test of anxiety in the rat. *Pharm. Biochem. Behav.*, 24, 525–529.

[44] Platt-Higgins A.M., Renshaw Ch. A., West Ch.R., et al. (2000) Comparison of the metastasis-inducing protein S100A4 (p9Ka) with other prognostic markers in human breast cancer. *Int. J. Cancer*, 89, 198-208.

[45] Porsolt R.D., Anton G., Blavet N. et al. (1978). Behavioral despair in rats: a new model sensitive to antidepressant treatment. *Eur. J. Pharm.*, 47, 379-391.

[46] Rommer B., Ingebritsen T., Kongstad P., Borgsen S.E. (2000). Traumatic brain damage: serum S-100 protein measurements related to neuroradiological findings. *J. Neurotrauma,* 17, 641-647.

[47] Sanger D.J., Perrault G., Morel E., et al. (1991). Animal models and recent developments in the search for novel anxiolytics. In: Animal Models in Psychopharmacology., *Adv. Pharmacol. Sci.* (Eds: Oliver B., Mos J., Slangen J.L.), Birkhauser Verlag Basel, p.3-14.

[48] Schmidt A.M., Yan S.D.,Yan S.F., Stern D.M. (2000). The biology of the receptor for advanced glycation end products and its ligands. *Biochem. Biophys. Acta*, 1498, 99-111.

[49] Sheng J.G., Mrak R.E., Bales K.R., et al. (2000). Overexpression of the neurotrophic cytokines S100 beta precedes the appearance of neurotic beta amyloid plaques in APPV717F mice. *J. Neurochem.,* 74, 295-301.

[50] Shtark M.B., Epstein O.I., Vorobyova T.M. (2002). Use of preparation proproten-100 for treatment of alcohol abstinence syndrome. In: Proproten-100. *Materia Medica Holding*, Moscow, 100-107.

[51] Triet D. (1985). Animal models for the study of anti-anxiety agents, a review. *Neurosci. Biobehav. Revs*, 9, 203-222.

[52] Vogel J.R., Beer B., Clody D.E. (1971). A simple and reliable conflict procedure for testing antianxiety agents. *Psychopharmacol*, 21, 1-7.

[53] Volodina O.P., Volodina O.V., Epstein O.I., Martyushev A.V. (2002). Proproten-100 in correction of anxiety symptoms in cardiovascular patients. In: Proproten-100. *Materia Medica Holding, Moscow*, 108-111.

[54] Voronina T.A. (1994) Dissociation of anxiolytic, amnestic and antiamnestic effects of GABA-benzodiazepine receptor ligands., In: *Biological basis of individual sensitivity to psychotropic drugs* (Eds: Seredenin S.B., Longo V., Gaviraghi G.), Graffham Press, Edinburgh, UK, p.39-46.

[55] Yu W.H., Frazer P.E. (2001). S100 β interaction with tau is promoted by zinc and inhibited by hyperphosphorylation in Alzheimer's disease. *J. Neurosci*, 21, 2240-2246.

In: Animal Models in Biological Psychiatry
Editor: Allan V. Kalueff, pp. 153-163
ISBN 1-59454-814-5

Chapter 9

Experimental Models in Epilepsy Research: Intranasal Human Interleukin-6 Increases the Severity of Seizures in Rats

Allan V. Kalueff
Medical School, Tampere University and Tampere University Hospital,
Tampere, Finland

I. Introduction

A pleiotropic cytokine interleukin-6 (IL-6), identified in 1985, is involved in inflammatory processes as a systemic mediator of the acute phase response in infection (Go, Nakamura, 2002; Lemke et al., 1998). In the periphery IL-6 has many important functions in the immune system. In addition, IL-6 has been found in the brain, including neuronal, glial and microglial cells (Lemke et al., 1998; Samland et al., 2003), where it plays an important modulatory and neuroprotective role (D'Arcangelo et al., 2000). IL-6 influences mesocorticolimbic dopamine and serotonin neurotransmission and also has activating effects on locomotion (Zalcman et al., 1994, 1998, 1999). High levels of IL-6 have been recognized to produce many behavioural symptoms collectively termed "sickness behaviour" (Bluthe et al., 2000). Recently IL-6 was reported to have neurotoxic effects and has also been suggested to play a significant role in various diseases of the central nervous system (D'Arcangelo et al., 2000; Sallmann et al., 2000).

Epilepsy is a common severe brain disorder with multiple pathogenic mechanisms (Peltola et al., 1998, 2000, 2002). There is a growing body of evidence linking IL-6 to epilepsy (Sallmann et al., 2000; Samland et al., 2003). Seizures are a common complication in patients with infectious diseases accompanied by elevated plasma and brain IL-6 levels (Go, Nakamura, 2002, Ichiyama et al., 1998; Kawada et al., 2003; Kimura et al., 2002). Elevated levels of IL-6 occur in the plasma and cerebrospinal fluid of patients with recent epileptic seizures, where the levels of IL-6 generally correlate with the severity of the seizures (Lehtimaki et al., 2003, 2004; Peltola et al., 1998, 2000, 2002). These elevated IL-6 levels were observed in patients without any infection or brain trauma, and are most likely a consequence of neuronal epileptic activity associated with seizures (Peltola et al., 1998, 2000, 2002).

In rodents, limbic seizures rapidly and transiently enhanced IL-6 in the hippocampus (De Simoni et al., 2000; Vezzani et al., 202). Elevated IL-6 levels are seen after *in vivo* administration of excitatory amino acids (Minami et al., 1991). Neuronal depolarisation and Ca^{++} influx have been shown to directly activate production of IL-6 in the neuronal cells *in vitro* (Sallmann et al., 2000). Finally, transgenic mice over-expressing IL-6 in the brain develop spontaneous behavioural seizures, increased hippocampal excitatory activity and increased sensitivity to glutamatergic-induced seizures (Campbell et al., 1993; Samland et al., 2003; Steffensen et al., 1994).

However, the role of IL-6 in epilepsy is still unclear and thus needs further experimental investigation. In the present study, we directly examined the effects of IL-6 on chemically induced seizures. In order to minimize pyrogenic and other unwanted side-effects of IL-6, and since this cytokine penetrates the blood-brain barrier poorly, we used intranasal administration shown to be effective in by-passing the blood-brain barrier for several other cytokines and similar polypeptides (Dufes et al., 2003; Huber et al., 2003; Lawrence, 2002; Liu et al., 2001). Indeed, numerous studies have shown that intranasal administration of the drugs produces high brain concentrations with minimal systemic exposure (Ross et al., 2004; Thorne et al., 2004).

Since the olfactory neuroepithelium is the only area of the body in which an extension of the CNS directly contacts the external environment (Liu et al., 2001), drug transport from the nasal cavity to the brain has been extensively investigated in the last decades. Intranasal administration provides a useful tool for a targeted delivery of drugs to the brain via olfactory and trigeminal pathways, and has been successfully used for a variety of substances, including peptides, neuromediators, hormones, etc. (Lawrence, 2002; Liu et al., 2001; Ross et al., 2004; Thorne et al., 2004; Reger et al., 2006). Since rat and human IL-6 possess a high degree of homology, we chose to use human recombinant IL-6 (hIL-6), a 20.9 kDa protein containing 184 amino acid residues, for our experiments.

Since our work is the first study to use IL-6 intranasally, we used 400 ng IL-6 for our studies, basing our choice on recent data (Zalcman et al., 1998, 1999) showing that at this dose IL-6 is able to cause central effects in rats following systemic administration. Choosing the pre-treatment time for our studies, we considered recent findings showing that:

1. cytokine-like molecules may appear in the brain within 20-30 min. following their intranasal administration (Dufes et al., 2003; Liu et al., 2001); and
2. IL-6 can cause its central effects 30-60 min following its systemic administration (Zalcman et al., 1998, 1999).

As such, 1 h pre-treatment time seemed appropriate for IL-6 at this dose to reach the brain and affect seizures.

Since pentylenetetrazole (PTZ), a potent blocker of the chloride ionophore at the gamma-aminobutyric acid GABA-A receptors, is the most frequently used chemoconvulsant in experimental models of epilepsy (Kalueff et al., 2005, 2006), we used this model in our experiments. In our recent study (Kalueff et al., 2004), we demonstrated that intranasally administered hIL-6 appears in the brain and leads to increased severity of seizures and higher mortality in the model of PTZ-induced seizures in rats.

II. Methods

Twenty two adult male Wistar rats (220-240 g; University of Tampere, Finland) were maintained in a standard virus/parasite-free facility and exposed to a 12-h light, 12-h dark cycle. Lights were turned off at 18.00 and on at 6.00. The animals were experimentally naïve and housed in pairs, with food and water freely available. The testing was always conducted between 14.00 and 18.00. On the days of the experiments animals were brought individually into the experiment room and immobilized in a vertical position, head up, for 5 min. in a specially designed plastic restraint box (Kalueff et al., 2004).

HIL-6 purchased from R & D Systems (USA; 10 μg diluted in 1 ml of sterile isotonic saline) was used in this study. Intranasal administration was performed in immobilized unanaesthetised animals using a 40 μl micropipette (Labsystems, Finland). Each animal received 10 μl of hIL-6 or isotonic saline at once in each nostril. This treatment was repeated after a 3-min. interval (total amount administered was 400ng/40 μl/rat). After the intranasal administration procedure the animals were returned to their cages for recovery. One hour later, each animal received a bolus of intraperitoneal injection of PTZ (Sigma, UK; 75 mg/kg) and was placed in a new clean cage for observation of seizure profile. Seizures and seizure latency times were observed visually over a 30-min. observation period by a trained experimenter blind to the treatment groups.

The following parameters of seizure-like activity were recorded: the time to onset of the first twitch; the number of rats having motor seizures; the duration of the ofo-facial, clonic and tonic components of seizures; the mortality rate, essentially as described elsewhere (Kalueff et al., 2004, 2005, 2006). The intensity of seizures was registered using a modified Racine's scoring system (Racine, 1972):

1. 0 (no response),
2. 1 (freezing),
3. 2 (head nodding or isolated twitches),
4. 3 (oro-facial seizure),
5. 4 (clonic seizure),
6. 5 (tonic seizure),
7. 6 (death).

Clonic seizures consisted of rhythmic contractions of forelimbs and/or hind limbs. Tonic seizures consisted of rigid extension of the fore- and/or hind limbs with or without posture loss. An animal was considered dead if the heart was not beating upon manual check.

Following decapitation, brains were removed and dissected on a cold plate. Frontal lobes (anterior to optic chiasma) were isolated and stored at –70 °C until the time of assay. Samples were weighted and homogenized in 50mM PBS (pH = 7.5) using a Potter homogenizer. Thereafter, they were centrifuged for 15 min (5000 rpm) and supernatant was removed and stored.

To investigate whether a drug is delivered to the brain (rather than to the systemic circulation), the drug uptake in brain tissue needs to be monitored. For this, commercial ELISA kit (R & D Systems, USA) was used to measure the level of hIL-6 in the frontal lobe of the brain. Animal care and experimental procedures were conducted in accordance with the European legislation and the guidelines of the National Institutes of Health. All animal experiments reported here were approved by the Ethical Committee of the University of Tampere. Statistics: All results are expressed as means ± S.E.M. Data were analysed by Student's t-test for independent samples. A probability of less than 0.05 was considered statistically significant.

III. Results

The results of the present study are summarized in Table 1. Overall, hIL-6 produces a dramatic increase in seizure severity in PTZ-treated rats. While the duration of relatively mild oro-facial seizures was similar in both groups (Table 1), the duration of more severe clonic/tonic components and the total duration of seizures were almost double in rats treated with hIL-6. Also, there was a significantly shorter latency to the first twitch (Table 1). Mortality rate (55%) was almost 3-fold higher in the hIL-6 treated group (18%), although not significantly.

Analysis of ELISA data shows that intranasal administration of hIL-6 results in a significant increase in IL-6 levels in frontal lobe (18.6 ± 5.4 pg/g brain tissue) compared to (2.2 ± 0.6 pg/g brain tissue) in saline-treated controls ($P < 0.05$), thus, correlating with an increased severity of seizures. Together, these data clearly indicate a pro-convulsant effect of exogenously applied hIL-6 in the brain following intranasal administration in a model of PTZ-induced seizures.

IV. General Discussion

In general, our findings are the first data that directly link exogenous IL-6 to increased seizure severity in rats. The chemoconvulsant drug PTZ used in the present study to induce seizures, is known to act in the brain through inhibition of gamma-aminobutyric acid (GABA) Sieghart, 1995). Many drugs that act on the GABAergic system are able to affect IL-6. For example, the antiepileptic drug sodium valproate, a stimulator of GABAergic transmission, inhibits IL-6 synthesis in several human cell lines (Abdul, Hoosein, 2001; Ichiyama et al., 1998). The anticonvulsant GABA-A agonist muscimol, injected into the brain, inhibits stress-induced elevation of plasma IL-6 (Song et al., 1998). Anticonvulsant benzodiazepines, known to stimulate GABA-A receptors, inhibit the ability of peripheral blood monocytes to synthesize IL-6 both in humans and mice (Fruscella et al., 2001) and decrease the secretion of IL-6 in human prostate cancer cells (Abdul, Hoosein, 2001).

In contrast, GABA-A antagonists, such as SR-95 531, increase both the basal and the restraint stress-induced plasma IL-6 levels (Song et al., 1998). This therefore demonstrates a clear negative correlation between GABAergic activity and IL-6 production. Although the biological meaning of this correlation has yet to be investigated, its existence confirms the interplay between the GABAergic and IL-6 systems. In line with this, a preferential neuronal localization of IL-6 in GABAergic neurons of the basal forebrain - an area actively involved in epilepsy pathogenesis – has recently been demonstrated (Lemke et al., 1998). Clearly, some other brain neurotransmitters, including glutamatergic and mesocortical dopaminergic systems, may also be involved in the modulation of IL-6 action and epileptogenesis (Samland et al., 2004; Zalcman et al., 1994). However, the important role of the GABAergic system in controlling seizure (Sieghart, 1995), and the link between GABA- and IL-6-related brain mechanisms may explain why IL-6 exacerbates PTZ-induced seizures.

Considering the existing data linking the IL-6 system to epilepsy, one can argue that IL-6 synthesis may represent a compensatory pathway activated after seizures in order to protect the brain, as does, for example, a well-studied anticonvulsant cytokine IL-1Ra (De Simoni et al., 2000; Lehtimaki et al., 2003; Vezzani et al., 2000). However, two other cytokines, IL-1β and TNFα, are also elevated after seizures along with IL-6 and IL-1Ra (Janowsky, Patterson, 2001; Lehtimaki et al., 2003). These cytokines both possess inflammatory and pro-convulsant properties (Shandra et al., 2002; Vezzani et al., 2000, 2002; Yuhas et al., 2003) and are known to stimulate the expression of IL-6 (Sallmann et al., 2000).

Furthermore, analysis of the time course of cytokine release after seizures shows that increase was first seen in pro-inflammatory convulsant cytokines IL-6, IL-1β and TNFα, while anti-inflammatory anticonvulsant cytokine IL-1Ra peaked much later (De Simoni et al., 2000; Janowsky, Patterson, 2001; Vezzani et al., 2002). Taken together, these observations indicate that IL-6 release after seizures resembles more that of IL-1β and TNFα, than of IL-1Ra, and are in line with the hypothesis linking pro-inflammatory cytokines to epilepsy.

It is therefore no surprise that many anti-inflammatory drugs generally have anticonvulsant effects. Thus, these findings give additional support to the pro-convulsant mode of action of IL-6 in the brain suggested in our study.

However, there are also data in the literature showing some anticonvulsant potential of IL-6. For example, IL-6 enhances expression of brain adenosine A1 receptors known to inhibit neuronal excitation (Biber et al., 2001) and inhibits the spread of excitation and glutamate release in the somatosensory cortex in rats (D'Arcangelo et al., 2000). Moreover, IL-6 knockout mice were reported to have increased susceptibility to kainic acid-induced seizures (Penkowa et al., 2001). Although these findings may seem to contradict the potential pro-convulsant role of IL-6, their exact mechanisms and biological implication remain unclear.

In general, several mechanisms may underlie these conflicting results. First, IL-6 may activate cascades of secondary mechanisms in the brain, some of which may be anticonvulsant. Furthermore, IL-6 may have different actions depending on different experimental models of epilepsy. For example, pro-convulsant effects of IL-6 hyper-production are seen in glutamatergic- but not cholinergic-induced seizures (Samland et al.,

2003). In addition, the difference between central vs. peripheral site(s) of action for IL-6 may contribute to such conflicting results as suggested by Bluthe et al. (2000). Clearly, such duality in the mechanisms of actions during epilepsy cannot be excluded for IL-6, which already shows dual effects in the brain with both neuroprotective and neurotoxic actions (D'Arcangelo et al., 2000; Penkowa et al., 2001; Sallmann et al., 2003; Steffensen et al., 1994).

Table 1. Increased susceptibility to PTZ-induced seizures in rats treated with intranasal hIL-6 (adapted from Kalueff et al., 2004)

Group	Number of rats with seizures					Onset of the twitch, sec	Seizure duration, sec		
	TW	O	C	T	D		O	C/T	Total
Saline	10/11	11/11	7/11	7/11	2/11	417± 59	9±3	27±6	36±7
IL-6	9/11	10/11	10/11	9/11	6/11	260± 56 *	8±3	51±8 *	59±10*

TW – twitches, O – oro-facial seizures, C – clonus, T – tonus (C/T – clonic or tonic seizures), D – death. Data are the means + S.E.M. Fractions represent the number of rats showing different stages of seizures of the total number of rats. The onset of the first twitch was reckoned as 1800 sec (total observation time) in the rats not showing this behaviour. * $P<0.05$ by t-test vs. saline control rats.

Furthermore, it will be of interest to examine the effects of intranasally applied IL-6 in epilepsy in more detail, using different doses and pretreatment times, especially (considering the pleotropic nature of IL-6 and multiplicity of its mechanisms of actions) since, like other cytokines (Yuhas et al., 2003), IL-6 may have different and even opposite effects at different doses and check-points. It will also be interesting to analyse CSF and plasma levels of IL-6 after intranasal administration, as well as its levels in other parts of the brain (in addition to frontal lobe). Finally, it may be necessary to further assess the role of IL-6 in different models of epilepsy by influencing its physiological effects (for example, blocking them using inhibitors of IL-6 signal transduction or neutralising antiserum). We suggest that such studies may represent very important directions for future research focusing on the role of IL-6 in epilepsy.

In summary, here we have demonstrated a clear pro-convulsant action of exogenously applied IL-6 in rats. Using the intranasal route for IL-6 delivery to the brain, we minimised possible peripheral side effects of IL-6, resolved the problem of by-passing the blood-brain barrier, and assessed the central effects of IL-6 during seizures induced by inhibition of the central GABAergic system. Our data show that intranasally administered hIL-6 (400 ng) leads to a rise in IL-6 levels in the frontal lobe and increases the susceptibility of rats to PTZ-induced seizures. IL-6 affected predominantly the more severe stages of seizures (Table 1), showing the pro-convulsant profile which is clinically relevant and may be of interest for potential application. Importantly, since behavioural activation and epilepsy are based on the same arousal-related neural pathways, the pro-convulsant profile of IL-6 in our study is consistent with earlier data on the general pro-activatory action of IL-6 on behaviour in rats (Zalcman et al., 1994; 1998; 1999). The results of our studies also confirm recent data showing increased sensitivity to glutamatergic-induced seizures in mice with elevated IL-6 levels in the brain (Samland et al., 2003).

Finally, a recent study by Xiaoqin et al. (2005) provided convincing evidence supporting the results of our pioneering study (Kalueff et al., 2004). Their experiments assessed the mechanism of epilepsy induced by IL-6, and analysed changes of glutamic acid and GABA immunoreaction in the cerebral cortex and hippocampus in rats. Rats were randomly divided into 2 groups: intracerebroventricularly injected with saline or IL-6. 120 min after the injection, behavioral changes were observed and Glutamate and GABA in the cerebral cortex and hippocampus were examined. Their results showed that no seizure developed in the control group, while moderate seizures were indeed observed in the IL-6 group. Compared with the controls, the immunoreaction of glutamate was significantly increased, while GABA was decreased in the IL-6 group 120 min after injection. In line with our hypothesis (Kalueff et al., 2004), this study suggested that IL-6 promotes and induces epilepsy by increasing glutamate and decreasing GABA in the cerebral cortex and hippocampus.

Taken together, these data and those reported in our study (Kalueff et al., 2004) prove that IL-6 has a marked pro-convulsant effect in several experimental models of epilepsy, and may therefore act in the brain as a pro-convulsant cytokine. These findings may point to a new area for the search of novel anti-epileptic drugs based on targeting the central IL-6 system. Furthermore, our study confirmed the important role of intranasal delivery of neurotropic agents, such as IL-6, as a fast, reliable and effective method of administration of drugs able to influence epilepsy-related mechanism in the brain. Our study shows the potential utility of this method for the epilepsy-oriented biomedical research.

In addition, given the utility of this approach in therapy of various brain disorders (see (Ross et al., 2004; Thorne et al., 2004) for review), it is also possible to suggest that intranasal administration of anti-epileptic drugs may have important clinical implications, leading to new highly effective strategies of anti-epileptic therapy.

Acknowledgements

This study was supported by the Medical Research Fund of Tampere University Hospital and the Centre for International Mobility (CIMO).

References

[1] M. Abdul, N. Hoosein, Inhibition by anticonvulsants of prostate-specific antigen and interleukin-6 secretion by human prostate cancer cells, *Anticancer Res.* 21 (2001) 2045-2048.

[2] K. Biber, B. Lubrich, B.L. Fiebich, H.W. Boddeke, D. van Calker, Interleukin-6 enhances expression of adenosine A(1) receptor mRNA and signaling in cultured rat cortical astrocytes and brain slices, *Neuropsychopharmacol.* 24 (2001) 86-96.

[3] R.M. Bluthe, B. Michaud, V. Poli, R. Dantzer, Role of IL-6 in cytokine-induced sickness behavior: a study with IL-6 deficient mice, *Physiol Behav.* 70 (2000) 367-373.

[4] L. Campbell, R.D. Abraham, E. Masliah, P. Kemper, J.D. Inglis, M.D. Oldstone, L. Mucke, Neurologic disease induced in transgenic mice by cerebral overexpression of interleukin 6, *Proc Natl Acad Sci* U S A. 90 (1993) 10061-10065.

[5] G. D'Arcangelo, V. Tancredi, F. Onofri, M. D'Antuono, S. Giovedi, F. Benfenati, Interleukin-6 inhibits neurotransmitter release and the spread of excitation in the rat cerebral cortex, *Eur J Neurosci.* 12 (2000) 1241-1252.

[6] M.G. De Simoni, C. Perego, T. Ravizza, D. Moneta, M. Conti, D. Marchesi, A. De Luigi, S. Garattini, A. Vezzani, Inflammatory cytokines and related genes are induced in the rat hippocampus by limbic status epilepticus, *Eur J Neurosci.* 12 (2000) 2623-2633.

[7] C. Dufes, J.C. Olivier, F. Gaillard, A. Gaillard, W. Couet, J.M. Muller, Brain delivery of vasoactive intestinal peptide (VIP) following nasal administration to rats, *Int J Pharm.* 255 (2003) 87-97.

[8] P. Fruscella, M. Sottocorno, M. Di Braccio, L. Diomede, N. Piccardi, A. Cagnotto, G. Grossi, M. Romano, T. Mennini, G. Roma, 1,5-Benzodiazepine tricyclic derivatives exerting anti-inflammatory effects in mice by inhibiting interleukin-6 and prostaglandin E(2) production, *Pharmacol Res.* 43 (2001) 445-452.

[9] V.V. Huber, B.P. Arulanandam, P.M. Arnaboldi, M.K. Elmore, C.E. Sheehan, B.V. Kallakury, D.W. Metzger, Delivery of IL-12 intranasally leads to reduced IL-12-mediated toxicity, *Int Immunopharmacol.* 3 (2003) 801-809.

[10] T. Go, K. Nakamura, Frequent seizures with elevated interleukin-6 at the eruptive stage of exanthema subitum, *Eur J Paediatr Neurol.* 6 (2002) 221-223.

[11] J.L. Jankowsky, P.H. Patterson, The role of cytokines and growth factors in seizures and their sequelae, *Prog Neurobiol.* 63 (2001) 125-149.

[12] T. Ichiyama, M. Nishikawa, T. Yoshitomi, T. Hayashi, S. Furukawa, Tumor necrosis factor-alpha, interleukin-1 beta, and interleukin-6 in cerebrospinal fluid from children with prolonged febrile seizures. Comparison with acute encephalitis/encephalopathy, *Neurology.* 50 (1998) 407-411.

[13] A.V. Kalueff, K.A. Lehtimaki, A. Ylinen, J. Honkaniemi, J. Peltola, Intranasal administration of human IL-6 increases the severity of chemically induced seizures in rats, *Neurosci. Lett.* 365 (2004) 106-110.

[14] A.V. Kalueff, A. Minasyan, P. Tuohimaa, Anticonvulsant effects of 1,25-dihydroxyvitamin D in chemically induced seizures in mice, *Brain Res. Bull.* 67 (2005) 156-160.

[15] A.V. Kalueff, A. Minasyan, T. Keisala, M. Kuuslahti, S. Miettinen, P. Tuohimaa, Increased severity of chemically induced seizures in mice with partially deleted Vitamin D receptor gene, *Neurosci. Lett.* 394 (2006) 69-73.

[16] J. Kawada, H. Kimura, Y. Ito, S. Hara, M. Iriyama, T. Yoshikawa, T. Morishima, Systemic cytokine responses in patients with influenza-associated encephalopathy, *J Infect Dis.* 188 (2003) 690-698.

[17] M. Kimura, M. Tasaka, H. Sejima, Y. Takusa, T. Ichiyama, S. Yamaguchi, Hemiconvulsion-hemiplegia syndrome and elevated interleukin-6: case report, *J Child Neurol.* 17 (2002) 705-707.

[18] D. Lawrence, Intranasal delivery could be used to administer drugs directly to the brain, *Lancet.* 359 (2002) 1674.

[19] K.A. Lehtimaki, J. Peltola, E. Koskikallio, T. Keranen, J. Honkaniemi, Expression of cytokines and cytokine receptors in the rat brain after kainic acid-induced seizures, *Brain Res Mol Brain Res.* 110 (2003) 253-260.

[20] K.A. Lehtimaki, T. Keranen, H. Huhtala, M. Hurme, J. Ollikainen, J. Honkaniemi, J. Palmio, J. Peltola, Regulation of IL-6 in cerebrospinal fluid and serum compartments by seizures: the effect of seizure type and duration, *J Neuroimmunol.* 152 (2004) 121-125.

[21] R. Lemke, W. Hartig, S. Rossner, V. Bigl, R. Schliebs, Interleukin-6 is not expressed in activated microglia and in reactive astrocytes in response to lesion of rat basal forebrain cholinergic system as demonstrated by combined in situ hybridization and immunocytochemistry, *J Neurosci Res.* 51 (1998) 223-236.

[22] X.F. Liu, J.R. Fawcett, R.G. Thorne, T.A. DeFor, W.H. Frey, Intranasal administration of insulin-like growth factor-I bypasses the blood-brain barrier and protects against focal cerebral ischemic damage, *J Neurol Sci.* 187 (2001) 91-97.

[23] M. Minami, Y. Kuraishi, M. Satoh, Effects of kainic acid on messenger RNA levels of IL-1 beta, IL-6, TNF alpha and LIF in the rat brain, *Biochem Biophys Res Commun.* 176 (1991) 593-598.

[24] J. Peltola, M. Hurme, A. Miettinen, T. Keranen, Elevated levels of interleukin-6 may occur in cerebrospinal fluid from patients with recent epileptic seizures, *Epilepsy Res.* 31 (1998) 129-133.

[25] J. Peltola, J. Palmio, L. Korhonen, J. Suhonen, A. Miettinen, M. Hurme, D. Lindholm, T. Keranen, Interleukin-6 and interleukin-1 receptor antagonist in cerebrospinal fluid from patients with recent tonic-clonic seizures, *Epilepsy Res.* 41 (2000) 205-211.

[26] J. Peltola, J. Laaksonen, A.M. Haapala, M. Hurme, S. Rainesalo, T. Keranen, Indicators of inflammation after recent tonic-clonic epileptic seizures correlate with plasma interleukin-6 levels, *Seizure.* 11 (2002) 44-46.

[27] M. Penkowa, A. Molinero, J. Carrasco, J. Hidalgo, Interleukin-6 deficiency reduces the brain inflammatory response and increases oxidative stress and neurodegeneration after kainic acid-induced seizures, *Neurosci.* 102 (2001) 805-818.

[28] R. Racine, Modification of seizure activity by electrical stimulation: II. Motor seizure, Electroenceph. *Clin. Neuropsysiol.* 32 (1972) 281-294.

[29] M.A. Reger, G.S. Watson, W.H. Frey, L.D. Baker, B. Cholerton, M.L. Keeling, D.A. Belongia, M.A. Fishel, S.R. Plymate, G.D. Schellenberg, M.M. Cherrier, S. Craft, Effects of intranasal insulin on cognition in memory-impaired older adults: modulation by APOE genotype, *Neurobiol Aging.* 27 (2006) 451-458.

[30] T.M. Ross, P.M. Martinez, J.C. Renner, R.G. Thorne, L.R. Hanson, W.H. Frey, Intranasal administration of interferon beta bypasses the blood-brain barrier to target the central nervous system and cervical lymph nodes: a non-invasive treatment strategy for multiple sclerosis, *J Neuroimmunol.* 151 (2004) 66-77.

[31] S. Sallmann, E. Juttler, S. Prinz, N. Petersen, U. Knopf, T. Weiser, M. Schwaninger, Induction of interleukin-6 by depolarization of neurons, *J Neurosci.* 20 (2000) 8637-8642.

[32] H. Samland, S. Huitron-Resendiz, E. Masliah, J. Criado, S.J. Henriksen, I.L. Campbell, Profound increase in sensitivity to glutamatergic- but not cholinergic agonist-induced seizures in transgenic mice with astrocyte production of IL-6, *J Neurosci Res.* 73 (2003) 176-187.

[33] A.A. Shandra, L.S. Godlevsky, R.S. Vastyanov, A.A. Oleinik, V.L. Konovalenko, E.N. Rapoport, N.N. Korobka, The role of TNF-alpha in amygdala kindled rats, *Neurosci Res.* 42 (2002) 147-153.

[34] W. Sieghart, Structure and pharmacology of gamma-aminobutyric acidA receptor subtypes, *Pharmacol Rev.* 47 (1995) 181-234.

[35] D.K. Song, H.W. Suh, S.O. Huh, J.S. Jung, B.M. Ihn, I.G. Choi, Y.H. Kim, Central GABAA and GABAB receptor modulation of basal and stress-induced plasma interleukin-6 levels in mice, *J Pharmacol Exp Ther.* 287 (1998) 144-149.

[36] S.C. Steffensen, I.L. Campbell, S.J. Henriksen, Site-specific hippocampal pathophysiology due to cerebral overexpression of interleukin-6 in transgenic mice, *Brain Res.* 652 (1994) 149-153.

[37] R.G. Thorne, G.J. Pronk, V. Padmanabhan, W.H. Frey, Delivery of insulin-like growth factor-I to the rat brain and spinal cord along olfactory and trigeminal pathways following intranasal administration, *Neurosci.* 127 (2004) 481-96.

[38] Vezzani, D. Moneta, M. Conti, C. Richichi, T. Ravizza, A. De Luigi, M.G. De Simoni, G. Sperk, S. Andell-Jonsson, J. Lundkvist, K. Iverfeldt, T. Bartfai, Powerful anticonvulsant action of IL-1 receptor antagonist on intracerebral injection and astrocytic overexpression in mice, *Proc Natl Acad Sci* U S A. 97 (2000) 11534-11539.

[39] Vezzani, D. Moneta, C. Richichi, M. Aliprandi, S.J. Burrows, T. Ravizza, C. Perego, M.G. De Simoni, Functional role of inflammatory cytokines and antiinflammatory molecules in seizures and epileptogenesis, *Epilepsia.* 43 Suppl 5 (2002) 30-35.

[40] Z. Xiaoqin, L. Zhengli, Z. Changgeng, W. Xiaojing, L. Li. Changes in behavior and amino acid neurotransmitters in the brain of rats with seizure induced by IL-1beta or IL-6, *J Huazhong Univ Sci Technolog Med Sci.* 25 (2005) 236-239.

[41] Y. Yuhas, A. Weizman, S. Ashkenazi, Bidirectional concentration-dependent effects of tumor necrosis factor alpha in Shigella dysenteriae-related seizures, *Infect Immun.* 71 (2003) 2288-2291.

[42] S. Zalcman, J.M. Green-Johnson, L. Murray, D.M. Nance, D. Dyck, A. Anisman, A.H. Greenberg, Cytokine-specific central monoamine alterations induced by interleukin-1, -2 and -6, *Brain Res.* 643 (1994) 40-49.

[43] S. Zalcman, L. Murray, D.G. Dyck, A.H. Greenberg, D.M. Nance, Interleukin-2 and -6 induce behavioral-activating effects in mice, *Brain Res.* 811 (1998) 111-121.

[44] S. Zalcman, I. Savina, I., R.A. Wise, Interleukin-6 increases sensitivity to the locomotor-stimulating effects of amphetamine in rats, *Brain Res.* 847 (1999) 276-283.

In: Animal Models in Biological Psychiatry
Editor: Allan V. Kalueff, pp. 165-182 ISBN 1-59454-814-5

Chapter 10

On the Problem of Memory-Anxiety Interaction: Anxiolytic Effects of Memory-Impoving Dipeptide GVS-111

Rita U. Ostrovskaya, Sergey B. Seredenin, Tatiana A. Voronina, Gennadiy M. Molodavkin and Tatiana A. Gudasheva
State Institute of Pharmacology RAMS, Moscow, Russia

I. Introduction

Although it is generally recognized that anxiety and cognitive processes are tightly linked, there is no consensus about the precise nature of this relationship. There are numerous experimental data demonstrating that memory-improving substances are anxiogenic, while many conventional anxiolytics are amnestic (see: Kalueff and Nutt, 1997 for details). Among the drugs displaying this type of memory-anxiety relationships are those directly affecting the central gamma-aminobutyric acid (GABA) neurotransmission. On the other hand, stress-induced disregulation of the hypothalamic-pituitary system followed by increased glucocorticoid secretion have been repeatedly reported to cause cognitive impairments including selective attentional and memory deficits, as well as impeded information processing (Wolkowitz et al., 1990; Bremner et al., 1993). Increased glucocorticoid levels are associated with a wide range of metabolic disorders since glucocorticoids induce cytotoxic damage of neurons making them more vulnerable to the endogenous glutamate, free radicals and Ca^{2+} (Armanini et al., 1990; Gold, 1988; Liu et al., 1994). Therefore, diminishing the metabolic consequences of stress can improve learning, memory and other cognitive functions. Thus, not only the reciprocal but also synergetic memory-anxiety inter-relationship may occur, enabling us to obtain new anxiolytics able to improve cognitive functions.

Stress-induced changes in structural and physico-chemical properties of neuronal membranes (first of all influencing the balance of pro- and antioxidant systems) may affect not only the GABA-ergic system, but also many other neurotransmitter and neuropeptide systems. This prompts the research of a wide spectrum of neurotropic medicines based on their potential modulatory effects on memory-anxiety interplay. As such, nootropic drugs (cognitive enhancers) may be a useful pharmacological tool to further study this problem.

All attempts to selectively affect the cognitive functions (memory, vigilance, orientation, cognitive performance, comprehension) originated from the pioneering studies of H. Giurgea (UCB, Belgium) coining the term “nootropics” in the early 1970s. He applied this term to the psychoactive substances able to facilitate attentional abilities and acquisition, storage and retrieval of information, and to attenuate the impairment of cognitive functions associated with brain trauma, stroke, and age-related cognition decline. While piracetam was the first compound of this group, a large number of piracetam congeners (e.g., aniracetam, oxiracetam, pramiracetam, nebracetam) have been developed in the last decades. The term "nootropics" is now used mostly to define this group, while a large number of investigators prefer the term "cognitive enhancers" (CE), referring to the wide spectrum of substances, including Ca^{++} channels blockers, free radical scavengers and antioxidants, cholino-positive substances, and mnemotropic peptides. Piracetam-like nootropics have never reached general acceptance because of low activity and the lack of convincing data on the mechanisms of action.

Endogenous peptides with pro-mnestic activity (arginine-vasopressine, ACTH, TRH) are known to be highly effective (compared to piracetam) and nontoxic (in contrast to a majority of the above-mentioned CE). Unfortunately, their clinical use is hindered by the failure to enter the brain, and by their low biological stability.

However, the design of dipeptides is one of the promising approaches in this area, since these short molecules demonstrate relatively high biological stability. Our search for dipeptides with CE-activity was based on the idea of imitating the structural and conformational features of piracetam. This approach has been used in the Institute of Pharmacology for 20 years, originating from the assumption that piracetam has a peptidergic mechanism of action, i.e. it might be considered as an exogenous agonist for hypothetical recognizing sites binding endogenous ligands including short peptides containing one of two pyrrolidine-carboxylic aminoacids, pyroglutamic acid or proline (Gudasheva, 1985; 1996 a). This drug-based peptide design led to the development of a novel group of nootropics, acylprolyl-containing dipeptides (Seredenin et al., 1995).

N-phenylacetylprolyl-glycine ethyl ester (GVS-111, Noopept) was first chosen from this series as a drug possessing pronounced antiamnestic activity in the passive avoidance test. Its advantages over a non-peptide prototype piracetam include: lower threshold doses (0.1-1 mg/kg vs. 200-500 mg/kg for piracetam); a wider spectrum of positive mnemotropic effect; and effectiveness of systemic administration (including per os); making this dipeptide a better medication compared to other mnemotropic peptides such as arginine-vasopressine and ACTH. Further studies of GVS-111 revealed its complex memory-restoring effects not only in passive avoidance paradigm but also in the active avoidance, water maze, contextual conditional freezing and habituation tests (Ostrovskaya et al., 2002). Given the uncertainty of the relationships between the cognition and emotional states, it is of interest to study whether the memory-improving drug GVS-111 may affect the levels of anxiety.

II. Materials and Methods

Subjects and Drugs

Experiments were performed on Wistar male rats (200-250 g), randomly bred male white mice or inbred male BALB/c and C57BL/6 mice (18-22 g; Stolbovaja Farm RAMS, Moscow, Russia). Animals were housed in their home cages and kept under 12L:12D cycle in a temperature controlled room (22±2.5 C). All behavioral tests were run during the light phase from 10.00 to 14.00 h. Food and water were available ad lib (except the conflict test, see below). All animals and experimental procedures were authorized and approved by the Institute Ethical Committee; procedures were performed in compliance with the NIH Guide for the Care and Use of Laboratory animals. In all experiments, freshly prepared GVS-111 solution with saline was administered intraperitoneally (i.p.) 15 min prior to testing.

Procedures

The Light-Dark (LD) Box Test

Two different LD apparatus were used in the present study. First, we used the LD initially described by Ader (1973), consisting of a hanging platform (25 x 7 cm) attached (through a 6 x 6 cm guillotine door) to the dark chamber (40 x 40 x 40 cm; Lafaette Instruments, USA). The platform was constantly illuminated with a 60-W lamp. The second LD apparatus (PACS-16) consisted of two equal compartments (25 x 25 x 25 cm; one illuminated with a 15-W lamp). Rat were placed individually either on the illuminated platform, or in the illuminated compartment and allowed to explore it and to enter the dark compartment. The latency of the first entry to the dark compartment was recorded for 3 min.

The Elevated Plus-Maze Test (EPM)

Three strains of mice were used in these experiments: BALB/c, C57BL/6 and outbred mice. The maze composed of four runways (45 x 5 cm) connected to a central platform (5 x 5 cm). Two of the runways had vertical walls (30-cm high) and were opposite to each other. The other two runways did not have walls. The apparatus was mounted 30 cm above the floor. Each mouse was placed individually on the central platform facing the open arm. Animals were observed for 3 min, recording their anxiety behaviours: the number of entries and the time spent in the open arms, time spent on the central platform. The ratio of open/total entries was calculated for each group. The total number of central platform transitions served as a measure of general motor activity (Pellow et al., 1985).

Conflict Test

This test was performed according to Vogel (1971) with some modifications (Molodavkin, 1996). Experiments were performed on male albino outbred rats. The apparatus consisted of experimental chamber supplied with a drinking bowl attached to the front wall, electrified floor, and the electronic block with the counting device. Conflict situation was produced by clashing of the two different motivations: thirst and fear. Experiments were carried out for 3 days. On Day 1, the animals were deprived of water. On Day 2, the training session (acquisition of water licking from a drinking bowl) was performed individually for each rat. Placed in the experimental chamber for 5 min, the animal would explore it, and after a while finds the drinking bowl and starts to drink. On this day, a very weak current not felt by a rat (50 μV) was delivered to a drinking bowl and the floor of the chamber (non-punished drinking). The rats that did not drink were excluded from the experiments. On Day 3, 30 min after GVS-111 (or saline) injection, the animals were placed into the experimental chamber for 10 min. After the first water lick, a direct current (0,25 mA) was delivered to the drinking bowl and the electrified floor for 10 sec (punished licking). The number of punished water intakes was recorded automatically during a 10-min period. The decrease in the number of punished water intakes was considered as an anxiogenic behavior; the increase in this measure was interpreted as the anxiolytic effect.

Behavior in the Brightly Lit Open Field Test

BALB/c and C57BL/6 strains used in these experiments were chosen for their genetically determined differences in responses to emotional stress (Seredenin et al., 1994; Seredenin 2003). Immediately before the test, each animal was placed into the dark box for 1 min for acclimation. Then the mouse was placed into the round open field arena illuminated with 4 60-W lamps symmetrically fixed 1 m above the arena. The open field was a circular arena 1 m in diameter (with the floor marked with three concentric circles and sectors) surrounded by 50-cm walls. The behavior of mice was registered by two independent observers, counting the number of peripheral and central sectors crossed and the number of rearing episodes for 3 min.

Screening of Locomotion, Muscle Tone and Motor Coordination

In order to test whether GVS-111 may be a selective anxiolytic agent with no sedative and muscle relaxant effects, its influence on locomotor activity, muscle tone and motor coordination was assessed in the present study. Spontaneous locomotor activity was studied using the multi-channel automatic analyzer Opto-Varimex (Columbus Instr., USA). A group of 10 animals was recorded in this chamber for 30 min. The number of horizontal and vertical movements, as well as nonambulatory activity was recorded using 5-min intervals. Scores obtained for the first 5 min were taken as a background activity. Habituation index - the ratio of horizontal scores for the last 5 min to the scores measured for the first 5 min (100%) - was calculated in each experiment. GVS-111 was injected 15 or 45 min prior to testing; control mice received 0.9% of NaCl.

Motor coordination was evaluated in the rota-rod test. Mice were placed individually on the rota-rod (3 cm in diameter, 3 rotation/min) for 2 min, and the number of animals falling from the rod was registered. Muscle relaxation was evaluated using the traction test. Briefly, each mouse was forced to hang for 2 min on its forelimbs on a horizontal wire (1,6 mm in diameter) elevated 30 cm from the floor. The number of animals remaining on the wire was registered for all groups.

Data Analysis

The Mann-Whitney U-test was used to analyze the statistical difference between the GVS-111 and saline-treated groups. All data are expressed as the mean +SEM; P less than 0.05 was considered statistically significant.

III. Results

Behavioural Effect of GVS-111 in the LD Test

Our results obtained in the Lafayette LD apparatus (having a hanging platform) revealed a short latency to enter the dark compartment in control animals (12.8±3.1 sec). The rats treated with GVS-111 at 0.5 mg/kg 15 min prior to testing did not display changes in these measures (14.2±4.6 sec). Paradoxically, the effect of GVS-111 in this test increased with a time: latency was 15.8±2.9 sec after 1 h and 25.1±4.36 sec ($P<0.05$ vs. the respective controls) after a 2-h interval. Lacking the hanging platform and bright lights, the PACS-16 apparatus was less stressogenic than the Lafayette Instruments test. In this "mild stress" LD modification, the latency to enter the dark compartment was longer in control rats (30±8.2 sec), whereas GVS-111 at 0.5 mg/kg significantly increased this measure (60.0±9.4 sec; $P<0,05$). Since anxiolytic drugs are known to increase this latency, our results therefore indicate anxiolytic-like effects of GVS-111.

Behavioural Effects of GVS-111 in the EPM

EPM has long been known as a highly reliable behavioural paradigm to test anxiolytic drugs (File, 1990). GVS-111 significantly affected the EPM performance in mice. In BALB/c mice (usually displaying "passive" stress reactions), GVS-111 altered all EPM measures, especially time spent in the center, total number of arms visits, percent of open visits, time in open arms (Table 1). At 0.5-3.5 mg/kg, GVS-111 produced clear dose-dependent effects. This activating effect fits the pattern of inverted U-shaped dose-dependent curve. The same treatment with GVS-111, however, did not affect C57BL/6 mice (Table 2).

Table 1. Effects of GVS-111 in the elevated plus maze in BALB/c mice (*P< 0.05 vs. saline)

Dose of GVS-111, mg/kg	Time in the open arms (sec)	Time in the center (sec)	Total number of entries	% of open entries
Saline n=80	21.7 ± 4.6	9.1 ± 1.5	5.4 ± 0.6	24.2 ± 3.3
0.25 n=30	36.2 ± 7.5	13.8 ± 3.9	9.7 ± 5.9	33.7 ± 6.5
0.5 n=30	80.2 ± 15.1*	12.3 ± 7.5	10.0 ± 2.5*	37.0 ± 5.9
1.5 n=30	101.4 ± 10.2*	24.2 ± 5.7*	13.6 ± 2.2*	46.2 ± 4.2*
2.5 n=30	90.7 ± 10.2*	18.2 ± 3.1*	13.8 ± 2.4*	52.6 ± 3.9*
3.0 n=30	97.3 ± 9.3*	28.8 ± 3.1*	13.5 ± 1.2*	45.1 ± 2.8*
3.5 n=30	43.6 ± 15.9*	24.9 ± 3.5*	9.0 ± 1.5*	25.8 ± 3.3

Table 2. Effects of GVS-111 in the elevated plus maze in C57BL/6 mice

Dose of GVS-111, mg/kg	Time in open arms (sec)	Time in center (sec)	Total number of visits to arms	% of visits to open arms
Saline n=80	7.6 ± 2.7	23.1 ± 3.3	7.5 ± 0.8	2.3 ± 0.8
0.5 n=30	8.9 ± 3.1	22.5 ± 4.6	9.2 ± 3.5	1.9± 0.5
1.5 n=30	11.4 ±4.8	20.8 ± 3.0	10.9 ± 4.9	2.6± 1.2
2.5 n=30	10.8 ±3.7	25.8 ± 3.5	9.8± 1.5	3.1 ± 1.4
3.0 n=30	8.7 ± 2.5	24.8± 4.0	10.4 ± 2.5	2.2 ± 0.6
3.5 n=30	9.5 ± 2.9	23.4 ± 3.7	12.5 ± 5.1	3.0 ± 0.9

Interestingly, outbred mice treated with 0.3 mg/kg GVS-111, did not show altered open time, although this parameter increased at 0.5-5.0 mg/kg, showing a clear dose-dependent increase – the phenomenon confirming anxiolytic action of the drug. Dose-activity relationship at these doses demonstrated a clear inverted U-curve, typical for peptidergic psychoactive substances. At 7.5 mg/kg, the open time scores returned to control values (Fig. 1). Also there was no difference between the groups in the number of central platform crossing. The latter result clearly indicates the absence of sedative and activating properties of GVS-111.

Effects of GVS- 111 in the Conflict Test

Control rats quickly ceased punished drinking and after brief exploration of the chamber reduced their activity and stayed immobile in one of the corners. The number of punishable water licks (0.25 mA) scored for 10 min in this group was 472.3 ± 126.4. In contrast, GVS-111 at 2.5 mg/ kg slightly increased punished liking (610±125; P>0.05), while its higher doses (5 mg/kg) exerted a pronounced anxiolytic action manifest in the statistically significant increase in the number of punished water licks (1147.6±329,1).

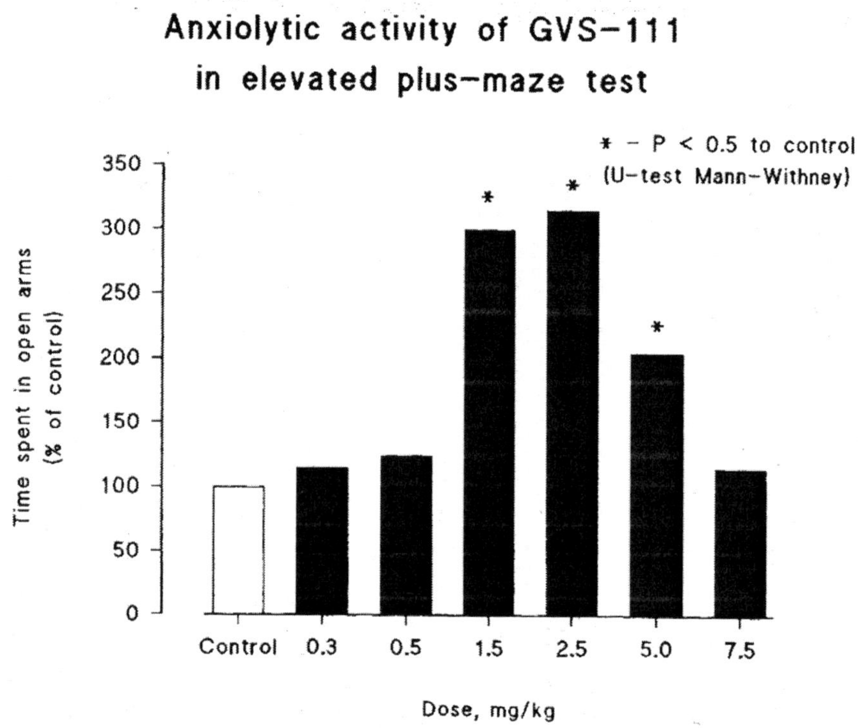

Fig. 1

Table 3. Effect of GVS-111 administered 30 min prior to the open-filed (BALB/c mice)

Dose mg/kg	Behavioral measures			
	Peripheral squares	Central squares	Rearing	Total
Saline (n = 30)	20.6±3.3	0.5±0.2	-	21.1±3.3
0.25 (n = 33)	23.9±6.7	0.9±0.9	-	24.8±7.3
0.50 (n = 35)	41.4±6.7	2.1±1.4	0.25±0.2	43.8±7.4*
1.50 (n = 38)	50.8±8.3	0.9±0.6	-	51.7±8.4*
2.50 (n = 35)	63.8±7.1	-	-	63.8±7.12*
3.50 (n = 34)	12.2±6.7	-	-	12.2±6.7
5.00 (n = 28)	5.9±1.7	-	-	5.9±1.7*

* P< 0.05- significant difference from control; n – number of animals

Effect of GVS-111 in the Open Field Test

Table 3 summarizes data obtained in BALB/c mice generally displaying a «passive» type of reactions to emotional stressors. GVS-111 activated the behavior in these mice when injected 30 min prior to testing at 0.5-2.5 mg/kg. Similar activation was also observed for a 15-min pretreatment time. The activation was mainly displayed as the increase in motor activity at the periphery of the apparatus.

At 5 mg/kg, the drug reduced motor activity to values below the control group (Fig. 2). In contrast, the C57BL/6 mice demonstrated a higher background activity, consistent with their active non-anxious phenotype. GVS-111 did not change either level or pattern of motor activity of these mice in a wide dose range (0.25-1.25 mg/kg), see Table 4.

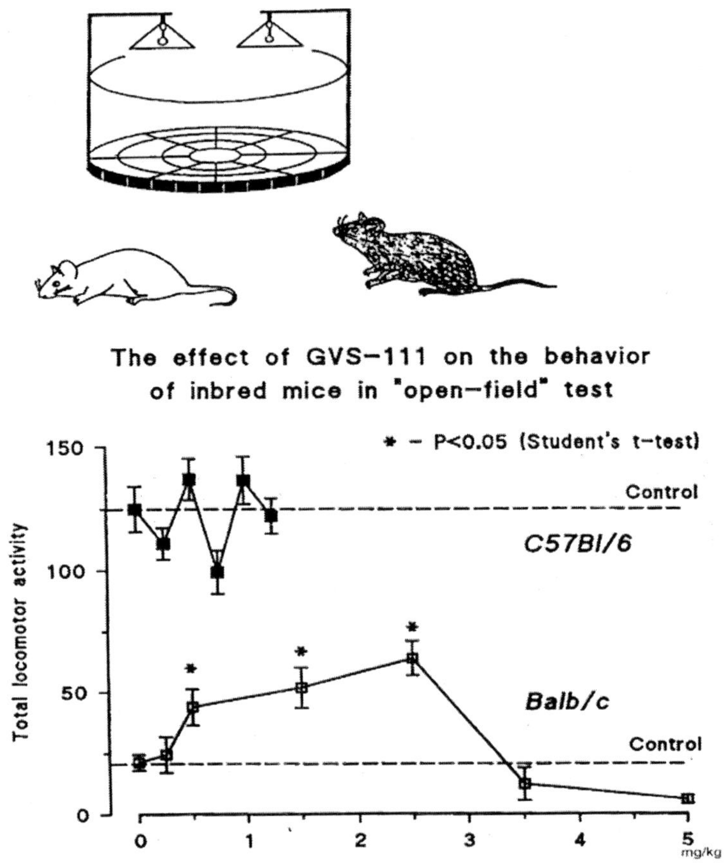

Fig. 2

Effects of GVS-111 on Locomotor Activity, Muscle Tone and Motor Coordination

Assessing the background activity (scored during the first 5 min), we noted that all groups did not differ in their locomotion. However, using a longer observation period, we revealed pronounced behavioural effects induced by GVS-111. While control animals actively explored the multi-channel activity analyzer chamber and each other for 10-15 min, then reducing their activity to 50-60% of the initial level by 30th min, the GVS-111-treated animals diminished their exploratory activity much faster, by 30th min showing activity levels much below their saline-treated counterparts. In addition, as can be seen in Table 5, this effect was clearly dose-dependent.

Table 4. Effects of GVS-111 administered 30 min prior to the open-field test (C57Bl /6 mice)

Dose mg/kg	Behavioral measures			
	Peripheral squares	Central squares	Rearing	Total activity
Saline (n = 35)	89.0±6.3	22.8±2.8	9.0±1.4	125.5±9.2
0.25 (n = 32)	84.1±6.8	19.5±1.1	7.3±1.4	110.9±6.5
0.50 (n = 38)	101.8±4.3	24.8±3.9	11.1±2.3	137.7±8.3
0.75 (n = 34)	79.0±8.2	15.0±3.3	5.2±1.0	99.2±9.8
1.00 (n = 29)	105.6±6.8	20.7±2.3	10.1±1.1	136.5±9.5
1.25 (n = 32)	92.2±2.3	21.7±0.9	8.1±1.1	122.1±7.2

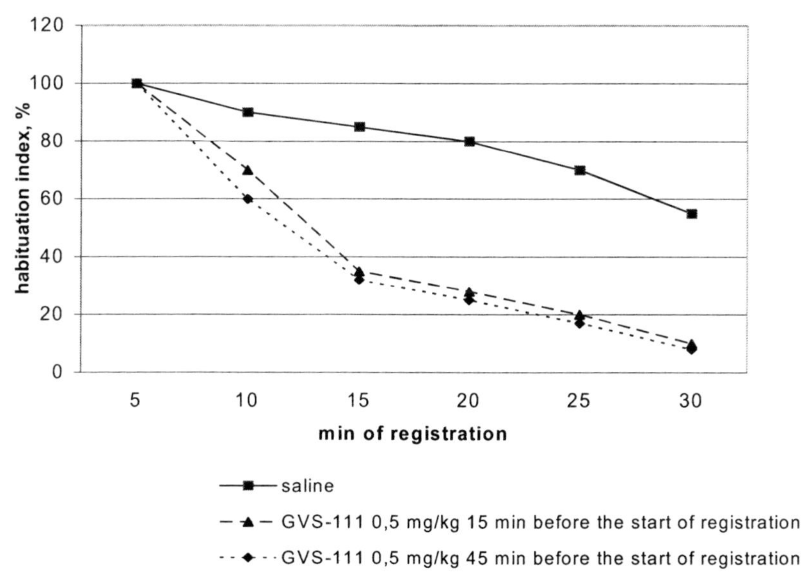

Fig. 3. Habituation in the saline-treated and the GVS-111-treated mice

As reported previously, various CE are able to facilitate habituation extinction of locomotory exploration (Ostrovskaya, Gudasheva, 1991). Habituation is known to be the result of animal' estimation of the environment as exerting neither positive nor negative influences, i.e. not provoking the active behavior. We suggest that following CE treatment, animals realize that there is no need to explore ("negative learning") much faster than do their saline-treated controls. However, the decrease in activity of GVS-111-treated animals may not only be due to its ability to facilitate habituation but also due to its sedative effects developing in the course of the time.

In order to discriminate between these two potential factors, an additional experiment was performed, in which GVS-111 was injected 45 (not 15) min prior to testing. Fig. 3 shows that the background activity in GVS-111-treated animals was similar to that of the control group, whereas for the next 30 min the decrease in the activity developed again more rapidly than in controls. Similar background activity observed in both experiments (using 15-min and 45-min intervals) allows us to assume that activity reduction observed here is due to increased habituation and not because of sedation. This conclusion is in a good agreement with the fact that GVS-111 (0.5-1000 mg/kg) produced no effects on the mouse ability to hang on the wire and did not disturb the rota-rod performance, i.e. neither induced muscle relaxation nor disturbed motor coordination.

Table 5. Effects of GVS-111 on habituation in mice

Dose of GVS-111, mg/kg	Habituation index (%)		P<
	Saline-treated group	GVS-111 treated group	
0.05	55	40	0.5
0.1	53	15	0.05
0.5	57	10	0.01
2.5	80	25	0.05
5.0	63	27	0.05
10.0	68	28	0.05

IV. General Discussion

The main aim of this study was to clarify whether GVS-111 (previously reported to be a highly effective CE), influences the level of anxiety. In order to evaluate the effect of GVS-111 on anxiety, a wide spectrum of methods was used, including both the conventional and novel behavioural models. Overall, GVS-111 increased the latency to enter the dark LD compartment (only in less anxiogenic PACS apparatus). GVS-111 also increased open time spent in the EPM.

An in-depth analysis of GVS-111 activity over a wide dose range revealed the inverted U-shaped dose-activity curve typical for peptidergic drugs. In the conflict behavior test, GVS-111 increased the number of punished water intakes. The distinguishing feature of our experiments was the use of relatively weak punishment (0.25 mA), since it has been shown previously that only highly active nonselective benzodiazepines are able to affect the reaction caused by a stronger stimuli, such as 1.0 mA (Molodavkin, 1996). Our results obtained in two LD tests, EPM, the conflict test as well as Opto-Varimex tests, show the inability of the drug to cause sedation, thus suggesting its selective anxiolytic effect.

Several important data to prove this profile of GVS-111 were obtained in pharmacogenetic studies (see details in: Seredenin et al. 1986, 1994, 2003). Numerous experiments using C57Bl/6 and Balb/c mice revealed marked differences in their behaviors in stessogenic open-field situation: active type of behavior in C57Bl/6 and "freezing" responses in Balb/c mice. These two strains also demonstrate different responses to benzodiazepine tranquillizers: dose-dependent activation in Balb/c and sedation in C57Bl/6 mice. In addition, these two strains exhibit marked metabolic differences closely related to the problem in question. Briefly, Balb/c mice are less resistant to pro-oxidant factors, demonstrating higher content of lipid peroxidation products in the brain, than C57Bl/6 mice (Durnev, Seredenin, 1998). These strain differences in the action of selective anxiolytics on the animals with various type of stress reactions (C57Bl/6 and Balb/c mice, MR and MNRA rats) have been confirmed in the experiments with a novel selective benzimidazol anxiolytic Afobasol (Seredenin et al., 2003). Consistent with this, GVS-111 produced inverted U-shaped behavioural activation (similar to those revealed in the EPM) in Balb/c mice.

Taken together, our results show that GVS-111 exerts a clear profile of a mild selective anxiolytic drug. At the same time, several our previously published studies have shown that GVS-111 is a highly effective CE able to facilitate different forms of learning, restore memories disturbed by brain trauma, ischemia and other damaging factors (Ostrovskaya et al., 2002), increase the amplitude of transcallosal response (Molodavkin et al., 2002), and augment hippocampal long-term potentiation (Chepkova A. et al., 1995), the synaptic equivalents of memory-improving effect. These combined nootropic and anxiolytic effects of GVS-111 were independently confirmed by other groups using active avoidance disturbed by stress (Ujanaev et al., 2003).

The fact that this CE also demonstrates anxiolytic effect represents an important difference of GVS-111 from many other memory-improving drugs. According to Kalueff and Nutt (1997), and Takamatsu et al. (2003), memory-improving substances usually provoke anxiogenic states, whereas anxiolytics exert clear amnestic effect. In both works, these authors analyze GABA-positive and GABA-negative substances, provoking anxiolytic and amnestic (e.g. muscimol) or anxiogenic and memory-improving (e.g. bicuculline) effects. GVS-111 in our experiments failed to antagonize the amnestic effect of diazepam and did not alter the effects of bicuculline. These findings allow us to suggest that GABA-related mechanisms may not be implicated in the GVS-111 profile.

Thus, the question arises as for whether there may be some other special mechanisms involved in the action of GVS-111, and whether the mechanisms contributing to its CE/anxiolytic effects overlap. At least two possible mechanisms may be suggested to explain the GVS-111 activity. First, pharmacokinetic studies of GVS-111 demonstrate that this linear dipeptide in vivo gives a rise to formation of cyclo-prolile-glycine (cPG) as a main metabolite. Notably, cPG is a natural endogenous metabolite of brain tissues (Gudasheva et al., 1996b; 1997). Administered exogenously (0.05-0.1 mg/kg), cPG (like GVS-111) exerts selective anxiolytic effect in a battery of punished and unpunished tests (Gudasheva et al., 2001). The content of endogenous cPG in Balb/c mice brain was lower than in C57Bl/6 mice. Finally, the increase of GVS-111 effect in the LD test with a 2-h interval also supports the assumption that cPG contributes to anxiolytic effect of the parental molecule, especially given previously published pharmacokinetic data showing the maximum brain cPG level at a 2-h checkpoint (Bojko et al., 2000). At the same time cPG, administered exogenously prior to learning, improves memory, although it does not imitate the effect of GVS-111 on the later stages of memory processing (Gudasheva et al., 1999). Taken together, these results suggest that cPG may be involved in both anxiolytic and memory-improving effects of GVS-111.

Another common aspect in cognition and anxiogenesis relates to nicotine-sensitive cholinergic mechanisms. Our previous electrophysiological experiments (Ostrovskasya et al., 2001) on the isolated neurons of *Helix lucorum* revealed that GVS-111 increases the amplitude of the neuronal response to acetylcholine (Ach) microiontophoretic application and to facilitate the endo-neuronal pacemaker activity. Taking into account that GVS-111 does not inhibit cholinesterase activity, and that the effects of GVS-111 were attenuated by the N-cholinolytic substance mecamilamine (n-Ach receptor antagonist), the hypothesis of nicotine-sensibilizing effects of this dipeptide may be suggested. A considerable body of evidence suggests that nicotine and nicotinic agonists have pronounced anxiolytic effects in experimental tests (Decker et al., 1994). Consistent with this, in humans, smoking–induced mood alteration, frequently associated with "calming" and even mild euphoric reactions in smokers (Warburton, 1988).

Moreover, there are numerous data showing cognitive and memory-enhancing properties of nicotine in animals and humans (Decker et al., 1995; Levin, Rezvani, 2000). An important role or nicotine in cognitive functions, including memory, becomes even more impressive given the significant loss of nicotinic receptors in hippocampus and frontal cortex, two brain regions crucial for cognitive function, in Alzheimer patients. Finally, a significant cognitive improvement in these patients after nicotine and positive modulators of n-Ach receptors has been reported in these patients. Collectively, this suggests that "nicotino-positive" effects of GVS-111 may be involved in its anxiolytic and CE-like effects.

Importantly, stressogenic influences have been repeatedly reported to increase the production of reactive oxygen species (ROS), damaging cellular macromolecules such as proteins, DNA and lipids. Therefore, anxiolytic effect may be coupled with cytoprotective action. Clearly, this notion is true for GVS-111, possessing pronounced neuroprotective effects (Ostrovsksaya et al., 1999, 2002). One of the important mechanisms of GVS-111' activity is its possible antioxidant action. Immobilization stress is known to provoke marked increase in both initial (diene conjugates) and terminal (Schiff's bases) products of lipid peroxidation. Pretreatment with GVS-111 lowered lipid peroxidation products in the brain and plasma, as well as prevented stress-induced extra-erythrocyte hemoglobin increase caused by the elevation of erythrocyte membrane permeability (Lysenko et al, 1997). Futher studies of GVS-111 revealed its ability to decrease ROS accumulation, and to increase the activity of antioxidant systems (superoxide-dismutase and catalase) in rats with high anxiety level (Mendzeherizkij et al, 2003). Strong evidences of anti-oxidant effects of this dipeptide have been obtained in the Department of Pharmacology of the University of Connecticut Health Center (Farmington, CT, USA) by J. Busciglio and his colleagues using primary culture of human neurons prepared from the brains after medical abortion (17 to 19-week pregnancy). In their experiments, a 1-h exposure to 50 μM H_2O_2 resulted in 38±3 % neuronal survival. When added to H_2O_2 treated cultures, GVS-111 dose-dependently increased neuronal survival (10 nM: 47±5; 100 μM: 85±9.; IC_{50} for GVS-111: 1.7±0.07 μM).

Notably, neither a free radical speen trap s-PBN nor anti-oxidants vitamin E, propyl gallate and piracetam caused significant protection in this concentration. GVS-111 capability for preventing the increase in DCFDA- and TBA-fluorescence after H_2O_2 exposure clearly shows that GVS-111 neuroprotection is related to its antioxidant properties. These data also show that GVS-111 is by 2-3 orders of magnitude a more efficient antioxidant than PBN, vitamin E or piracetam (Pielsman et al., 2003). Considering ROS as important pathogenic membrane-damaging factors, it is worth to note that pronounced antioxidant activity of GVS-111 may contribute to its membrano-stabilizing effect which, in turn, may underlie both anxiolytic and neuroprotective effects of the drug.

Given the fact that GVS-111 combines nootropic, neuroprotective and anxiolytic profiles, it was therefore possible to test this compound in clinical conditions in patients with psychoorganic symptoms, including chronic cognitive deficit and cerebro-asthenic disorders. Since chronic treatment is more compatible with peroral (p.o.) administration, it was necessary to examine whether GVS-111 preserves its activity following p.o. administration. Notably, peptides generally fail to re-produce their effects following p.o. administration due to rapid metabolization in the stomach and intestine. However, dipeptides are the only exception from this rule, since due to ATP-dependent transport systems they are able to absorb from the intestine to the blood (Friecker, Drewe, 1996). The presence of the substitutions in N- and C- positions was an additional factor for the increased biological stability of GVS-111. Indeed, behavioral experiments demonstrated that GVS-111 maintains the activity following its p.o. administration. These results are consistent with pharmacokinetic data showing good GVS-111 p.o. absorbtion. In addition, these studies showed that GVS-111 enters the blood and penetrates into the brain, where its concentrations are higher than in plasma, thus confirming highly specific bioavailability of this dipeptide in the brain. These pharmacodynamic and pharmacokinetic studies led to the development of a pharmaceutical form of GVS-111 (trade name Noopept) in tablets containing 5 or 10 mg of this substance.

Clinical trials with Noopept were carried out at two clinical centers in 60 patients suffering from chronic cerebro-vascular insufficiency or brain trauma (F.06.7, F.06.6, F.07.2). The clinical program (second phase) examined the effect of Noopept in patients with mild psychoorganic symptoms caused by cerebrovascular disorder or traumatic brain injury.

Chronic treatment with Noopept (28 days, three 5-mg intakes daily) produced clear therapeutic effects in these patients improving their major psychoorganic symptoms. Noopept showed robust cognito-tropic properties, manifest in its positive influence on the basic cognitive parameters: memory, attention, senso-motor activity, goal-directed intellectual activity. These effects directly suggest nootropic component in the spectrum of GVS-111 pharmacological activity. The results of psychophysiological study of its effects further support clinical data suggesting its potency to improve cognitive functions, especially attention. Noopept also produced statistically significant reduction in cerebro-asthenic disorders (exhaustion, apathy, etc.), anxiety, irritability, hyperesthesia, affective instability, night sleep disorders, and various vegetative dysfunctions. The pharmaco-EEG analysis of acute and chronic (28 days) treatment with Noopept revealed EEG-responses typical for traditional nootropic drugs, including increased power of alpha-rhythm and decreased power of slow rhythms and beta-rhythms.

These clinical data show that therapeutic potency of Noopept combines nootropic, anxiolytic, vegeto-normalizing and "mild" activating effects. The drug has no genuine hypnotic effect, but was capable to produce marked sleep-normalizing effects (probably, due to its anxiolytic activity and reduction of other negative symptoms). Specific nootropic effects of the drug developed 2-3 weeks after the beginning of the therapy, which is in agreement with typical dynamic characteristics of nootropic drugs (Neznamov et al., 2002). Therefore, Noopept is efficient for the therapy of psychoorganic disorders with predominant cognitive and cerebro-asthenic dysfunctions. Importantly, the drug was well-tolerated, and therefore may be recommended as a prospective nootropic drug to treat psychoorganic disorders of traumatic and vascular genesis with mild-to-moderate cognitive disorders. Moreover, further studies of Noopept effectiveness in patients with severe cognitive deficit will provide an important area for its clinical investigation.

V. Concluding Remarks

Notably, stress-induced disregulation of the hypothalamo-pituitary-adrenocortical system has long been known to cause cognitive impairments. Various stressogenic factors, including chronic restraint stress (Bowman et al., 2002), brain trauma (Brandes et al., 2002), long-term prednisone administration (Ramos-Remus et al., 2002), neonatal maternal separation (Huot et al., 2002), were reported to impair learning and memory due to increased glucocorticoid secretion. These impairments include deficits in acquisition in the Morris watermaze (Huot et al., 2002) and the radial-arm maze performance (Bowman et al., 2002). Corticotropin–releasing hormone (CRH) was shown to impair spatial discrimination in a two-choice watermaze (Steckler et al., 2001), whereas chronic administration of prednisone (5 mg/kg/day, equivalent to moderate doses used in clinical settings) has been shown (Ramos-Remus et al., 2002) to disturb learning and memory retention, produce neuronal degeneration and cerebral glial changes, cytoplasmic transformation of astrocytes and microglia cells in the prefrontal cortex and the CA1 area of hippocampus, i.e. in cerebral regions directly involved in cognitive functions.

Moreover, there are numerous data showing that stress can improve selective attention due to reduced task-irrelevant cognitive processes (Chajut, Algom, 2003). In general, as already mentioned, the relationships between stress responses and cognitions are rather ambiguous. The nature, intensity and duration of stress, as well as the form of the cognition in question (e.g., attention, perception, memory), may cause either negative or positive interplay. Perhaps, the best generalization of these two determinants was given by Mc Namura and Skelton (1993) noting that "optimal level of anxiety is required for learning, while shifts in either direction resulting in the worsening of performance". It is therefore possible to assume that GVS-111 with its mild selective (non-sedating) anxiolytic profile may indeed be a substance "tuning" the anxiety to such "optimal" level.

Importantly, in clinical situations anxiety and cognitive impairments usually co-exist. All forms of cognitive deficits (e.g., cerebro-vascular insufficiency, post-traumatic pathology, age-dependent cognitive and neurodegenerative dysfunctions, alcohol-induced encephalopathy, etc.) typically co-occur with more or less pronounced affective disorders, such as anxiety (Errico et al., 2002; Brandes, 2002). Therefore, the search of substances possessing both cognitive-improving and anxiolytic activity represents an important area of psychopharmacological research. A better understanding of complex interplay between stress and cognition opens avenues for creation of such principally new therapeutic agents, and Noopept (GVS-111) clearly holds great promise in this respect.

Acknowledgements

This study was supported by the Russian Foundation for Basic Research (03-04-49049).

References

[1] Ader R., Weijnen J.A.W.M., Moleman P. Retention of a passive avoidance responses as a function of the intensity and duration of electric shock. *Psychol. Sci.* 1972, 26(3), 125-128.

[2] Armanini M.P., Hutchins C., Stein B.A., Sapolsky R.M. Glucocorticoid endangerment of hippocampal neurons is NMDA-receptor dependent. Brain Research 1990; 532, 7-12.

[3] Bojko S.S., Ostrovskaya R.U., Zherdev V.P. et al., Pharmacokynetics and blood-brain permeability of the novel acylproline dipeptide with nootropic properties in case of its peroral administration. *Bull. Experim. Biol. Med.* 2000, 129 (4), 426-429.

[4] Bowman R.E., Ferguson D., Luine V.N. Effects of chronic restraint stress and estradiol on open field activity, spatial memory, and monoaminergic neurotransmitters in ovariectomized rats. *Neurosci.* 2002, 113, 401-410.

[5] Brandes D., Ben-Schachar G., Gilboa A. et al. PTSD symptoms and cognitive performance in recent trauma survivors. *Psychiatry Res.* 2002, 110(3), 231-238.

[6] Bremner D.J., Scott T.M, Delaney R.C. et al. Deficits in short-term memory in posttraumatic stress disorders. *Am. J. Psych.* 1993, 150, 1015-1019.

[7] Chajut E., Algom D. Selective attention improves under stress: implications for theories of social cognition. *J. Pers. Soc. Psychol.* 2003, 85, 231-248.

[8] Chepkova A.N., Trofimov S.S., Ostrovskaya R.U. The damage of the rat hippocampal plasticity caused by prenatal hypoxia and its treatment with nootropic dipeptides. *Bull. Exp. Biol. Med.* 1995, 120, 592-595.

[9] Decker M.W., Brioni J.D., Bannon A.W., Arneric S.P. Diversity of neuronal nicotinic acetylcholine receptors: lessons from behavior and implications for CNS therapeutics. *Life Sci.* 1995, 56, 545-570.

[10] Durnev A.D., Seredenin S.B. Mutagens. Screening and pharmacological prophylaxis of action. Medicine, Moscow 1998 .

[11] Errico A.L., King A.C., Lovallo W.R., Parsons O.A. Cortisol dysregulation and cognitive impairment in abstinent male alcoholics. Alcohol Clin. Exp. Res. 2002, 26(8), 1198-1204.

[12] File S.E. The history of benzodiazepine dependence: a review of animal studies. Neurosci. Biobehav. Revs 1990, 14, 135-146.

[13] Friecker G., Drewe J. Current concepts in intestinal peptide absorption. *J. Pept. Sci.* 1996, 2 (4), 194-211.

[14] Giurgea C. Vers une pharmacologie de l'active integrative du cerveau. Tentative du concept nootrope en psychopharmacologie. *Act. Pharmacol.* 1972, 25, 115-156.

[15] Gold P.E., Stone W.S. Neuroendocrine factors in age-related memory dysfunctions: studies in animals and humans. *Neurobiol. Aging* 1988, 9, 709-717.

[16] Gudasheva T.A., Ostrovskaya R.U., Trofimov S.S. et al. Peptide analogues of Piracetam as a ligands of the proposed nootropic receptors. Chim.-Farm. Zh. 1985, 11, 1322-1329.

[17] Gudasheva T.A., Voronina T.A., Ostrovskaya R.U. et al. Synthesis and antiamnesic activity of a series of N-acylprolyl-containing dipeptides. *Eur. J. Med. Chem.* 1996a, 31, 151-157.

[18] Gudasheva T.A., Boyko S.S., Akparov V.Kh. et al. Identification of a novel endogenous memory facilitating cyclic dipeptide cyclo-prolyl-glycine in rat brain. FEBS Lett. 1996b, 391, 149-152.

[19] Gudasheva T., Bojko S., Voronina T. et al. The major metabolite of dipeptide piracetam analogue GVS-111 in rat brain and its similarity to endogenous neuropeptide cyclo-L-prolylglycine. *Eur. J. Drug Metabol. Pharmacokin.* 1997, 22, 245-252.

[20] Gudasheva T.A., Ostrovskaya R.U., Trofimov S.S.et al., Structuro-functional similarity of the brain peptide, cyclo-Pro-Gly and nootropic drug Piracetam. *Bull. Exp. Biol. Med.* 1999, 116, 411-413.

[21] Gudasheva T.A., Konstantinopolsky M.A., Ostrovskaya R.U., Seredenin S.B. Anxiolytic action of endogenous nootropic dipeptide cyclo-Pro-Gly in elevated plus maze test. *Bull. Exp. Biol. Med.* 2001, 131, 547-550.

[22] Huot R.L., Plotsky P.M., Lenox R.H. et al. Neonatal maternal separation reduces hippocampal mossy fiber density in adult Long Evans rats. *Brain Res.* 2002, 950, 52-63.

[23] Kalueff A.V., Nutt D.J. Role of GABA in memory and anxiety. Depress. Anxiety, 1997, 4, 100-110.

[24] Levin E.D., Rezvani A. Development of nicotinic drug therapy for cognitive disorders. *Eur. J. Pharm.* 2000, 393, 141-146.

[25] Liu J., Mori A. Involvement of reactive oxygen species in emotional stress: a hypothesis based on the immobilization stress-induced oxidative damsge and

antioxidant defense changes in rat brain, and the effect of antioxidant treatment with reduced glutathione. *Int. J. Stress Manag*. 1994, 1, 249-263.

[26] Lysenko A.V., Uskova E.I., Gudasheva T.A., Voronina T.A. Dipeptide nootropic substance GVS-111 prevents the accumulation of the free oxygen radicals caused by the immobilization in rats. *Exp. Clin. Farm*. 1997, 60, 15-18.

[27] Mendzeritsky A.M., Lysenko A.V., Demianenko S.V. et al. Lipid peroxidation in a cerebral cortex and blood plasma of young rats with high level of anxiety under emotional stress: protective effect of nootropic dipeptide GVS-111. Neurochem. 2003, 20(4), 281-286.

[28] McNamara R.K., Skelton R.W. The neuropharmacological and neurochemical bases of place learning in the Morris water maze. *Brain Res. Rev*. 1993, 18, 33-49.

[29] Molodavkin G.M., Borlicova G.G., Voronina T.A. et al. The effect of the novel dipeptide cognitive enhancer Noopept and its metabolite cyclo-Pro-Gly on the transcallosal evoked potential in the rat neocortex. *Exp. Clin. Pharm*. 2002, 65, 3-5.

[30] Molodavkin G.M., Voronina T.A. The dependence of the anxiolytic activity in conflict behavior test on the anxiety level. *Bull. Exper. Biol. Med*. 1996, 121(1), 63-66.

[31] Neznamov G., Seredenin S., Siuniakov S. et al. Novel notropic drug Noopept; results of pilot clinical trials. *Pharmacologist*. 2002, 44 Suppl. 1, A 164.

[32] Ostrovskaya R.U., Gudasheva T.A. The acute extinction of the explorative behavior as a test for the revealing of the cognitive enhancing activity. *Bull. Exp. Biol. Med*. 1991, 3(5), 644-647.

[33] Ostrovskaya R.U., Romanova G.A., Gudasheva T.A. et al. Memory restoring and neuroprotective effects of the proline containing dipeptride, GVS-111, in a photochemical stroke model. *Behav. Pharmacol*. 1999, 10, 549-553.

[34] Ostrovskaya R.U., Mirzoev T.Kh., Firova F.A. et al. Behavioral and electrophysiological analysis of the cholino-positive effect of the nootropic acyl-prolyn containing dipeptide GVS-111. Exp. *Clin. Farm*. 2001, 64(2), 11-14.

[35] Ostrovskaya R.U., Gudasheva T.A., Voronina T.A., Seredeninn S.B. Novel nootropic and neuroprotective medicine, Noopept. *Exp.Clin. Farm*. 2002, 5, 66-73.

[36] Pellow S., Chopin P., File S., Briley M. Validation of open: closed arm entries in an elevated plus-maze as a measure of anxiety in the rat. *J. Neurosci. Methods* 1985, 14, 149-167.

[37] Pelsman A., Hoyo-Vadillo C., Tatiana A. Gudasheva T.A. et al. GVS-111 prevents oxidative damage and apoptosis in normal and Down's syndrome human cortical neurons. *Int. J. Dev. Neurosci*, 2003, 21, 117–124.

[38] Ramos-Remus C., Gonzalez-Castaneda R.E., Gonzalez-Perez O. et al. Prednisone induces cognitive dysfunction, neuronal degeneration, and reactive gliosis in rats. *J. Investig. Med*. 2002, 50(6), 458-464.

[39] Seredenin S.B., Viglinskaya I.V., Kashevskaya O.B. The pharmacogenetic approach to the evaluation of the effect of tranquillisers. In: Seredenin S.B., Longo V., Gaviraghi G., eds. *Biological Basis of Individual Sensitivity to Psychotropic Drugs*. Edinburgh: Graffham Press, 1994. P. 47-56.

[40] Seredenin S.S., Voronina T.A., Gudasheva T.A. et al. Biologically active N-acylprolyldipeptides having antiamnestic, antihypoxic and anorexigenic effects. *US Patent* 5, 439, 930. 1995.

[41] Seredenin S.B. Genetic differences in response to emotional stress and tranquilizers. *Psychopharm. Biol. Narcol.*, 2003, 1-2, 494-509.

[42] Steckler Th, Holsboer F. et al. Interaction between the cholinergic system and CRH in the modulation of spatial discrimination learning in mice. *Brain Res.*, 2001, 906, 46-59.

[43] Takamatsu H., Noda A., Kurumaji A. et al. A PET study following treatment with a pharmacological stressor, FG7142, in conscious rhesus monkeys. *Brain Res.*, 2003, 980(2), 275-280.

[44] Trullas R., Skolnick P. Differences in fear motivated behaviors among inbred mouse strains. *Psychopharmacol.* 1993, 111, 323-331.

[45] Ujanaev A.A., Fisenko V.P., Hitrov N.K. The influence of noopept and afobazole on the dynamics of neurotic state in learned helplessness test in rats. *Bull. Exp. Biol. Med.* 2003, 136(8), 187-189.

[46] Vogel J., Beer B., Clody D. A simple and reliable conflict procedure for testing antianxiety agents. *Psychopharmacol.* 1971, 21, 1-7.

[47] Warburton D. The puzzle of nicotine use. In: Lader M., ed. *The psychopharmacology of addiction*. Oxford: Oxford University Press; 1988, 27-49.

[48] Wolkowith O.M., Reus V.I., Weigartner H. et al. Cognitive effects of corticosteroids. *Am. J. Psych.* 1990, 147(10), 1297-1303.

In: Animal Models in Biological Psychiatry
Editor: Allan V. Kalueff, pp. 183-196
ISBN 1-59454-814-5

Chapter 11

Mouse Grooming Microstructure is a Reliable Behavioural Index in Anxiety Psychopharmacology: GABA-ergic Drugs

Allan V. Kalueff and Pentti Tuohimaa
Medical School of the University of Tampere,
Tampere University Hospital, Tampere, 33014, Finland

I. Introduction

Self-grooming is an ancient innate behaviour that is represented across most animal species (Berridge et al., 1987; Aldridge and Berridge, 1998). It is an important, complex and hierarchically ordered part of rodent behavioural repertoire (Berridge and Aldridge, 2000) generally proceeding in cephalo-caudal direction: paw licking - nose and face wash - head wash - body wash and fur licking - leg licking - tail/genitals licking and wash (Fentress, 1977; Berridge and Whishaw, 1992; Cromwell and Berridge, 1996). In rodents, grooming is particularly sensitive to stress and various endo- and exogenous manipulations (Van Erp et al., 1994, 1995; Moyaho et al., 1995; Moyaho and Valencia, 2002). It has long been known that rodents' grooming activity can be generally increased in two opposite situations: in high and low stress (Kalueff and Tuohimaa, 2004a). Low-stress comfort grooming is a spontaneous body care ritual which occurs as a transition from rest to activity; it is a typical behavioural marker of low or no stress, usually going uninterrupted in a "relaxed fashion" from paw licking to tail/genitals wash (Fentress, 1977). Similarly, stress has long been known to induce grooming in rodents (Moyaho et al., 1995; Moyaho and Valencia, 2002). However, this stress-evoked grooming ethologically differs from low-stress comfort grooming, and is characterised by frequent bursts of rapid short grooming activity with abnormal progression and frequent incomplete and interrupted bouts (Fentress, 1977).

Many neuromediators and hormones as well as multiple brain regions are involved in the regulation of comfort and stress-evoked grooming (Dunn et al., 1987; Van Erp et al, 1994; Cromwell et al., 1998; Eguibar et al., 2003). Importantly, several peptides released under stress conditions (e.g., adrenocorticotropic hormone (ACTH), corticoliberin (CRH), prolactin, vasopressin, oxytocin, bombesin) stimulate grooming in rodents, mimicking the effects of stressors on grooming behaviour (Drago et al., 1980, 1983; Gispen and Isaacson, 1981; Caldwell et al., 1987; Bertolini et al., 1988; Dunn et al., 1988; Traber et al., 1988; Lumley et al., 2001; Amico et al., 2004). These observations further strengthen the link between stress and grooming behaviour in rodents.

Gamma-aminobutyric acid (GABA) is the primary mediator of inhibitory transmission in the mammalian central nervous system (Sieghart et al., 1999). It has complex interactions with other neurotransmitter systems and acts through ionotropic A and metabotropic B type receptors which play important role in the brain and are a target for a variety of endogenous and exogenous modulators (Nutt and Malizia, 2001; Korpi et al., 2002; Mombereau et al., 2004). GABA-A receptors are ligand-gated ion channels (Inbox I). Binding of GABA opens up a Cl^- channel, which is part of the protein structure. GABA-A receptors contain binding sites for many positive modulators including barbiturates, benzodiazepines, steroids and ethanol (Sieghart et al., 1999; Korpi et al., 2002).

Inbox I. The GABA-A benzodiazepone receptor complex: schematic representation of the binding sites

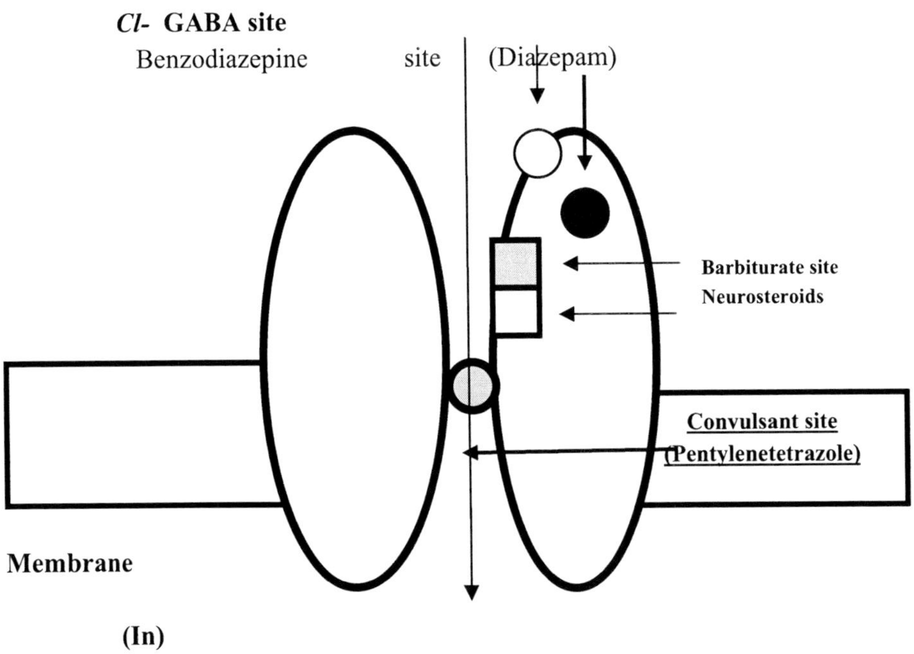

See (Kalueff and Nutt, 1997; Nutt and Malizia, 2001; Kutsenko, 2002; Korpi et al., 2003) for details. Note: Diazepam binds to benzidiazepine site, pentylenetetrazole binds to convulsant site (located near the ionophore).

GABA and its $GABA_A$ receptors are involved in the regulation of a number of normal and pathological brain mechanisms, such as sleep, epilepsy, memory, emotions and various behaviours (Kalueff and Nutt, 1997; Sieghart et al., 1999; Nutt and Malizia, 2001), including grooming (Barros et al., 1992; 1994). At the same time, dysfunctions of the GABAergic system have long been associated with stress and anxiety spectrum disorders (Nutt and Malizia, 2001). In both humans and animals, positive modulators of $GABA_A$ receptors, such as benzodiazepines, possess robust anxiolytic activity while negative modulators, such as chloride channel blockers, have been reported to produce anxiogenic effects (Kalueff and Nutt, 1997; Belzung, 2001; Korpi et al., 2002). Given the role of GABA in the regulation of anxiety and grooming, and the influence of stress on grooming behaviours, it is therefore of interest to assess the effects of GABAergic anxiolytic and anxiogenic drugs on grooming behaviours.

Although grooming in rodents plays a very important role, in many anxiety studies this behaviour has merited little scrutiny, frequently addressed only cursorily among other measures (for details, see Kalueff and Tuohimaa, 2004a; Kalueff et al., 2004). In general, traditional grooming measures include the latency to onset, the number of bouts and the duration of grooming bouts. Although several GABAergic drugs have been reported to affect the duration and frequency of grooming (Barros et al., 1992; 1994), we note that grooming is a complex ethologically "rich" behaviour (Fentress, 1977), and therefore its behavioural organization (patterning), in addition to activity measures, also needs experimental investigation in detail. The present study sought to extend the available literature on the behavioural pharmacology of anxiety by presenting a detailed ethological analysis of the effects of GABAergic anxiolytic and anxiogenic drugs on grooming in mice. In the present study, we used as reference compounds anxiolytic benzodiazepine diazepam and anxiogenic chloride channel blocker pentylenetetrazole (Inbox I) at systemic doses traditionally known to induce specific anxiolytic and anxiogenic effects in rodents, respectively.

Since our work was the first study to analyse the effects of these drugs on grooming sequencing, and given its high sensitivity to various manipulations, we wanted to avoid possible non-specific effects of these drugs (Kalueff and Tuohimaa, 2005). For example, C57BL/6 mice used in the present study have long been known as a mouse strain highly sensitive to diazepam. Indeed, acute i.p. administration of 1 mg/kg diazepam produced strong sedative effects in these mice (Ohl et al., 2001a). Therefore, we chose a non-sedating 0.5 mg/kg dose as a maximal diazepam dose for our experiments (also see (Hascoet and Bourin, 1998) noting that anxiolytic effects of diazepam at 1 mg/kg coincide with the onset of sedation in mice). Importantly, at this dose of diazepam has been reported to exert reliable anxiolytic non-sedating effects in many rodent anxiety tests, including the light-dark and social defeat tests in mice (Lepicard et al., 2000; Lumley et al., 2000), elevated plus maze in hamsters and rats (Yannielli et al., 1996; Bert et al., 2001), devibrissation and the open field tests in rats (Kozlovskii and Prakh'e, 1995; Bert et al., 2001). Moreover, Merali et al. (2003) have recently reported a robust anxiolytic effect of 0.25 mg/kg diazepam in a novel sensitive palatable food consumption mouse paradigm. Collectively, these data justify the doses of diazepam used in the present study (0.1 and 0.5 mg/kg) to reduce anxiety in C57BL/6 mice without affecting locomotory functions in mice (which are crucial for grooming). The doses of pentylenetetrazole (5 and 10 mg/kg) were chosen based on its strong anxiogenic profile in the elevated plus maze in mice at 15-20 mg/kg (Rodgers et al., 1995), and on our own data showing that both doses used here elicited marked anxiogenic effects in the elevated plus-maze and the light-dark tests in rats (Kalueff, 2002).

Choosing the observation period for our study (5 min), we note that grooming is the immediate rodents' response to stress (Moyaho et al., 1995; Moyaho and Valecia, 2002), and therefore anxiety-related grooming alterations have to be analysed shortly after the stressor (novelty) is applied. Furthermore, given the impact of within-trial habituation on grooming (File et al., 1988), and since both drugs might affect grooming, habituation or both, we wanted to minimize the role of these additional factors in our study. Therefore, a short 5-min test (rather than a longer observation period) seemed to be appropriate to assess grooming in the present study. Finally, the pre-treatment time for our experiments (45 min) has been chosen based on numerous data showing that both drugs are able to exert their clear-cut behavioural effects 30-45 min after i.p. administration (Rodgers et al., 1995; Bert et al., 2000; Lumley et al., 2000; Ohl et al., 2001a; Kalueff, 2002).

Overall, here we analyse 1) grooming traditional cumulative measures and 2) grooming behavioural microstructure, following treatment with reference anxiolytic and anxiogenic GABAergic compounds, and using our grooming analysis algorithm already reported to be a reliable tool in neurobehavioural stress research in mice and rats (Kalueff and Tuohimaa, 2004a,b; 2005).

II. Materials and Methods

Animals

Experiments were carried out on adult C57BL/6 male mice (25-30 g; Tampere University, Finland). All animals were experimentally naïve, housed 4 per cage and kept in a controlled environment maintained at a constant temperature (24±1 °C) and humidity (60%), with free access to food and water. Lights were turned on at 6.00 h and off at 18.00 h. Animal care procedures were conducted in accordance with guidelines set by the European Community Council Directives (86/609/EEC).

Apparatus and Procedures

Behavioural testing was always conducted between 14.00 and 18.00 h. On test days, the animals were transported to the dimly lit laboratory and left undisturbed for 2 h prior to testing. The mice were administered the drugs intraperitoneally, placed individually in the clean plastic box (30 x 30 x 30 cm), and observed by an experienced investigator (intra-rater reliability >0.9) for a period of 5 min. The observer was blind to the treatment groups tested in a counter-balanced, random order. Between subjects, the box was thoroughly cleaned with wet and dry cloths. Non-grooming behavioural measures included vertical exploration (the number of vertical rears) and defecation (the number of defecation boli deposited).

Grooming Ethological Analysis

The observer recorded the duration and the number of grooming behaviours, using specially designed protocol sheets. In addition, the following grooming stages were recorded for each bout: paw licking, nose/face grooming (strokes along the snout), head washing (semicircular movements over the top of the head and behind ears), body grooming/scratching (body fur licking and scratching the body with the hind paws), leg licking and tail/genitals grooming (licking of the genital area and tail). Overall, five ethological measures of grooming activity were evaluated in our experiments: frequency (the number of grooming bouts); duration (total time spent grooming, s); average duration of a single grooming bout (s) calculated as total time spent grooming divided by the number of bouts; total number of transitions between grooming stages and average number of transitions per bout, calculated as total number of transitions divided by the number of bouts. To analyse grooming patterning, the following scaling system was used in the present study: no grooming (0), paw licking (1), nose/face/head wash (2), body grooming (3), leg licking (4), and tail/genitals grooming (5). A grooming bout was considered "interrupted" if at least one interruption was recorded within its transitions. Interruptions greater than 6 s determined separate grooming bouts. Grooming interruptions and correct vs. incorrect transitions between stages were analysed using the transition matrix, according to (Moyaho et al., 1995; Kalueff and Tuohimaa, 2004a). Correct transitions between grooming stages included the following progressive transitions: 0–1, 1–2, 2–3, 3–4, 4–5, 5–0. Incorrect transitions were chaotic and characterised by skipped (e.g. 0–5, 1–5, etc.) or reversed (e.g. 3–2, 4–1, 5–2, etc.) stages. Overall, two ethological measures of grooming behavioural patterning were evaluated in our experiments: the percentage of incorrect transitions (of total transitions) and the percentage of interrupted grooming bouts (of total number of bouts), according to (Kalueff and Tuohimaa, 2004a,b; 2005). The procedures used in this study were in strict accordance with the European legislation (86/609/EEC) and approved by the Ethical Committee of the University of Tampere.

Drugs

Diazepam and pentylenetetrazole were obtained from Sigma-Aldrich (Finland). Diazepam was dissolved in saline (to which a drop of Tween 80 per 5 ml saline had been added) 1 h prior to administration. Pentylenetetrazole was dissolved in saline 1 h prior to administration. Injection volumes of all drugs were 5 ml/kg body weight. Diazepam (0.1 and 0.5 mg/kg) and pentylenetetrazol (5 and 10 mg/kg) were injected intraperitoneally 45 min prior to testing. Control groups received the appropriate vehicle treatment.

Statistical Analysis

All results are expressed as mean ± S.E.M. Data were analysed by Kruskal-Wallis followed by a post-hoc Mann-Whitney tests for comparisons between control and experimental groups. A probability of less than 0.05 was considered statistically significant.

III. Results

Effects of Diazepam on Grooming

Diazepam exerted clear anxiolytic effects on non-grooming behaviours, significantly increasing vertical rears (14±3 (saline) vs. 26±4 (0.1 mg/kg, P<0.05) and 36±5 (0.5 mg/kg; P<0.05)) and predictably decreasing defecation boli (5+1 (saline) vs. 2+0.4 (0.1 mg/kg, P<0.05) and 2+0.2 (0.5 mg/kg, P<0.05); Kalueff and Tuohimaa, 2005.

Figure 1 shows grooming activity of mice following diazepam administration. In this experiment, the number of grooming bouts, the duration of grooming and total transitions between grooming stages were not altered by diazepam at any dose given. The drug also did not change the average duration of a single bout and the number of transitions per bout (Fig. 1). However, using a detailed grooming ethological analysis, we found that diazepam at both non-sedating anxiolytic doses produced a robust shift in grooming, "normalizing" its behavioural microstructure by decreasing the percentages of incorrect transitions (diazepam: 24±5% (0.1 mg/kg); 21±4% (0.5 mg/kg); saline: 48±7%; P < 0.05) and interrupted bouts (diazepam: 15±3% (0.1 mg/kg); 20±5% (0.5 mg/kg); saline: 36±5%; P < 0.05) (Fig. 1).

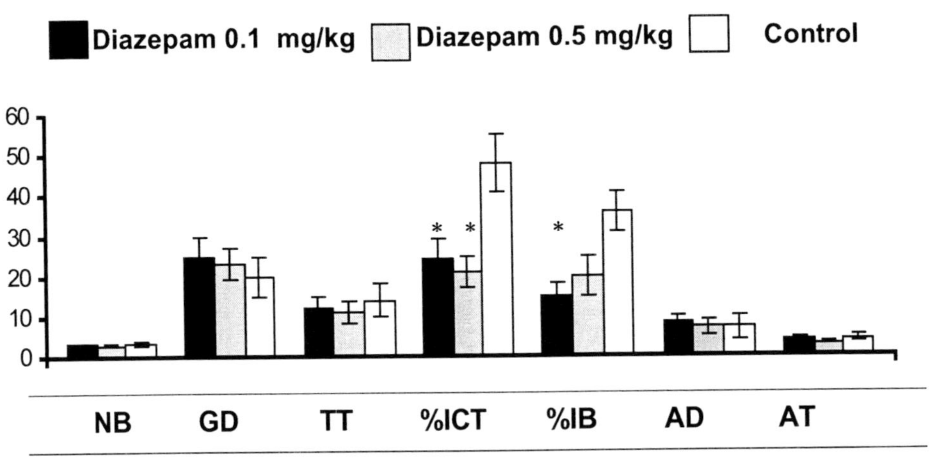

Fig. 1. Effects of diazepam on grooming behaviour in mice (n = 8), adapted from Kalueff and Tuohimaa, 2005. Data are expressed as mean ±S.E.M. *P<0.05, compared to control group. NB – number of grooming bouts; GD – total duration of grooming activity, (s); TT – number of transitions between grooming stages; %ICT – percentage of incorrect transitions (of total transitions); %IB – percentage of interrupted bouts (of total grooming bouts); AD – average duration of a single bout, AT – average number of transitions per bout.

Effects of Pentylenetetrazole on Grooming

Pentylenetetrazole exerted clear anxiogenic effects on non-grooming behaviours in mice, significantly decreasing vertical rears (18±4 (saline) vs. 9±1 (5 mg/kg, P<0.05) and 8±1 (10 mg/kg; P<0.05)), while predictably increasing defecation boli (4±1 (saline) vs. 7±2 (5 mg/kg, NS) and 8+1 (10 mg/kg, P<0.05).

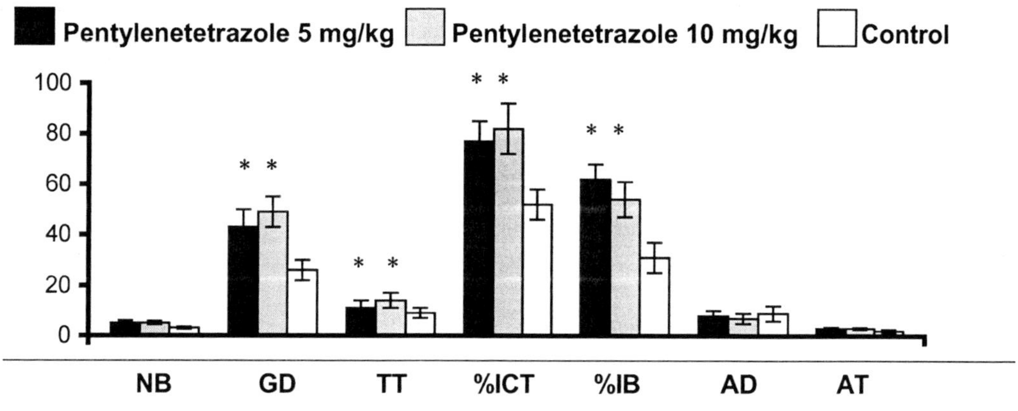

Fig. 2. Effects of pentylenetetrazole on grooming behaviour in mice (n = 8) (adapted from Kalueff and Tuohimaa, 2005). Legend as in Fig. 1.

Figure 2 shows the behavioural effects of pentylenetetrazole on mouse grooming activity. In this experiment, the drug-treated mice showed similar number of grooming bouts but spent significantly more time engaged in grooming activity than did their control counterparts (pentylenetetrazole: 43±7 s (5 mg/kg); 49±6 s (10 mg/kg); saline: 26±4 s; P < 0.05). The drug also had no effects on the average duration of a single bout and the number of transitions per bout (Fig. 2). However, a detailed ethological analysis of grooming microstructure in this experiment showed that pentylenetetrazole-treated mice, compared to the control group, generally display "high arousal" grooming patterns, including frequent incorrect transitions (pentylenetetrazole: 77±8% (5 mg/kg); 82±10% (10 mg/kg); saline: 52±6%; P < 0.05) and interrupted bouts (pentylenetetrazole: 62±6% (5 mg/kg); 54±7% (10 mg/kg); saline: 31±6%; P < 0.05).

IV. Discussion

The main aim of these studies was to pharmacologically assess the mouse grooming behavioural microstructure by testing standard anxiolytic and anxiogenic GABAergic drugs. The experiments with two classical reference compounds, diazepam and pentylenetetrazole, show that grooming behavioural sequencing, rather than its general "activity" measures, can effectively measure pharmacologically induced anxiolytic and anxiogenic-like effects. Indeed, diazepam did not alter grooming activity measures, but decreased the percentage of incorrect transitions and uninterrupted bouts. In contrast, both doses of pentyleneterazole, increasing the duration of grooming, also predictably increased the percentages of incorrect transitions and interrupted bouts. In addition, both drugs affected non-grooming behavioural indices of anxiety (vertical rears, defecation boli), producing clear anxiogenic (pentylenetetrazole) or anxiolytic (diazepam) effects.

Notably, these results differ from several previously published studies examining the effects of some GABAergic drugs on rodent novelty-induced grooming. For example, anxiolytic drugs that increase GABAergic function (aminooxiacetic acid, valproate, barbital and chlorazepam), have been shown to decrease grooming activity measures in the open field (Barros et al., 1992; 1994). Non-sedating anxiolytic doses of diazepam and chlordiazepoxide inhibited novelty-induced grooming and blocked the increase in grooming produced by i.c.v. administration of stress-related peptides bombesin and $ACTH_{1-24}$ (Crawley and Moody, 1983; Moody et al., 1988). In the open field test, diazepam inhibited mouse grooming in the "thigmotactic" areas - corners and walls (Choleris et al., 2001), while doramectin, a novel compound with GABAergic anxiolytic/anticonvulsant properties, reduced grooming duration and frequency in rats (De Souza Spinosa et al., 2000). In contrast, several anxiogenic drugs that inhibit central GABAergic transmission, have been shown to increase grooming activity. For example, $GABA_A$ receptor chloride channel blockers pentylenetetrazole, picrotoxin and benzylpenicillin all dose-dependently elicited grooming activity in rats (Adams et al., 1993; Kalueff, 2002; Giorgi et al., 2003). Together, this allowed Barros et al. (1994) to suggest that grooming scores can be useful to detect the effects of GABAergic anxiolytic/anxiogenic drugs and manipulations. Supporting this notion, recent drug-free factor analysis studies have shown that grooming cumulative measures in the holeboard and the elevated plus maze positively correlate with "anxiogenic" arousal and negatively – with "low anxiety" exploratory motivation (Ohl et al., 2001b).

However, there are numerous published data contradicting this "high GABA - low stress – low grooming" theory. For example, microinjection of anxiogenic $GABA_A$ receptor antagonist bicuculline (50-100 μg/μl) into the rat brain produced a decrease in spontaneous grooming (Perier et al., 2002); also see similar dose-dependent trend in the elevated plus maze in mice (Dalvi and Rodgers, 1996). Perfusion of the preoptic area with $GABA_A$ receptor agonist, anxiolytic muscimol (10-100 μM) induced a dose-dependent increase in grooming activity which was attenuated by co-perfusion with bicuculline (Osborne et al., 1993). In mice, the anxiolytic drug ethanol increased grooming (see (File et al., 1988) for details), whereas a dramatic 10-fold increase was observed in the elevated plus maze following anxiolytic treatment with 15 mg/kg chlordiazepoxide (Rodgers et al., 2002). In line with this, diazepam has been recently shown to increase grooming in aversive "non-thigmotactic" areas of the open field (Choleris et al., 2001) in mice. Collectively, these data clearly negate the hypothesis that activation of GABAergic system always leads to reduced grooming activity.

Does anxiety always lead to increased grooming frequency or duration? Although this is a widely accepted view, there are many data showing the opposite phenomena. For example, "anxiolytic" sudden darkness (Nasello et al., 2003) is seen together with increased time spent grooming, while Lawler and Cohen (1988) reported pawgrooming activation induced by positive stimuli in rats. In line with this, our recent studies in mice have shown no clear correlation between grooming scores and anxiety. For example, lower grooming activity was seen in more anxious 129S1 mice, compared to non-anxious C57BL/6 mice (Kalueff and

Tuohimaa, 2004c), see also similar data in (Hossain et al., 2004), whereas essentially the same grooming activation was seen in C57Bl/6 mice in both low-stress (novel box) and high-stress (social encounter with an unfamiliar male) situations (Kalueff and Tuohimaa, 2004a). Finally, more stressful situation (exposure to the elevated plus maze) produced less grooming in mice than did a relatively weak stressor such as exposure to a familiar box (Kalueff and Tuohimaa 2004a). Taken together, these findings indicate that the effects on grooming behaviours produced in rodents by stress, as well as GABAergic anxiolytic and anxiogenic drugs, are rather complex and not yet fully understood; see also (File et al., 1988; Moyaho and Valencia, 2002) for discussion.

In contrast, while grooming levels varied inconsistently in these studies, the behavioural microstructure of grooming was consistently impaired in more anxious animals: 129S1 vs. non-anxious C57BL/6 mice, anxious Vitamin D receptor knockouts vs. 129S1 wild type mice, stressed vs. non-stressed C57BL/6 mice (Kalueff and Tuohimaa, 2004a,c). Collectively, this confirms that behavioural patterning of grooming is indeed a very sensitive marker of stress in rodents; see similar data obtained in rats (Komorowska and Pellis, 2004; Kalueff and Tuohimaa, 2004b) using different ethological approach. Therefore, it is possible to assume that "qualitative" characteristics of grooming may also be sensitive to various anxiogenic or anxiolytic pharmacological manipulations. As such, it is necessary to more fully assess GABAergic behavioural pharmacology of grooming and its relation to anxiety.

As already mentioned, all previously published works analysed the effects of GABAergic drugs on grooming by measuring changes in its traditional "quantitative" parameters, such as the frequency and the duration. To the best of our knowledge, the present work is the first study focusing on detailed "in-depth" ethological analyses of changes in grooming patterning ("quality") following administration of reference GABAergic anxiolytic and anxiogenic drugs. Overall, our data show that the number of bouts and, at a lesser extent, the duration of grooming, may not detect anxiety, if taken alone. In contrast, grooming behavioural microstructure is particularly sensitive to GABAergic anxiolytic/anxiogenic drugs, and can therefore represent a reliable grooming-related behavioural marker of anxiety[9].

In general, the idea of analysing grooming separately instead of focusing on grooming demonstrated only during other anxiety tests (such as the open field or elevated plus maze, as done in the majority of studies (Barros et al., 1994; Moyaho and Valencia, 2002; Rodgers et al., 2002)) is important for several reasons. Grooming scores taken during these tests are generally low (being masked by alterations in other, non-grooming behaviours), and their analysis can therefore be extremely difficult. In contrast, more specific analysis of mouse grooming in an observation box enables not only higher grooming scores, but also the identification of more "pure" stress- or drug-evoked grooming, not confounded by other (non-grooming) behaviours (Kalueff and Tuohimaa, 2004a). In general, this allows obtaining several parallel sets of data, including: (a) behavioural measures taken in these initial anxiety

---

[9] For example, it may be suggested that anxiolytic drugs such as diazepam exert general "behaviour-normalizing" effects reducing the portion of "chaotic" arousel-evoked behaviours, including grooming. The latter is in line with numerous clinical observations showing (in addition to "direct" anxiolytic action minimizing anxious thoughts and worries) general behaviour-normalizing "calming" effects of therapy with benzodiazepine tranquilizers.

tests, and (b) grooming measures obtained using this current protocol, which can then both be used for a detailed behavioural analysis, such as reported here.

Importantly, the attractiveness of the present approach is the ease of behavioural analysis and its potential good predictive validity in respect to GABAergic drugs, although future studies using other GABAergic agents are necessary to further examine this notion. Moreover, clear neurobiological rationale behind stress-evoked "high-arousal" alterations in grooming behavioural microstructure (Kalueff and Tuohimaa, 2004a,b) indicates that this approach to measure anxiety may also have good construct validity. Indeed, similar phenomenon of stress-evoked disruption of the cephalo-caudal patterning of grooming has been recently reported in rats (Komorowska and Pellis, 2004), further supporting the utility of our approach to assess stress-evoked alterations in grooming patterning, including testing anxiolytic and anxiogenic drugs. Furthermore, we can suggest that our approach is also suitable for use with rats and other laboratory rodents, given the similarity in patterning of their grooming behaviours (Kalueff and Tuohimaa, 2004a,b). Finally, although not directly tested in this study, it is possible to speculate that our method may be sensitive to other, non-GABAergic anxiotropic pharmacological agents. Given earlier data showing that antidepressant (amitriptyline, nomifensine, mianserin) and neuroleptic (haloperidol, clozapine) drugs influence stress-evoked grooming in rats (Traber et al., 1988), it is possible to assume that these drugs may also affect grooming patterning in rodents. Clearly, this promising research direction will almost certainly require further investigation, and may represent an important potential application of our findings.

Given the results of our study, assessment of grooming may also be useful in assisting with more accurate interpretation of other (non-grooming) behavioural data, especially in situations when conflicting data have been obtained, and there is a need for more detailed and in-depth behavioural analysis. For example, it may be extensively used when studying different pharmacological manipulations with mixed or unclear effects, or interpreting drug-induced behaviours of novel mutant mice with unknown or unclear behavioural phenotype.

In conclusion, our results not only confirm the link between the GABAergic system, anxiety and grooming, but also pharmacologically validate the shifts in grooming behavioural microstructure as a sensitive measure of anxiety in mice (Kalueff and Tuohimaa, 2004a; 2005). This grooming-oriented ethological approach can be a novel tool in behavioural pharmacology of anxiety, used to complement the existing mouse tests. We can also suggest that ethological dissection of grooming, such as reported here, may be used for the search of novel antianxiety antistress psychotropic drugs.

Acknowledgements

This research was supported in part by the grants from the University of Tampere, the Medical Research Council of the University Hospital, and the Academy of Finland.

References

[1] Adams, D.B., Boudreau, W., Cowan, C.W., Kokonowski, C., Oberteuffer, K., Yohay, K., 1993. Offense produced by chemical stimulation of the anterior hypothalamus of the rat. *Physiol. Behav.* 53, 1127-1132.

[2] Aldridge, J.W., Berridge, K.C., 1998. Coding of serial order by neostriatal neurons: a "natural action" approach to movement sequence. *J. Neurosci.* 18, 2777-2787.

[3] Amico, J.A., Vollmer, R.R., Karam, J.R., Lee, P.R., Li, X., Koenig, J.I., McCarthy, M.M., 2004. Centrally administered oxytocin elicits exaggerated grooming in oxytocin null mice. *Pharmacol. Biochem. Behav.* 78, 333-339.

[4] Barros, H.M., Tannhauser, S.L., Tannhauser, M.A., Tannhauser, M., 1992. Effect of sodium valproate on the open-field behavior of rats. *Braz. J. Med. Biol. Res.* 25, 281-287.

[5] Barros, H.M., Tannhauser, S.L., Tannhauser, M.A., Tannhauser, M., 1994. The effects of GABAergic drugs on grooming behaviour in the open field. Pharmacol. Toxicol. 74, 339-344.

[6] Belzung, C., 2001. The genetic basis of the pharmacological effects of anxiolytics: a review based on rodent models. *Behav. Pharmacol.* 12, 451-460.

[7] Berridge, K.C., Aldridge, J.W., 2000. Super-stereotypy I: enhancement of a complex movement sequence by systemic dopamine D1 agonists. Synapse 37, 194-204.

[8] Berridge, K.C., Fentress, J.C., Parr, H., 1987. Natural syntax rules control action sequence of rats. *Behav. Brain Res.* 23, 59-68.

[9] Berridge, K.C., Whishaw, I.Q., 1992. Cortex, striatum and cerebellum: control of serial order in a grooming sequence. *Exp. Brain Res.* 90, 275-290.

[10] Bert, B., Fink, H., Sohr, R., Rex, A., 2001. Different effects of diazepam in Fischer rats and two stocks of Wistar rats in tests of anxiety. *Pharmacol. Biochem. Behav.* 70, 411-420.

[11] Bertolini, A., Poggioli, R., Vergoni, V., 1988. Cross-species comparison of the ACTH-induced behavioral syndrome. *Ann. N.Y. Acad. Sci.* 525, 114-129.

[12] Caldwell, J.D., Drago, F., Prange, A.J., Pedersen, C.A., 1986. A comparison of grooming behavior potencies of neurohypophyseal nonapeptides. *Regul. Pept.* 14, 261-271.

[13] Choleris, E., Thomas, A.W., Kavaliers, M., Prato, F.S., 2001. A detailed ethological analysis of the mouse open field test: effects of diazepam, chlordiazepoxide and an extremely low frequency pulsed magnetic field. *Neurosci. Biobehav. Rev.* 25, 235-260.

[14] Crawley, J.N., Moody, T.W., 1983. Anxiolytics block excessive grooming behavior induced by ACTH1-24 and bombesin. *Brain Res. Bull.* 10, 399-401.

[15] Cromwell, H.C., Berridge, K.C., 1996. Implementation of action sequences by a neostriatal site: a lesion mapping study of grooming syntax. *J. Neurosci.* 16, 3444-3458.

[16] Cromwell, H.C., Berridge, K.C., Drago, J., Levine, M.S., 1998. Action sequencing is impaired in D1A-deficient mutant mice. *Eur. J. Neurosci.* 10, 2426-2432.

[17] Dalvi, A., Rodgers, R.J., 1996. GABAergic influences on plus-maze behaviour in mice. *Psychopharmacol.* 128, 380-397.

[18] De Souza Spinosa, H., Gerenutti, M., Bernardi, M.M., 2000. Anxiolytic and anticonvulsant properties of doramectin in rats: behavioral and neurochemistric evaluations. Comp. Biochem. *Physiol. C. Toxicol. Pharmacol.* 127, 359-366.

[19] Drago, F., Canonico, P.L., Bitetti, R., Scapagnini, U., 1980. Systemic and intraventricular prolactin induces excessive grooming. *Eur. J. Pharmacol.* 65, 457-458.

[20] Drago, F., Bohus, B., Gispen, W.H., Scapagnini, U., De Wied, D., 1983. Prolactin-enchanced grooming behavior: interaction with ACTH. *Brain Res.* 263, 277-282.

[21] Dunn, A.J., Berridge, C.W., Lai, Y.I., Yachabach, T.L., 1987. CRF-induced excessive grooming behavior in rats and mice. *Peptides* 8, 841-844.

[22] Dunn, A.J., Berridge, C.W., Lai, Y.I., Yachabach, T.L., File, S.E., 1988. Excessive grooming behavior in rats and mice induced by corticotropin-releasing factor. *Ann. N.Y. Acad. Sci.* 525, 391-393.

[23] Eguibar, J.R., Romero-Carbente, J.C., Moyaho, A., 2003. Behavioral differences between selectively bred rats: D1 versus D2 receptors in yawning and grooming. *Pharmacol. Biochem. Behav.* 74, 827-832.

[24] Fentress, J.C., 1977. The tonic hypothesis and the patterning of behaviour. Ann. N.Y. *Acad. Sci.* 290, 370–394.

[25] File, S.E., Mabbutt, P.S., Walker, J.H., 1988. Comparison of adaptive responses in familiar and novel environments: modulatory factors. Ann. N.Y. *Acad. Sci.* 525, 69-79.

[26] Giorgi, O., Lecca, D., Piras, G., Driscoll, P., Corda, M.G., 2003. Dissociation between mesocortical dopamine release and fear-related behaviours in two psychogenetically selected lines of rats that differ in coping strategies to aversive conditions. *Eur. J. Neurosci.* 17, 2716-2726.

[27] Gispen, W.H., Isaacson, R.L., 1981. ACTH-induced excessive grooming in the rat. *Pharmacol. Ther.* 12, 209-246.

[28] Hascoet, M., Bourin, M., 1998. A new approach to the light/dark test procedure in mice. *Pharmacol. Biochem. Behav.* 60, 645-653.

[29] Hossain, S.M., Wong, B.K., Simpson, E.M., 2004. The dark phase improves genetic discrimination for some high throughput mouse behavioral phenotyping. *Genes Brain Behav.* 3, 167-177.

[30] Kalueff, A.V., 2002. Psychotropic effects of benzylpenicillin and related compounds in a battery of experimental models of stress. Published Doctoral dissertation. Avix, Kiv.

[31] Kalueff, A.V., Nutt, D.J., 1997. Role of GABA in memory and anxiety. Depress. Anxiety 4, 100-110.

[32] Kalueff A.V., Tuohimaa, P., 2004a. Grooming analysis algorithm for neurobehavioural stress research. *Brain Res. Protocols* 13, 151-158.

[33] Kalueff A.V., Tuohimaa, P., 2004b. The grooming analysis algorithm discriminates between different levels of anxiety in rats: potential utility for neurobehavioural stress research. *J. Neurosci. Methods*, 143, 169-177.

[34] Kalueff A.V., Tuohimaa, P., 2004c. Contrasting grooming phenotypes in C57BL/6 and 129S1/SvImJ mice. *Brain Res.,* 1028, 75-82.

[35] Kalueff, A.V., Lou, Y.-R., Laaksi, I., Tuohimaa, P., 2004. Increased grooming behavior in mice lacking vitamin D receptors. *Physiol. Behav.* 82, 405-409.

[36] Kalueff A.V., Tuohimaa P., 2005. Mouse grooming microstructure is a reliable anxiety marker bidirectionally sensitive to GABAergic drugs. *Eur J. Pharmacol.* 508, 147-153.

[37] Komorowska, J., Pellis, S.M., 2004. Regulatory mechanisms underlying novelty-induced grooming in the laboratory rat. *Behav. Processes* 67, 287-293.

[38] Korpi, E.R., Grunder, G., Luddens, H., 2002. Drug interactions at GABA(A) receptors. *Prog. Neurobiol.* 67, 113-159.

[39] Kozlovskii, V.L., Prakh'e, I.V., 1995. Diazepam eliminates the anxious state induced by amputation of the vibrissae (a model for assessing anxious behavior). *J. High. Nerv. Activity* 45, 1057-1061.

[40] Kutzenko S.A. *Fundamentals of toxicology*. St-Petersburg, 2002, 343.

[41] Lawler, C.P., Cohen, P.S., 1988. Pawgrooming induced by intermittent positive reinforcement in rats. *Ann. N.Y. Acad. Sci.* 525, 417-419.

[42] Lepicard, E.M., Joubert, C., Hagneau, I., Perez-Diaz, F., Chapouthier, G., 2000. Differences in anxiety-related behavior and response to diazepam in BALB/cByJ and C57BL/6J strains of mice. *Pharmacol. Biochem. Behav.* 67, 739-748.

[43] Lumley, L.A., Charles, R.F., Charles, R.C., Hebert, M.A., Morton, D.M., Meyerhoff, J.L., 2000. Effects of social defeat and of diazepam on behavior in a resident-intruder test in male DBA/2 mice. *Pharmacol. Biochem. Behav.* 67, 433-447.

[44] Lumley, L.A., Robison, C.L., Chen, W.K., Mark, B., Meyerhoff, J.L., 2001. Vasopressin into the preoptic area increases grooming behavior in mice. *Physiol. Behav.* 73, 451-455.

[45] Merali, Z., Levac, C., Anisman, H., 2003. Validation of a simple, ethologically relevant paradigm for assessing anxiety in mice. *Biol. Psychiatry* 54, 552-565.

[46] Moody, T.W., Merali, Z., Crawley, J.N., 1988. The effects of anxiolytics and other agents on rat grooming behavior. *Ann. N.Y. Acad. Sci.* 525, 281-290.

[47] Moyaho, A., Eguibar, J.R., Diaz, J.L., 1995. Induced grooming transitions and open field behaviour differ in high- and low-yawning sublines of Sprague-Dawley rats. *Anim. Behav.* 50, 61-77.

[48] Moyaho, A., Valencia, J., 2002. Grooming and yawning trace adjustment to unfamiliar environments in laboratory Sprague-Dawley rats (Rattus norvegicus). *J. Comp. Psychol.* 116, 263-269.

[49] Nasello, A.G., Sassatani, A.S., Ferreira, F.S., Felicio, L.F., Tieppo, C.A., 2003. Modulation by sudden darkness of apomorphine-induced behavioral responses. *Physiol. Behav.* 78, 521-528.

[50] Nutt, D.J., Malizia, A.L., 2001. New insights into the role of the GABA(A)-benzodiazepine receptor in psychiatric disorder. *Br. J. Psychiatry* 179, 390-396.

[51] Ohl, F., Sillaber, I., Binder, E., Keck, M.E., Holsboer, F., 2001a. Differential analysis of behavior and diazepam-induced alterations in C57BL/6N and BALB/c mice using the modified hole board test. *J. Psychiatr. Res.* 35, 147-154.

[52] Ohl, F., Toschi, N., Wigger, A., Henniger, M.S., Landgraf, R., 2001b. Dimensions of emotionality in a rat model of innate anxiety. *Behav. Neurosci.* 115, 429-436.

[53] Osborne, P.G., Mataga, N., Onoe, H., Watanabe, Y., 1993. Behavioral activation by stimulation of a GABAergic mechanism in the preoptic area of rat. *Neurosci. Lett.* 158, 201-204.

[54] Perier, C., Tremblay, L., Feger, J., Hirsch, E.C., 2002. Behavioral consequences of bicuculline injection in the subthalamic nucleus and the zona incerta in rat. *J. Neurosci.* 22, 8711-8719.

[55] Rodgers, R.J., Cole, J.C., Aboualfa, K., Stephenson, L.H., 1995. Ethopharmacological analysis of the effects of putative 'anxiogenic' agents in the mouse elevated plus-maze. *Pharmacol. Biochem. Behav.* 52, 805-813.

[56] Rodgers, R.J., Davies, B., Shore, R., 2002. Absence of anxiolytic response to chlordiazepoxide in two common background strains exposed to the elevated plus-maze: importance and implications of behavioural baseline. *Genes Brain Behav.* 1, 242-251.

[57] Sieghart, W., Fuchs, K., Tretter. V., Ebert, V., Jechlinger, M., Hoger, H., Adamiker, D., 1999. Structure and subunit composition of GABA(A) receptors. *Neurochem. Int.* 34, 379-385.

[58] Traber, J., Spencer, D.G., Glaser, T., Gispen, W.H., 1988. Actions of psychoactive drugs on ACTH- and novelty-induced behavior in the rat. *Ann. N.Y. Acad. Sci.* 525, 270-280.

[59] Van Erp, A.M., Kruk, M.R., Meelis, W., Willekens-Bramer, D.C., 1994. Effect of environmental stressors on time course, variability and form of self-grooming in the rat: handling, social contact, defeat, novelty, restraint and fur moistening. *Behav. Brain Res.* 65, 47-55.

[60] Van Erp, A.M., Kruk, M.R., Willekens-Bramer, D.C., Fermont, P.C., Nijsen, M.J., 1995. PVH lesions do not inhibit stressor-induced grooming in the rat. *Physiol. Behav.* 57, 887-892.

[61] Yannielli, P.C., Kanterewicz, B.I., Cardinali, D.P., 1996. Daily rhythms in spontaneous and diazepam-induced anxiolysis in Syrian hamsters. *Pharmacol. Biochem. Behav.* 54, 651-656.

In: Animal Models in Biological Psychiatry
Editor: Allan V. Kalueff, pp. 197-211 ISBN 1-59454-814-5

Chapter 12

Neurotransplantation Approaches in Biological Psychiatry

Irina V. Ermakova, Elena V. Loseva and Maria A. Aleksandrova
Institute of Higher Nervous Activity and Neurophysiology,
Institute of Developmental Biology, Moscow, Russia

I. Introduction

Diffuse dystrophy and death of neurons in the cerebral cortex, hippocampus and other brain regions generally accompany neurological and mental disorders. Experimental studies on intracerebral grafts of immature nervous tissue and their influence on functioning of animal-recipients are widely performed to model different pathologies of the central nervous system. The attempts have been made to use neurotransplants (NT) in clinical trials to treat Parkinson and Alzheimer diseases, schizophrenia, epilepsy, infant cerebral palsy, Down's syndrome, brain trauma, etc. (Tsymbaliuk et al., 1989; Lindvall et al., 1992; Widner et al., 1992; Freed, 1993; Rasskazov et al., 1994; Bersnev et al., 1998; Sukhikh et al., 1998; Kulakov et al., 1998; Turner, Shetty, 2003). NT can positively influence the host brain, rendering modulating or stimulating influences, promoting the synthesis of different chemical substances (neurotransmitters, peptides, hormones, neurotrophic factors, etc.) or the formation of new neurons and/or glia from both the brain stem cells of the transplants and the host brain (Dunnett, Bjorklund, 1994; Sinden et al., 1992, 1997; Stein, Glasier, 1995; Cotman, Kesslak, 1998; Gray et al., 1999; Hodges et al., 2000; Dobrossy, Dunnett, 2001; Englund et al., 2002).

Transplantation of the nervous tissue appears to be one of the most interesting directions to study the mechanisms underlying both brain pathology and its recovery. It is also possible to study the differentiation, development and interaction of nervous cells by using the neurotransplantation (Nottebhom, 1985; Aleksandrova, 2001). However, for successful application of the neurotransplantation in clinic, it is important to know mechanisms of graft's influence on compensatory-recovery processes in the host brain by studying various experimental models of CNS disorders.

Different experimental models are currently used to examine the ability of NT to normalize the functions of pathologically altered brain. Here we employ several different experimental models of brain pathology, including hypoxia (model of Alzheimer disease, infantile cerebral paralysis), seizures (model of epilepsy), brain trauma (model of various brain injuries), to demonstrate the effects of NT on brain functions and their recovery.

II. Hypoxic Hypoxia

A number of pathologies affecting human brain and leading to diffuse dystrophy and death of neurons include Alzheimer disease, infantile cerebral paralysis and various brain traumas (Bondareff et al., 1982; Gross, 1982; Arendt et al., 1983; Gash, 1987). Despite different etiologies, these diseases are characterized by similar morphological dystrophic-like changes of the neurons. To investigate whether regeneration of the dystrophic neurons is feasible by means of the embryonic nervous tissue transplantation, a model of hypoxic hypoxia in rats has been extensively used (Polezhaev, Aleksandrova, 1986; Aleksandrova, 1990). Hypoxic hypoxia is known to result in severe pathological changes in the CNS (Jabotinsky, 1965; Polezhaev, Aleksandrova, 1986). This model was also used to study possible stimulating/compensatory restorative processes in the dystrophic neurons following allotransplantation of the embryonic nervous tissue.

Hypoxic hypoxia in rats was induced in a special pressure chamber (Bogolepov, 1979). Rats were kept for 3 min at 180 mm Hg with a corresponding reduction of oxygen content. Some exposed rats (30-35%) died following clonic spasms. The surviving rats received transplants of embryonic tissue (cortical, cerebellar and hippocampal). The animals with grafts were sacrificed 4, 60, 100 and 365 days after the surgery. A comprehensive study of the histological, histochemical, autoradiographic, biochemical and physiological parameters was carried out. Cross sections containing NT were obtained from cerebral hemispheres and fixed in 10% formalin; 7-mm paraffin sections were stained with cresyl-violet (Nissle technique).

Synaptic interneuronal connections between the host and the transplant were studied histochemically utilizing retrograde axonal transport of HRP. To assess DNA, RNA and protein synthesis, the autoradiographic and radioisotopic biochemical assays were employed. To elucidate the role of injury per se, we punctured the brain with a syringe needle in the same region, injecting saline (~0,01 ml) as control. Parts of the host hemispheres without NT were taken for biochemical estimation of brain proteins using polyacrylamide gel electrophoresis. The permeability of the blood-brain barrier (BBB) was investigated by the Coor's immunological method. The behavioral experiments included two-way active avoidance of electric shock (shuttle box test).

The first aim of this research was to elucidate whether it is possible to perform a successful transplantation of the embryonic nervous tissue into the rat brain (subjected to hypoxia causing diffuse dystrophy of neurons). The experiments established the feasibility of transplantation of solid tissue pieces from cerebellum, hippocampus and the cerebral cortex, taken from 17-day-old embryos (Polezhaev and Aleksandrova, 1984, 1986; Aleksandrova, 1990).

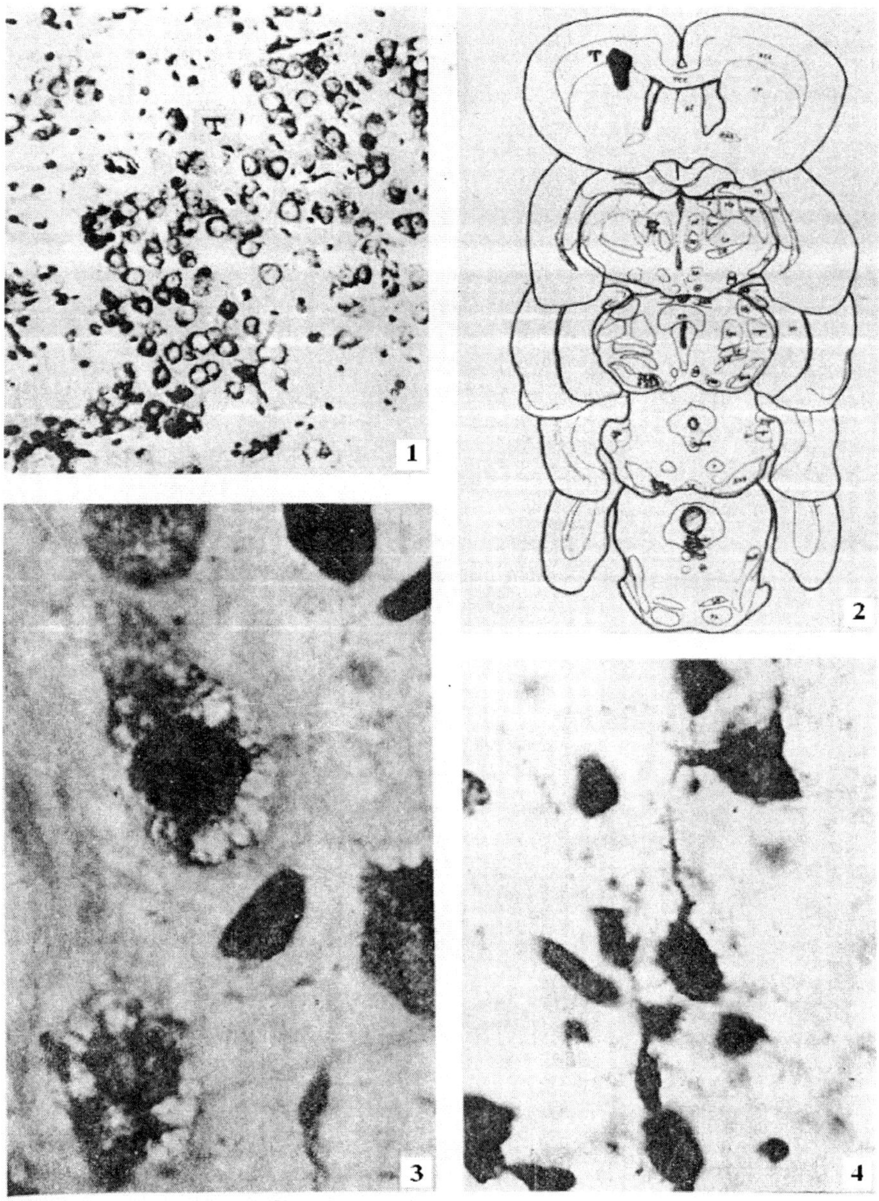

Fig. 1: deep frozen transplanted embryonic cortex cells (T) normally differentiated in the host hypoxia-subjected brain. Fig. 2: schematic representation of afferent connection between transplant (T) and neurons of various brain regions of an adult hypoxia treatment rat HRP labeled neurons are marked by large dots. Fig. 3: vacuolyzed neurons in the rat cortex after hypoxia treatment. Cresyl-violet (x400). Fig. 4: wrinkled and lysed neurons in the hypoxia-subjected rat cerebral cortex. Cresyl-violet (x400).

The NT differentiated and survived in the pathologically changed brain of the adult recipient. The cortical grafts showed no overt pathology even a year after the transplantation into the brain of adult hypoxia-subjected rats. Besides the solid pieces of the embryonic nervous tissue, the dissociated cells also successfully developed in the hypoxia-treated rat brain.

Labeled with H^3T, the transplanted cells were easily seen in the host brain. Cortical grafts cryopreserved for a long time were also seen to survive in the host brain. The neurons of the transplants established active afferent and efferent connections with the host brain (Fig. 1). Thus, we show that the NT can survive and form interneuronal connections with the neurons of the hypoxia-subjected recipients.

Our data also show that hypoxia caused mass dystrophy and death of the neocortical neurons accompanied by a decline of the DNA, RNA and protein synthesis. It also damaged the BBB and affected memory and learning in rats. In summary, here we show that:

1. NT developed well in the brain with hypoxia-exposed rats (Fig. 1);
2. The neurons of transplants formed afferent and efferent links with those of the recipient; there was no rejection or death of the transplants (despite the fact that they were developing in dystrophic tissue of the recipient, previously exposed to hypoxia, which damages the BBB);
3. Embryonic nervous tissue transplantation stimulated the repair of hypoxia-damaged BBB, prevented dystrophy and death of neurons in the cortex and hippocampus of the recipient, and normalized their structure;
4. Neurotransplantation stimulated protein, RNA and DNA biosynthesis in the affected cortical neurons;
5. NT also markedly normalized the behavior of rats, as assessed by the conditioned reflex in the two-way avoidance of the electric shock in the shuttle box test.

Taken together, these results imply that NT stimulate and normalize the dystrophic nervous tissue by providing neurotrophic factors and also as a result of interneuronal interactions.

II. Seizures

Numerous studies have demonstrated that it is feasible to suppress epileptic seizures in animals using embryonic grafts. The main concepts of epilepsy include the reduction or the lack of inhibition and/or the increase of excitation in the presence of an intact inhibitory system (van Gelder, 1988). Therefore, two possible experimental approaches to the study of seizure suppression may be used: first, to restore the inhibitory system by transplantation of the structures producing inhibitory neurotransmitters; second, to decrease the level of excitatory transmitter activity by implantation of cultured astrocytes (known to up-take an abundance of excitatory neurotransmitters). The seizure-suppressing effects of NT may therefore affect the recovery of the disturbed balance between excitatory and inhibitory neurotransmitters in the epileptic brain.

The suppressive action of intracerebral grafting has been shown in chemically-induced seizures and in electrical kindling mainly by transplantation of noradrenergic (NA) or GABAergic neuronal structures (Lindvall et al., 1994, review). Reduction of the seizure severity has been found in genetically epilepsy prone rats (GEPRs) with primary generalized seizures after intraventricular or intrahippocampal grafting of some fetal structures such as locus coeruleus, neocortex, dorsal pontine tissue, hippocampus or septum (Aleksandrova et al., 1995; Clough et al.,1991, 1994; Savchenko et al., 1993).

Two anatomical systems are believed to be involved in the expression of generalized convulsions: forebrain and brain stem structures (Browning, 1986). A major role for the inferior colliculus in the genesis of audiogenic seizures has also been reported (Garcia-Cairasco, 1993; Ribak and Morin, 1995). However, transplantation of NA- rich locus coeruleus or GABA-rich cerebellar tissue into the inferior colliculus in GEPRs has revealed a rather weak suppressive effect (Holmes et al., 1992; Stevens et al., 1988). Changes in monoaminergic regulation and in amino acid neurotransmitters level in GEPRs have been reported in numerous studies, see (Jobe et al., 1993) for a detailed review.

Moreover, the role of GABAergic deficit and NMDA enhancement as a main cause of the epilepsy-prone state in GEPR has been supported by many investigations (Roberts et al., 1985; Avoli, 1988; Faingold et al.,1994; Meldrum, 1994). Some authors suggested that epilepsy might be associated with the changes in the balance of glutamatergic and GABAergic neurotransmission (Roberts, 1984; Meldrum, 1992; Bradford, 1995). A deficiency in striatal and cortical taurine concentrations has also been indicated (Lehmann, 1989). At the same time, Ribak et al. (1988) showed significant increases in the levels of GABA, taurine and glutamate in inferior colliculus, cerebellum and cortex of GEPRs.

Synchronous spike-wave discharges (SWD) in cortical EEG accompanied by behavioural arrest are observed in the genetically-absence epilepsy rat (GAER) as a model of non-convulsive epilepsy (Jobe et al., 1993). It has been shown that dopaminergic and noradrenergic deficits facilitate SWD (Micheletti et al., 1987; Warter et al., 1988). Following studies of GABAergic transmission, a direct role of GABA in generating SWD has been suggested (Vergnes et al., 1990). It was shown that in WAG/Rij rats (van Luijtelaar and Coenen, 1986), belonging to the GAER-like animal group, systemic administration of the GABA-A agonist - muscimol (Peeters et al., 1989) and injection of the GABA reuptake inhibitor, tiagabine (Coenen et al., 1995), as well as the dopaminergic (DA) antagonists haloperidol, flupentixol and pimozide, markedly increased SWD (Warter et al., 1988). At the same time, the GABA-B antagonists and DA agonists suppressed SWD (Depaulis et al., 1990; van Luijtelaar et al., 1996).

Importantly, a role for glial cells in the genesis of epilepsy has also been discussed in the literature. A deficit of glial mechanisms controlling neuronal excitation has been found in the spreading of paroxysmal activity from the brain stem to the cortex (Guillaume, 1988). Glutamate playing a critical role in epileptogenesis (Meldrum, 1994) is up-taken by astrocytes (Shao et al., 1994). In line with this, cultured hippocampal astrocyte-like glia are able to protect neurons against both natural and excitatory amino acid induced neuronal death (Matison and Rychlik, 1990).

In our studies, the effects of different neuronal and glial cell grafts in a kainate model of epilepsy and in genetic animal seizures were assessed in detail. Grafting of embryonic cerebellar tissue into the kainate-lesioned amygdala was found to decrease seizure susceptibility. Embryonic striatal grafts increased benzodiazepine binding. Transplantation of striatal as well as cerebellar tissue decreased the host brain damage in various structures and normalized some behavioural functions in the kainate lesion model (Ermakova et al., 1989, 1993). Combined transplantation of cerebellum+striatum (cer+str) tissue, taken from the newborn brain, into parietal cortex led to the suppression of audiogenic seizures (AS) in Wistar rats from 83% to 50% incidence vs. the combined transplantation of hippocampal and amygdala tissue (hip+am) and the control group after saline injection (Fig. 5; Ermakova et al., 1997; 1998; 2000).

Rats' audiogenic seizure activity was tested 20-24 weeks after transplantation using the following 4-point scale:

1. no seizures;
2. paroxysmal motor excitation in response to the sound stimulus (headlong running and chaotic jumping);
3. motor excitation followed by clonic seizures in a position on the belly;
4. turns from the belly to one side during clonic seizures,
5. three previous phases followed by tonic seizures (Krushinsky, 1960).

Similar results were found in Krushinsky-Molodkina rats (KM) with severe AS susceptibility after transplantation of cer+str tissue into cortex and inferior colliculus simultaneously (Ermakova et al, 2000). Suppressive effects of the grafts were seen 1 week after transplantation and lasted for several months. An imbalance in amino acid transmitters (GABA, taurine, glycine, aspartate and glutamate) in various brain structures has been shown in KM rats vs. the control rats insusceptible to sound stimulation (Rayevsky et al., 1995). Based on these data, it has been suggested that suppressive graft effects seen in the combined cer+str group of rats may be mediated by the normalization of amino acid balance.

At the same time, the transplantation of newborn cer+str tissue into parietal cortex in the AS-WAG/Rij rat substrain with mixed forms of epilepsy (AS and SWD) led to the reinforcement of AS (75% animals). Suppression of AS in these rats (62% rats) was registered after transplantation of newborn tissue of substantia nigra (SN) into the parietal cortex (Ermakova et al., 1997). Suppressive graft effects of SN grafts in WAG/Rij seem to be mediated by the recovery of DA levels. We concluded that for each type of epilepsy it is necessary to search for an adequate scheme of transplantation promoting the stable suppressive graft effect. This effect, possibly, was mediated by restoration of the disturbed balance of certain neurotransmitters in the structures involved in the genesis of definite forms of epilepsy.

An alternative approach to this problem is the use of glial transplantation. The positive influence of glial grafts on spatial memory tasks and passive avoidance performance has been shown in rats with damage to the forebrain cholinergic projection system (Ermakova et al., 1993; Bradbury et al., 1995). Behavioural and histological effects of grafted primary purified fetal hippocampal astrocytes were studied after unilateral kainic acid lesions (Ermakova et al., 1997; 2002; Sidorenkov et al., 2000). The astrocyte grafts compared to the lesioned and sham (vehicle) graft groups reduced the amount of kainic acid-induced brain damage when grafted several days after the lesion (Ermakova et al., 1997; Sidorenkov et al., 2000).

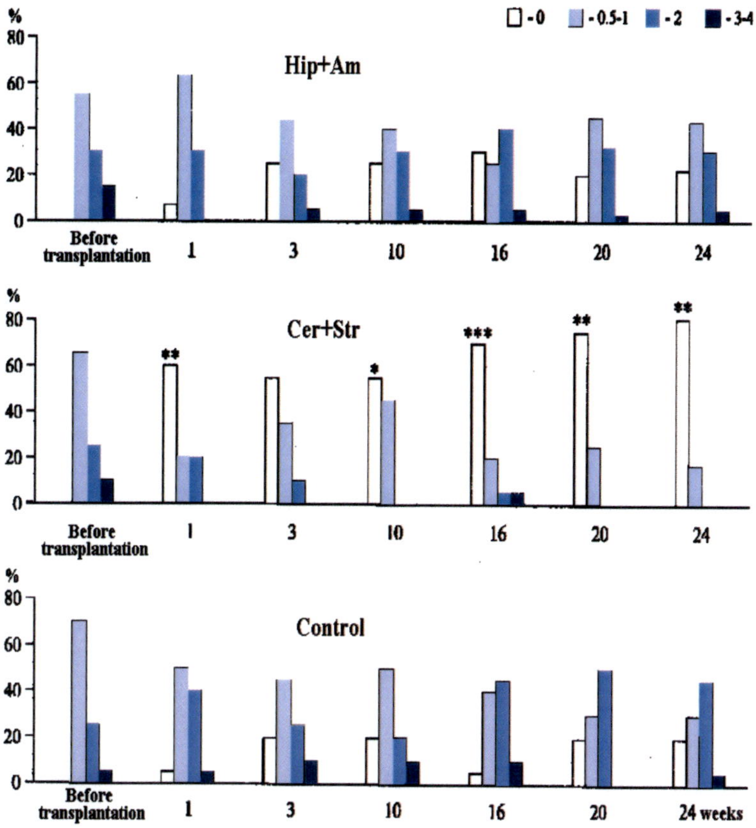

Fig. 5. Audiogenic seizures in different groups of AS-Wistar rats: Hip+Am – combined transplantation of hippocampal and amygdala tissue into parietal cortex; Cer+Str - combined transplantation of cerebellar and striatal tissue into parietal cortex; control – injection of saline into parietal cortex. Levels of audiogenic seizures: 0 – no seizures; 1 - paroxysmal motor excitation in response to the sound stimulus (headlong running and chaotic jumping); 2 - motor excitation followed by clonic seizures in a position on the belly; 3 - the rat turns from the belly to one side during clonic seizures, 4 - three previous phases followed by tonic seizures. *$P<0.05$; **$P<0.01$; *** $P<0.001$.

However, little is known about the mechanisms of suppressive graft effects on seizure activity. It is hypothesized that the main effect of neurotransplants is directed to the recovery of the disturbed balance between excitatory and inhibitory neurotransmitters and their receptor density in the epileptic brain.

Possible mechanisms underlying this phenomenon may be summarized as follows:

1. brain tissue grafts may produce required inhibitory amino acids in the host brain after transplantation;
2. the astrocytes in grafts up-take the abundance of excitatory amino acids which induced seizure activity and neuronal death;
3. the grafts affect the density of GABA and NMDA receptors in specific brain structures (for example, administration of NMDA receptor antagonists significantly decreased AS in GEPR; De Sarro and De Sarro, 1992; Faingold et al., 1993);

4. NT may influence the balance of glutamatergic and/or GABAergic neurotransmission;
5. two calcium-binding proteins, parvalbumin and calbindin (expressed in the GABAergic neurons of striatum, cerebellum and cortex) may regulate Ca++ and Mg++ balance (Celio, 1990) and play an important role in the seizure suppression after combined transplantation of cerebellar and striatal tissue.

IV. Skull-Brain Trauma

A model of severe brain trauma (skull-brain trauma, SBT) was used in these experiments. SBT was caused by a hard strike upon the head, leading to the destruction of the skull (by introduction of the bone splinters into the brain), numerous hematomes and other damages to the brain. Surgical processing (SP) of the trauma focus was used at clinic.

The aim of our experiments was to study the influence of allografts on the host brain after SBT. Solid pieces of E18 were transplanted into the cavities, formed after SP in parietal cortex. In one group, SP and transplantation were performed immediately after SBT (SBT+SP+Tr0 groups), in the second group – 5 days after SBT (SBT+SP+Tr5 group). SP and transplantation were performed under Nembutal (40 mg/kg) anesthesia. Histological analysis of perifocal zones and graft survival was performed 3 months after the transplantation by IBAS microscope (OPTON, Germany).

Histological analyses of the preparations (Nissle staining) have shown that powerful gliofibrosis excrescencies were developed in perifocal zones in the SBT and the SBT+SP groups. The transplants in the SBT+SP+Tr0 group filled the cavities made by surgery treatment. Scars and unscarred zones were seen on the border between transplant and brain parts, and characterized by different degrees of gliosis. In perifocal zones, the NT preserved stratification and normal neurons. The structure of the glia and neurons and their ratio in the NT were similar to normal samples, although orientation of their neurons was atypical. Transplants in rats of the SBT+SP+Tr5 group only partially filled the cavity made by the surgery, also showing a multi-layer gliofibrosis scar. The gliosis in the transplants of the SBT+SP+Tr5 animals was more expressed than in transplants of the SBT+SP+Tr0 group, showing a first stage of its resorption (Fig. 6).

Slices were treated by Goldgy-Coks method. We found that transplants in the SBT+SP+Tr0 group generally have atypical neurons with branches lacking any direct orientation (compared to the normal controls). The number of dendritic spikes in different transplants varied widely. In most cases, thickness of the spikes did not differ from normal controls, although dendrites with rare spikes were numerous in these NT. In NT from the SBT+SP+Tr5 group, the number of spikes on dendrites' stems was usually low. Extensive "dead zones" (containing no neurons around the cavity made by SP) appeared in all rats of SBT+SP group. At the same time, "dead zones" were absent in perifocal zones in the SBT+SP+Tr0 and the SBT+SP+Tr5 rats. Preservation of the neurons in perifocal zone was common for the SBT+SP+Tr0 group.

Notably, all known methods of neurosurgery in the animal SBT model have several important imperfections. Namely, in damaged and SP-treated brains, neuronal and vessels connections were broken, the thick gliofibrosis scares developed, and the "dead zones" were formed in perifocal areas. Using NT, it was possible to avoid these problems, allowing us to suggest that neurotransplantation may be successfully used in combination with the surgery in medical practice in patients with SBT.

V. Conclusion

In general, both short-term and long-term positive influences of neurotransplantation on a functional condition of animals depend on a number of factors, including age, the nature of a donor tissue, site of neurotransplantation, character and degree of damages in the host brain, type of the brain function in question, etc. Therefore, in order to receive positive effects of neurotransplantation, the application of the adequate graft scheme is necessary in each case.

In conclusion, it is necessary to note the dual influence of NT on the host brain: absence of connections between the NT and the host brain at early stages, and active synaptogenesis at the later stages. It is possible to explain the mechanism of early influences, probably, by volume transmission, i.e. diffusive distribution of neurotransmitters and other biologically active substances on intercellular spaces from transplants to remote receptors of a host brain (Agnati et al., 1995; Saulskaya, 1997). This may also explain numerous literary data showing positive effects of grafts implanted into the ventricles of the host brain (Polezhaev and Aleksandrova, 1986), and also general biochemical changes after neurotransplantation (Gulyaeva et al., 1990).

Overall, our present results indicate that both specific and non-specific effects of NT on the pathological brain may occur. Non-specific positive action of neurografts does not depend of the graft's site or the nature of a donor tissue, and correlates with the influence of neurotrophic factors. The specific positive effect of NT depends on the nature or location of grafts, and is related to the action of neurotransmitters. In the present study, non-specific positive graft effects were found in rats after hypoxic hypoxia and brain trauma (SBT model), whereas specific effects were found in rats in the model of epilepsy (AS experiments).

Clearly, neurochemical influence of the grafts from abortive material may represent a potential treatment of some brain disorders. Recently, a special attention has been given to the use of stem cells (polypotent cells of blastocysts and multipotent cells of endo-, ecto- and mesoderma) as donor material for neurotransplantation. Stem cells have also been found in the brain of the adult mammals, including humans. Clearly, isolation and culturing in vitro of the brain stem cells allows researchers to use them for intracerebral neurotransplantation. However, neural grafting and transplantation of stem cells also require further experimental investigation. From this point of view, our study shows that the neural transplantation opens many opportunities to study the disturbed function recovery and the compensatory processes in the pathologically changed brain, as well as to understand in detail both normal and pathogenic mechanisms of the brain.

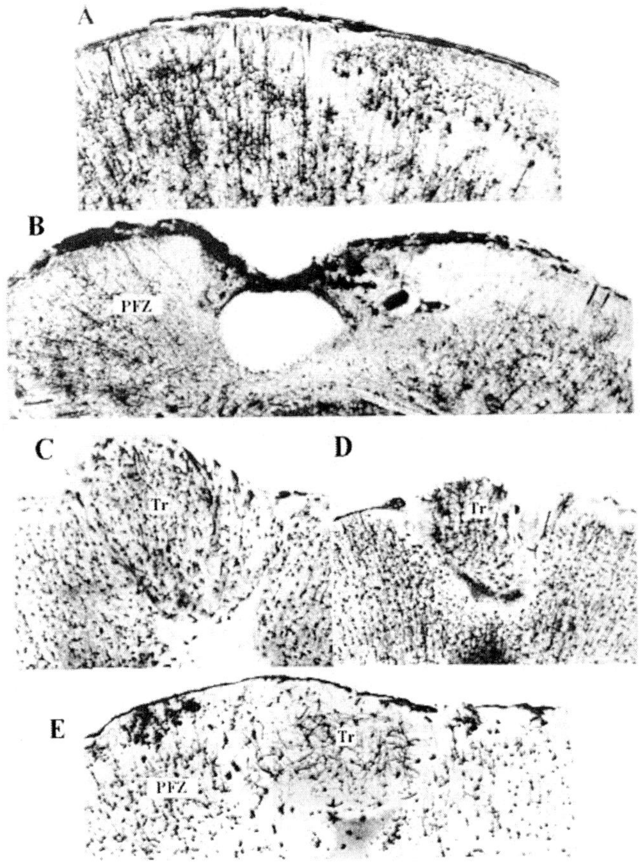

Fig. 6. Slices of parietal cortex in following groups: A – normal; B - SBT+SP group; C, D - SBT+SP+Tr0 and E - SBT+SP+Tr5 groups with transplants (Tr). PFZ – perifocal zone. See text for details.

References

[1] Agnati L.F., Zoli M., Stromberg I., Fuxe K. (1995). Intercellular communication in the brain: wiring versus volume transmission. *Neurosci.,* 69. 711- 726.

[2] Aleksandrova M.A. (1990). Transplantation of embryonic nervous tissue stimulates compensatory-restorative processes in the brain mammals with diffuse dystrophy of neurons. *Proc. Ind. Natl. Sci. Acad.*, 56 (1). 85-94.

[3] Aleksandrova M.A., Girman S.V., Poletaeva I.I., Korochkin L.I. (1995). Trophical effects of neural transplants on ingibition of seizure activity in rats with genuine epilepsy. *Reports RAS*, 341(3). 412-415.

[4] Aleksandrova M.A. (2001). Biological foundation of neurotransplantation. Ontogenez, 32(2). 106-113.

[5] Arendt T., Bigl V., Arendt A., Tennstedt A. (1983) Loss of neurons in the nucleus of Meynert in Alzheimer's desease, paralysis agitans, and Korsakoff's desease. *Acta Neuropathol.,* 61. 101-108.

[6] Avoli M. (1988). GABAergic mechanisms and epileptic discharges. In: Neurotransmitters and cortical function: from molecules to mind. Eds. M. Avoli, T.A. Reader, R.W.Dykes, P.Gloor. N.Y.-London: *Plenum Press.* 187-205.

[7] Bogolepov N. N. (1979). The ultrastructure of brain in hypoxia. Moscow: *Meditcina.* 168 p.

[8] Bondareff W., Mountjoy C., Roth M. (1982). Loss of neurons or origin of the adrenogenic projection to cerebral cortex (nucleus locus ceruleus) in senile demencia. *Neurol.*, 32., 164-168.

[9] Bradbury E.J., Kershaw T.R., Marchbanks R.M., Sinden, J.D. (1995). Astrocyte transplants alleviate lesion induced memory deficits independently of cholinergic recovery. *J. Neurosci.*, 65 (4). 955-972.

[10] Bradford H.F. (1995). Glutamate, GABA and epilepsy. *Prog. Neurobiol.*, 47(6). 477-511.

[11] Browning R.A. (1986). Neuroanatomical localization of structures responsible for seizures in the GEPR: lesion studies. *Life Sci.*, 39. 857-867.

[12] Celio M.R. (1990). Calbindine D-28 and parvalbumine in the rat nervous system. *Neurosci.*, 35. 375-475.

[13] Clough R.W., Browning R.A., Maring M.L., Jobe P.C. (1991). Intracerebral grafting of fetal dorsal pons in genetically epilepsy-prone rats: effects on audiogenic-induced seizures. *J. Exp. Neurol.*, 112 (2). 195-199.

[14] Clough R.W., Browning R.A., Maring M.L., Statnick M.A., Wang C., Jobe P.C. (1994). Effects of intraventricular locus coeruleus transplants on seizure severity in genetically epilepsy-prone rats following depletion of brain norepinephrine. *J. Neural Transpl. Plast.,* 5 (1). 65-79.

[15] Coenen A.M.L., Blezer E.M.H., van Luijtelaar E.L.M. (1995). Effects of the GABA-uptake inhibitor tiagabine on electroencephalogram, spike-wave discharges and behaviour of rats. *Epilepsy Res.*, 21. 89-94.

[16] Cotman C.W., Kesslak J.P. (1988). The role of trophic factors in behavioral recovery and integration of transplants. *Prog. Brain Res.*, 78. 311-319.

[17] De Sarro G. and De Sarro A. (1992). Anticonvulsant activity of competitive antagonists of NMDA receptor in genetically epilepsy-prone rats. *Eur. J. Pharm.*, 215. 221-229.

[18] Depaulis A., Liu Z., Vergnes M., Marescaux C., Micheletti G., Warter J.M. (1990). Suppression of spontaneous generalized non-convulsive seizures in the rat by microinjection of GABA antagonists into the superior colliculus. *Epilepsy Res.*, 5. 192-198.

[19] Dobrossy M.D., Dunnett S.B. (2001). The influence of environment and experience on neural grafts. Nat. *Revs Neurosci.*, 2. 871-879.

[20] Dunnett S.B., Bjorklund A. (1994). Mechanisms of function of neural grafts in the injured brain. *Funct. Neural Transpl.,* 2. 531-565.

[21] Englund U., Bjorklund A., Wictorin K. (2002). Migration patterns and phenotypic differentiation of long-term expanded human neural progenitor cells after transplantation into the adult rat brain. *Dev. Brain Res.*, 134. 123-141.

[22] Ermakova I.V. (1998). Correction of impaired behavioral functions by neurotransplantation. *Bull. Exp. Biol. Med.* 126. 82-86.

[23] Ermakova I.V., Fulop Z., Geller H.M., Chachaj J., Mody N., Stein D.G. (1993). Cultured astrocytes implanted into damaged NBM 48 hours after ibotenic acid lessions facilitate passive avoidance performance in rats. *Proc. Soc. Neurosci. III Ann. Conf.*, 189.

[24] Ermakova I.V., Kuznetsova G.D., Loseva E.V., Sidorenkov A.E., Ioffe M.E. (2000). The use of neural transplantation for suppression of seizure activity in genetically epilepsy-prone rats. *Bull. Exp. Biol. Med.* 130 (9), 852-856.

[25] Ermakova I.V., Loseva E.V., Bradbury E.J., Hodges H., Sinden J.D. (1997). Effects of primary astrosyte grafts on extent of brain damage and behavioural deficits in rats with kainate lesions of hippocampus. Focus on Epilepsy IY. Ste-Adele. Canada. 25.

[26] Ermakova I.V., Loseva E.V., Valouskova V., Bures J. (1989). The effect of embryonal amygdala grafts on the impairment of spatial working memory elicited in rats by kainate-induced amygdaloid damage. *Physiol. Behav.*, 45. 235-241.

[27] Ermakova I.V., Zhulin V.V. (1996). Recovery of behavioral functions following the transplantation of the embryonal striatum into the damaged amygdala of the rat brain. *Neurosci. Behav. Physiol.*, 26. 11-12.

[28] Faingold C.L., Marcinczyk M.J., Casebeer D.J., Randall M.E., Arneric S.P., Browning R.A. (1994). GABA in the inferior colliculus plays a critical role in control of audiogenic seizures. *Brain Res.*, 640. 40-47.

[29] Gulyaeva N.V., Ermakova I.V., Kurbatova M.B., Loseva E.V., Lushekina E.A., Obidin A.B., Khonicheva N.M. (1990). Lipid peroxidation induced by damage of amygdala and transplantation of embryonic brain tissue into damage area. *Neurohimia*, 9(1), 68-75.

[30] Garcia-Cairasco N., Terra V.C., Doretto M.C. (1993). Midbrain substrates of audiogenic seizures in rats. *Behav. Brain Res.*, 58. 57-67.

[31] Gash D. (1987). Neural transplantation: potential therapy for Alzheimer desease. *Neural Transm., Suppl.* 24. 301-308.

[32] Gray J.A., Hodges H., Sinden J. (1999). Prospects for the clinical application of neural transplantation with the use of conditionally immortalized neuroepithelial stem cells. Phil. Trans. Royal Soc. London, *Biol. Sci*, 354(1388). 1407-1421.

[33] Gross J., Lun A., and Odarjuk I. (1982). Eienflus von perinataler Hipoxia auf die Entwicklung zellularer und subzellularer Parameter des ZNS: in Hypoxia und Hypoxiakriterieneds G. Kramer, Berlin: *Humb. Univers.* 2. 68-76.

[34] Guillaume D. (1988). Brain cortical (Na+ K+)-ATPase in epilepsy. A biochemical study in animals and humans. *Acta Neurol. Belg.*, 88 (5). 257-280.

[35] Hodges H., Veizovic T., Bray N., French S.J., Rashid T., Chadwick A., Patel S., Gray J.A. (2000). Conditionally immortal neuroepithelial stem cell grafts reverse age-associated memory impairments in rats. *Neurosci.,* 101(4). 945-955.

[36] Holmes G.L., Thompson J.L., Huh K., Stuart J.D., Carl G.F. (1992). Effects of neural transplantation on seizures in the immature genetically epilepsy-prone rat. *Exp. Neurol.,* 116(1). 52 - 63.

[37] Jabotinsky Yu.M. (1965). Normal and pathological morphology of neuron. Leningrad, *Medcine*. 323 p.

[38] Jobe P.C., Mishra, P.K., Ludvig N., Dailey L.W. (1993). Genetic models of the epilepsies, *Epilepsy: models, mechanisms and concepts*. Cambridge University Press. 94-140.

[39] Krushinsky L.V. (1960). The forming of animal behavior in normal and pathological state. Moscow University Press. Moscow. 285 p.

[40] Lehmann A. (1989). Abnormalities in the levels of extracellular and tissue amino acids in the brain of the seizure-susceptible rat. *Epilepsy Res.*, 3 (2). 130-137.

[41] Lindvall O., Bengzon J., Elmer E., Kokaia M., Kokaia Z. (1994). Grafts in models of epilepsy. *Funct. Neural Transplantat.*, 1994. 2. 387 p.

[42] Loseva E. V., Tsymbalyk V. I., Pichkur L. D., Bragin A. G. (1995). Effect of embrionic tissue transplantation on structural changes in the rat brain after craniocerebral trauma. *Neurophysiol.,* 27 (5/6). 350-360.

[43] Matison M. P., Rychlik B. (1990). Glia protect hippocampal neurons against excitatory amino acid-induced degeneration: involvement of fibroblast growth factor. *J. Dev. Neurosci.,* 8(4). 399-415.

[44] Meldrum, B.S. (1992). Excitatory amino acids in epilepsy and potential novel therapies. *Epilepsy Res.,* 12 (2). 189-196.

[45] Meldrum B.S. (1994). The role of glutamate in epilepsy and other CNS disorders. *Neurol.,* 44 (11). S14-23.

[46] Micheletti G., Warter J.M., Marescaux C., Depaulis A., Tranchant C., Rumbach L., Vergnes M. (1987). Effects of drugs affecting noradrenergic neurotransmission in rats with spontaneous petit mal-like seizures. *Eur. J. Pharm.*, 135 (3). 397-402.

[47] Nottebhom F. (1985). Neuronal replacement in adulthood. *Ann. N. Y. Acad. Sci.* 475. 143-161.

[48] Peeters B.W.M.M., van Rijn C.M., Vossen J.M.H., Coenen A.L.M. (1989). Effects of GABA-ergic agents on spontaneous non-convulsive epilepsy, EEG and behaviour in the WAG/Rij inbred strain of rats. *Life Sci.,* 45. 1171-1176.

[49] Polezhaev L., Aleksandrova M. (1984). Transplantation of embryonik brain tissue in to the brain of adult rats in hypoxic hypoxia. *J. Hirnforschung*. 25. 99-106.

[50] Polezhaev L., Aleksandrova M. (1986). The transplantation of brain tissue in the norm and pathology. Moscow, *Nauka*. 152.p

[51] Rayevsky K.S., Bashkatova V.G., Kudrin V.S., Malikova L.A., Kosacheva E.S., Vitskova G.Yu., Semiokhina A.F., Fedotova L.B. (1995). Neurotransmitter amino acids and lipid peroxidation products in brain of rats genetically proned to audiogenic seizures. *Neurohimia*, 12(4). 47-54.

[52] Ribak C.E., Morin C.L. (1995). The role of the inferior colliculus in a genetic model of audiogenic seizures. *Anat. Embryol.*, 191(4). 279-295.

[53] Ribak C.E., Byun M.Y., Ruiz G.T., Reiffenstein R.J. (1988). Increased levels of amino acid neurotransmitters in the inferior colliculus of the genetically epilepsy-prone rat. *Epilepsy Res.*, 2 (1). 9-13.

[54] Roberts E. (1984). GABA-related phenomena, models of nervous system function, and seizures. *Ann. Neurol.,* 16. S77-89.

[55] Saulskaya N.B. (1997). Volume transmission as constituent of the intercellular communication in the striatum. Zh. *VND,* 47(2). 362-373.

[56] Savchenko Yu.N., Ereniev S.I., Genne R.I., Semchenko V.V. (1993). The dynamics of phenotypically and genotypically determined high brain seizure activity in the intracerebral allografting of embryonic nerve tissue. Zh. *Nevropatol. Psykh.*, 93. 3-7.

[57] Sinden J.D., Marsden K.M., Hodges H. (1992). Neural transplantation and recovery of function: animal studies. *In Recovery from brain damage: Reflections and Directions* (eds Rose F.D. and Johnson D.A.). Plenum Press. New-York. 35-65.

[58] Sinden J.D., Rashid-Doubell F., Kershaw T.R., Nelson A., Chadwick A., Jat P.S., Noble M.D., Hodges H., Gray J.A. (1997). Recovery of spatial learning by grafts of a conditionally immortalized hippocampal neuroepithelial cell line into the ischaemia-lesioned hippocampus. *Neuroscience,* 81(3). 599-608.

[59] Shao, Y., Enkvist M.O., McCarthy K.D. (1994). Glutamate blocks astroglial stellation: effect of glutamate uptake and volume changes. *Glia,* 11 (1). 1-10.

[60] Sidorenkov A.E., Ermakova I.V., Lermontova N.N. (2000). Influence of astrocyte grafts on the behaviour of rats with kainate lesioned amygdala. Proc. 2nd Int. Conf. *Glial Interfaces Nerv. Syst. Dev. Repair*, 28.

[61] Stein D.G., Glasier M.M. (1995). Some practical and theoretical issues concerning fetal brain tissue grafts as therapy for brain dysfunctions. *Behav. Brain Sci.*, 18(1). 36-45.

[62] Stevens J.R., Phillips I., Freed W.J., Poltorak M. (1988). Cerebral transplants for seizures: preliminary results. *Epilepsia,* 29. 731-737.

[63] Turner D.A., Shetty A.K. (2003). Clinical prospects for neural grafting therapy for hippocampal lesions and epilepsy. *Neurosurg., 52*(3). 632-644.

[64] Van Gelder N.M. (1988). H.H.Jasper: Modern concepts of epilepsy, Neurotransmitters and cortical function. From molecules to mind. *Plenum Press.* New York. 15-25.

[65] Van Luijtelaar E.L.J.M., Coenen A.M.L. (1986). Two types of electrocortical paroxysms in an inbred strain of rats. *Neurosci. Lett.*, 70. 393-397.

[66] Van Luijtelaar E.L.J.M., Dirksen R., Vree T.B., van Haaren F. (1996). Effects of acute and chronic cocaine administration on EEG and behaviour in intact and castrated male and intact and ovariectomized female rats. *Brain Res. Bull.*, 40. 43-50.

[67] Vergnes M., Marescaux C., Depaulis, A. (1990). Mapping of spontaneous spike and wave discharges in Wistar rats with genetic generalized non-convulsive epilepsy. *Brain Res.,* 523 (1). 87-91.

[68] Warter J.M., Vergnes M., Depaulis A., Tranchant C., Rumbach L., Micheletti G., Marescaux C. (1988). Effects of drugs affecting dopaminergic neurotransmission in rats with spontaneous petit mal-like seizures. *Neuropharmacol.*, 27 (3). 269-274.

Index

A

B

C

D

E

F

G

H

I

J

K

L

O

P

S

T

U

V

W

Y

Z